*tiO Techniques in Orthopaedics*

# Editorial Board

# *Techniques in Orthopaedics*

## Volume 5

# Arthroscopic Surgery Update

Edited by

**John B. McGinty, M.D.**

*Professor and Chairman*
*Department of Orthopaedic Surgery*
*Medical University of South Carolina*
*Charleston, South Carolina*

AN ASPEN PUBLICATION®

Aspen Systems Corporation
Rockville, Maryland
Royal Tunbridge Wells
1985

Aspen Systems Corporation
1600 Research Boulevard
Rockville, Maryland 20850



This publication was developed by University Park Press, Baltimore, Maryland.



ISBN 0-87189-262-6

*Printed in the United States of America*

1 2 3 4 5

# Contents

# Preface

The growth of arthroscopy in the last decade has been truly remarkable. By 1975 arthroscopy, as a diagnostic procedure in North America, was finally established in spite of the skepticism of some experienced knee surgeons. This growth opened the door for the development of arthroscopic surgery.

Through the pioneering efforts of the late Dr. Richard O'Connor and his operating arthroscope, meniscal surgery was shown to be effective. It has rapidly progressed with triangulation techniques, new instrumentation, and alternate energy sources. It is now apparent that in some lesions meniscal repair or reattachment is preferable to partial menisectomy. Clinical data is accumulating to substantiate basic laboratory observations regarding meniscal blood supply.

Through the use of mortorized instrumentation, the management of articular cartilage lesions has been adapted to arthroscopic techniques, with some reinforcement by the accumulation of clinical data. Some intra-articular fractures have been shown to be effectively managed by arthroscopic techniques. Repair and reconstruction of the anterior cruciate ligament with or without prosthetic replacements have entered the arena of arthroscopic surgery.

Arthroscopy is now being used in the surgery of joints other than the knee. We are witnessing an explosive growth of technique, a growth that sometimes exceeds logical indications. It is vital that careful statistical analysis of clinical data be performed on a continuing basis. We must be critical of our results before accepting a procedure as standard.

It is the purpose of this book to present current methods in the field of arthroscopic surgery. The presentation of these methods does not represent an endorsement but rather a review of the work being done. It should be read with careful criticism.

JBMcG

# Contributors

**James R. Andrews, M.D.**
*Hughston Orthopaedic Clinic, P.C.*
*6262 Hamilton Road*
*Columbus, Georgia 31995*

**Steven Arnoczky, D.V.M.**
*Director, Laboratory of Comparative Orthopaedics*
*The Hospital for Special Surgery*
*535 E. 170th Street*
*New York, New York 10021*

**Anna Marie Cable**
*Orthopaedic Specialty Nurse*
*Operating Room*
*Children's Hospital*
*Pittsburgh, Pennsylvania 15261*

**William Carson, M.D.**
*Tampa Orthopaedic Clinic*
*602 South Howard Avenue*
*Tampa, Florida 33606*

**Richard B. Caspari, M.D.**
*Tuckahoe Orthopaedic Associates, Ltd.*
*Tuckahoe Medical Center*
*8919 Three Chopt Road*
*Richmond, Virginia 23229*

**S. Ward Casscells, M.D.**
*1205 Gilpin Avenue*
*Wilmington, Delaware 19806*

**David Drez, Jr., M.D.**
*Clinical Professor of Orthopaedics*
*Louisiana State University Medical School*
*New Orleans, Louisiana; McNeese State University-Team Physician*
*Lake Charles, Louisiana 70609*

**John W. Ewing, M.D.**
*Orthopaedic Surgeons, Inc.*
*The Professional Center*
*75 Arch St., Suite 102*
*Akron, OH 44304;*
*Senior Staff Physician*
*Akron City Hospital*
*Associate Professor*
*Northeastern Ohio Universities*
*College of Medicine*
*Akron, Ohio*

**James M. Fox, M.D.**
*Southern California Sports Medicine and Orthopaedic Medical Group*
*15211 Vanowen Street, Suite 300*
*Van Nuys, California 91405*

**Douglas L. Gollehon, M.D.**
*20 Creekwood Square*
*Cincinnati, Ohio 45246;*
*Cincinnati Sports Medicine*
*Center for Orthopaedics*
*One Lytle Place*
*Cincinnati, Ohio*

**James F. Guhl, M.D., S.C.**
*5757 West Oklahoma Avenue*
*Milwaukee, Wisconsin 53219*

**Richard B. Hawkins, M.D.**
*John Fitch Orthopaedic Associates*
*1480 John Fitch Hwy.*
*Fitchburg, Massachusetts 01420*

**Charles E. Henning, M.D.**
*Mid-America Center for Sports Medicine*
*320 N. Hillside*
*Wichita, Kansas 67214*

**Ben L. Jolly, M.D.**
*Mid-America Center for Sports Medicine*
*320 N. Hillside*
*Wichita, Kansas 57214*

**Mary A. Lynch, M.D.**
*Mid-America Center for Sports Medicine*
*320 N. Hillside*
*Wichita, Kansas 67214*

**J. Lorin Mason, Jr., M.D.**
*Pee Dee Orthopaedic Associates*
*417 S. Dargan St.*
*P.O. Drawer 1771*
*Florence, South Carolina 29503*

**John B. McGinty, M.D.**
*Professor and Chairman*
*Department of Orthopaedic Surgery*
*Medical University of South Carolina*
*171 Ashley Avenue*
*Charleston, South Carolina 29425*

**Robert W. Metcalf, M.D.**
*Professor of Orthopaedic Surgery, The University of Utah School of Medicine, Div. of Orthopaedic Surgery*
*50 N. Medical Drive*
*Salt Lake City, Utah 84132*

**David Pevsner, R.P.T.**
*The Center for Sports Medicine and Fitness*
*15211 Vanowen Street*
*Van Nuys, California 91405*

**Gary A. Scott, M.D.**
*Mid-America Center for Sports Medicine*
*320 N. Hillside*
*Wichita, Kansas 67214*

**Orrin H. Sherman, M.D.**
*333 East 56th Street*
*New York, New York 10022*

**Joe W. Tippett, M.D.**
*4203 E. Southcross Blvd.*
*San Antonio, Texas 78222*

**Terry L. Whipple, M.D., F.A.C.S.**
*Assistant Clinical Professor, Orthopaedic Surgery*
*The Medical College of Virginia*
*President, Orthopaedic Research of Virginia*
*Consultant, Hand and Sports Medicine Division*
*Department of Orthopaedics*
*School of Medicine*
*University of Virginia at Charlottesville*
*Charlottesville, Virginia 22908*

**Tuckahoe Medical Center**
*8919 Three Chopt Road*
*Richmond, Virginia 23229*

# The Place of Arthroscopy in the Armamentarium of the Orthopaedic Surgeon

# 1

S. Ward Casscells

Although there are no reliable figures, it is becoming increasingly evident that, at the present time, arthroscopy is the most commonly performed elective orthopaedic procedure in the United States and Canada. Several years ago at the Canadian orthopaedic meeting, this was reported to be true of the province of Ontario. In the United States one only has to look at hospital surgery schedules to be convinced. In our own medical center during a 5-year period, from 1979 through 1983, 635 arthrotomies of the knee were performed, an average of 63 every 6 months. From January through June, 1984, at the same institution, 248 arthroscopic procedures of the knee were done. Media attention given this procedure plus the fact that it can be done on an outpatient basis, creates only a small scar, and has low morbidity account for the patient's willingness to accept this form of surgery and the orthopaedic surgeon's willingness to perform it. Like many new surgical procedures, the indications are often not clear-cut, and there is a tendency toward overutilization. The purpose of this paper is to outline what I consider the indications and relative contraindications for arthroscopy. If there is no clearcut indication for arthroscopy, then this is considered a relative contraindication.

## Diagnostic Arthroscopy

### Age

Although arthroscopy can be performed at almost any age, it finds its greatest use between the ages of 15 and 50 years. It is rare that a child under the age of 15 years needs to be arthroscoped, as discoid and torn menisci at that age are infrequent. Unfortunately, there have been reports of very young children with Legg-Perthes disease of the hip whose knees were arthroscoped before the real diagnosis was made.

At the other end of the age spectrum, patients over 50 years are generally not good candidates for arthroscopy. The most common diagnosis in this group is degenerative arthritis secondary to malalignment of the leg, and weight-bearing x-rays (Figure 1–1) usually supply all the necessary information. It has been my consistent observation that pain is a late phenomenon. By the time the patient presents himself, the disease is fairly well advanced. The argument has been made that it is necessary to look at the opposite side of the joint to ensure that there is good articular cartilage; however, experience at the Mayo Clinic and elsewhere has shown that this is not necessary. Recently, in an article in the *Journal of Bone and Joint Surgery,* Keene and Dyreby came to the same conclusion (4). It is my opinion, as well as Keene's that meniscal changes in patients who are candidates for osteotomy can usually be ignored.

There is one exception to the above statement, and that concerns the occasional middle-aged patient seen with pain in the knee in whom the weight-bearing films are negative. It is a little-known fact that some patients can have considerable loss of articular cartilage over a relatively small area, and because the surrounding good articular cartilage supports the joint space, nothing is seen on the weight-bearing films. Such patients, especially if they have angular deformity, should be arthroscoped to make a diagnosis relatively early in the stage of the disease. The best results from osteotomy are obtained in those in whom the joint is not too badly destroyed and who still have a good range of motion.

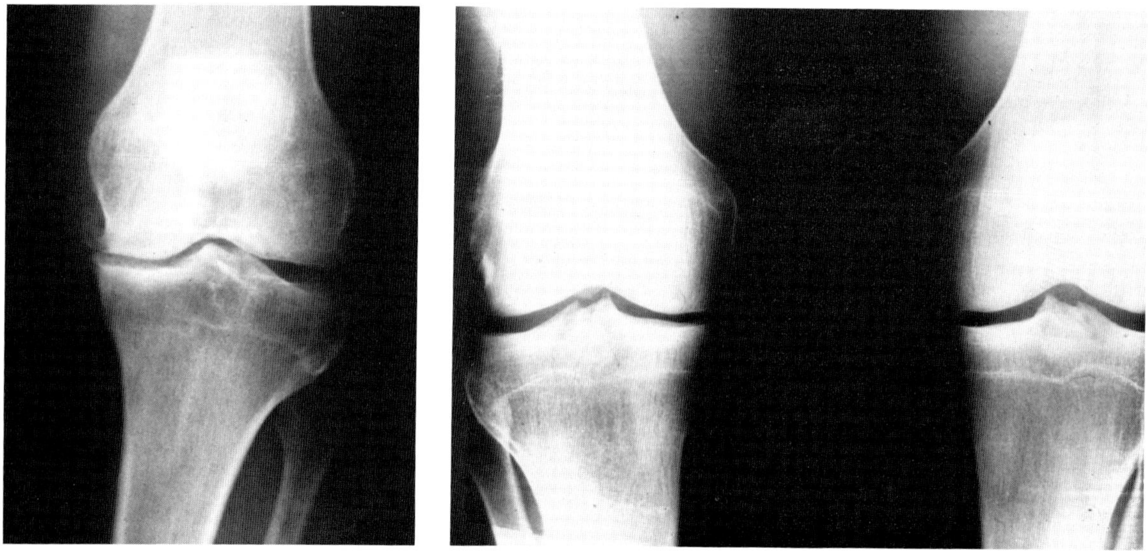

A B

**Figure 1–1** **A** Obvious varus alignment of the knee with marked narrowing of the medial joint space. **B** Erect T film of both knees, 14 × 17 film of this left knee showed approximately neutral alignment with loss of the normal valgus alignment. Despite the very mild narrowing of the medial joint space, arthroscopy showed a large area of articular cartilage degeneration, about 3 cm in diameter, with some bone exposed. It is unusual to see patients at this relatively early stage of the disease.

## Pain

More arthroscopies are being done for the complaint of pain than for any other reason. In the young person, it is frequently attributed to chondromalacia of the patella despite the fact that there is no physiological basis for chondromalacia being painful, and studies have shown that chondromalacia is often present in the absence of any significant discomfort. In my own review of 1000 arthroscopies (1) done several years ago, there was no pathology found in 160 of these patients who were quite young. Chondromalacia was suspected but not found. In retrospect, these patients should not have been arthroscoped because pain is a very common symptom among teenagers, and experience has shown that the source of the pain is rarely found inside the knee joint.

Another supposedly painful condition is "lateral compression syndrome," although there is no clear-cut pathological explanation for the pain. The presence of unmyelinated nerve fibers in the lateral retinaculum has been described and thought to be the cause of this pain (J. P. Fulkerson, unpublished data presented at the International Arthroscopy Association Meeting, London, September, 1984), but no investigation was carried out on similar tissue in patients who have no pain.

Some of these patients with a diagnosis of lateral compression syndrome have chondromalacia and some do not, and there is no consistency in the clinical findings. In our office we routinely take tangential views of the patella and often find some degree of lateral patellar displacement in patients in whom there are no painful symptoms (Figure 1–2). We have even seen patients with fairly marked lateral tracking of the patella who have no pain; this malalignment is likely to result in degenerative arthritis in later years. The patellofemoral joint can be evaluated very accurately, and it should be a part of every arthroscopic examination (Figure 1–3). There are other ways, however, of examining the patellofemoral area, and often patients will not profit by having this done arthroscopically.

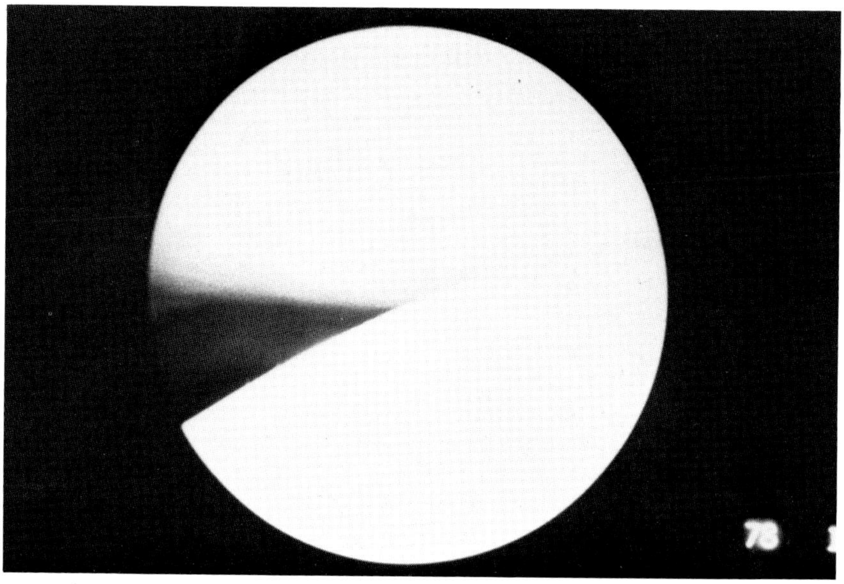

**Figure 1–2** A 24-year-old patient with fairly marked lateral tracking of the patella with no symptoms. This picture was taken with the knee flexed approximately 45 degrees.

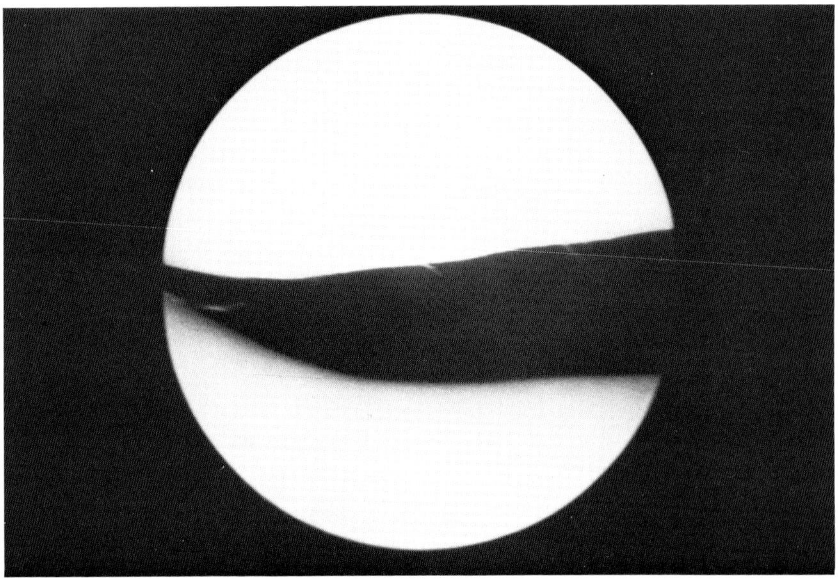

**Figure 1–3** A silent lesion of the patella in a patient who had meniscal problems.

Chronic pain is not a symptom that is characteristic of most meniscal tears, and pain has resulted in the loss of thousands of normal menisci in past years. Occasionally, one sees a patient with a long flap of meniscus (Figure 1–4) that is trapped under the condyle, the tip of which presents under the medial collateral ligament. These patients do have a chronic ache in their knees that is even troublesome at night. The majority of patients with meniscal tears, however, experience pain at the time of the injury when the tear suddenly displaces inside the joint; such patients have in addition a history of clicking or locking and usually some increased joint fluid.

The important thing to realize about chronic pain in its relationship to arthroscopy is that if the x-rays are negative, the source of pain is very likely outside of the joint. It may be in the femur, as reported by Joyce and Mankin (3). All of these patients had bone tumors diagnosed only after their knees had been arthroscoped. Pain may also be the result of pathology in the hip joint or even the lower back. Pain itself in the absence of any other findings is a poor indication for arthroscopy.

## Timing

Timing is another factor to be considered when faced with the decision of whether or not to operate on a patient. Young patients who have had an acute injury and in whom the diagnosis is obscure probably should have arthroscopy done promptly, especially if they are college or professional athletes. Most of these patients with an acute hemarthrosis have torn anterior cruciate ligaments, and a high percentage have concomitant meniscal tears, both of which can sometimes be treated by open or closed arthroscopic suture.

In older patients who are not as active physically, the decision for arthroscopy can be delayed, sometimes indefinitely. In a study by Noble and Erat (5), 250 patients were diagnosed as having meniscal tears and surgery was recommended. For one reason or another, an operation was not performed in 50 of these patients, and in 35 the symptoms had subsided when they were reevaluated some years later.

There is no evidence that a torn meniscus when left untreated is a great threat to the knee joint, which has been suggested by Watson-Jones (7), Smillie (6), and others.

## Ability And Experience Of The Arthroscopist

As with any operative procedure, the ability and experience of the surgeon bears some relationship to the decision to arthroscope a patient. This is especially true of arthroscopists because it has been long evident that in the ability to perform arthroscopic surgery, "all men are not created equal." It has been my experience over the past 15 years that some surgeons learned very rapidly and in a relatively short period of time become good and innovative arthroscopic surgeons. Others learn very slowly or not at all and don't seem to have the potential for advancing beyond diagnostic arthroscopy, and some are not very capable in this respect, either. By and large, the fast learners are young, patient, skilled in the use of both hands, and possess some indefinable ability to assemble in their minds a composite picture of the interior of the joint based on seeing successive small areas of the joint. As it is difficult, if not impossible for the peer review process to monitor an arthroscopic surgeon, it becomes a matter of conscience whether or not a surgeon does diagnostic arthroscopy and arthroscopic surgery, or perhaps leaves it all to one of his colleagues.

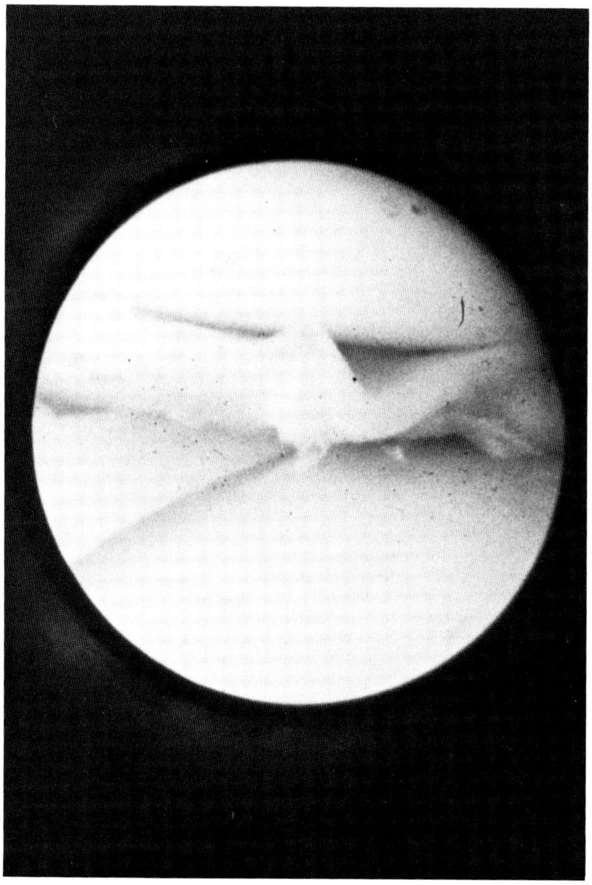

**Figure 1–4** Large flap of torn medial meniscus presenting slightly lateral to the femur under the medial collateral ligament.

## Arthroscopic Surgery

The magic of arthroscopic surgery has become so firmly embedded in the minds of patients as well as orthopaedic surgeons that it is difficult, if not impossible, to consider the possibility that the patient may be better served by having an arthrotomy rather than arthroscopic surgery. The one indisputable advantage of arthroscopy over arthrotomy is the difference in the length of the scar. Today this difference is not very great since the era of the long utility incision has passed, and meniscectomies can now be done through a 3-cm arthrotomy incision.

The other advantage, rightfully claimed for arthroscopy, is the lowered morbidity, assuming that the intra-articular surgery being performed is no different whether done by arthroscopy or arthrotomy. The difference in the morbidity is roughly proportional to the difference in the length of the scars. Surgeons have done arthrotomies on an outpatient basis. Gillquist et al. (2), in a recent article, stated that there is a difference in morbidity between arthroscopy and arthrotomy, but the difference is not nearly as great as has been claimed by some.

Arthroscopy is usually compared favorably with arthrotomy; rarely are the occasional unfavorable aspects mentioned. Danger of damage to the articular cartilage certainly is greater with arthroscopy. In the hands of the average arthroscopist, the time required to perform a meniscectomy is greater, sometimes considerably greater, with arthroscopy than with arthrotomy. There are numerous reports from all over the country of three or four hours being spent in the operating room attempting to do a meniscectomy arthroscopically. This, of course, is not good for the patient, and the likelihood of anesthetic and other complications is increased. I have seen records of one case in which too vigorous of an effort to remove a meniscus arthroscopically resulted in transection of the popliteal artery.

Another advantage claimed for arthroscopy is lowered cost. In patients in whom arthroscopy is done on an outpatient basis, this is certainly true, but in many places in the country, patients remain in the hospital for 1 or 2 days for a diagnostic arthroscopy. When one considers that a higher fee is usually charged for doing a meniscectomy arthroscopically, and with a longer operating time, many of the economic advantages are lost.

Rather than compare arthroscopy and arthrotomy, it is of more value to compare individual procedures that can be done either arthroscopically or by arthrotomy, and to do so one has to stipulate whether a diagnostic arthroscopy does or does not precede an arthrotomy.

### Loose Body

In the removal of a loose body, arthroscopy enjoys a great advantage over arthrotomy because often it is not easy to locate a loose body by arthrotomy without making a fairly substantial incision. Even if the loose body is first located arthroscopically, it may not be in that spot when the arthrotomy is performed, thus, necessitating a much larger incision to find it. Loose bodies can be difficult to find even arthroscopically.

### Synovectomy

Great advantages accrue to having a synovectomy done arthroscopically if it can be conclusively shown that it is possible to do a complete synovectomy this way. The morbidity is far greater with arthrotomy, especially when one long or sometimes even two fairly substantial incisions have to be made to do the synovectomy. When done arthroscopically, it is a time-consuming and often difficult procedure, and it is necessary to use the new high-speed shaver equipment with its various cutting attachments.

## Meniscectomy

As mentioned previously, the relative advantages of arthroscopy are dependent upon the skill of the arthroscopic surgeon and the type of meniscectomy being done. As Gillquist et al. (2) have shown the difference in morbidity between arthroscopy and arthrotomy when doing a total meniscectomy is virtually nil. When performing a partial meniscectomy, the advantages do lie with what is done arthroscopically, but these advantages are relatively small when compared with a miniarthrotomy. It is most important to do a diagnostic arthroscopy first and pinpoint the pathology; then the meniscectomy can be performed through a limited incision if not done arthroscopically.

## Shaving The Patella

The best you can say about shaving a patella is that it does no harm to the patella. Perhaps there are some temporary benefits that result from removing damaged tissue that may release undesirable lysosomal enzymes into the knee joint, such as cathepsin. On the other hand, it is an expensive and often unnecessary procedure. If one is looking into the knee joint for other reasons and discovers loosened, damaged patellar cartilage, there is no reason not to remove it arthroscopically (Figures 1–5 and 1–6). If chondromalacia is suspected on the basis of patellar crepitus, I believe one should hesitate before recommending patellar shaving because the benefits to the patient are doubtful and the cost is great. There probably have been more patellae shaved arthroscopically in the last 2 or 3 years than shaved with a knife in the preceding 50 years. It has yet to be shown that shaving the patella with a knife has beneficial long-term results, and there is no reason to think that the better results can be anticipated by shaving arthroscopically.

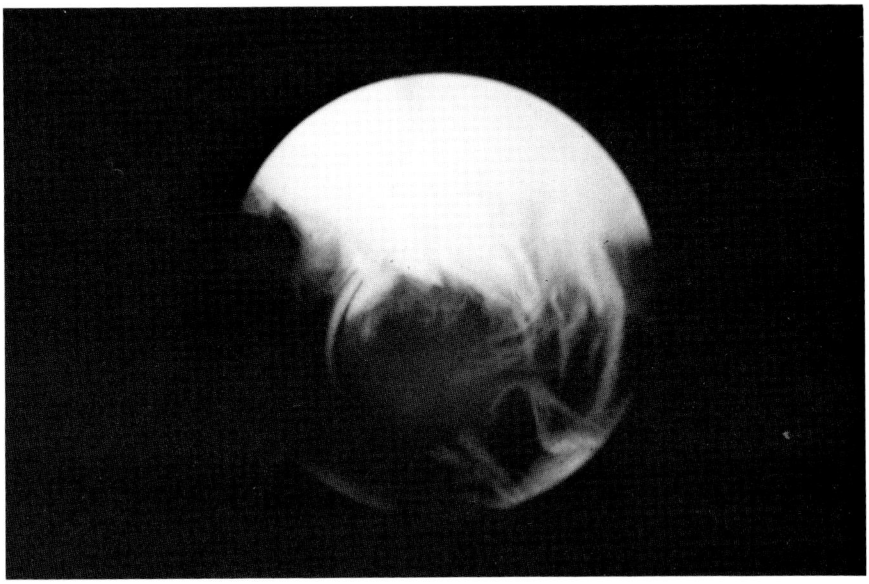

**Figure 1–5** Typical area of chondromalacia of the patella.

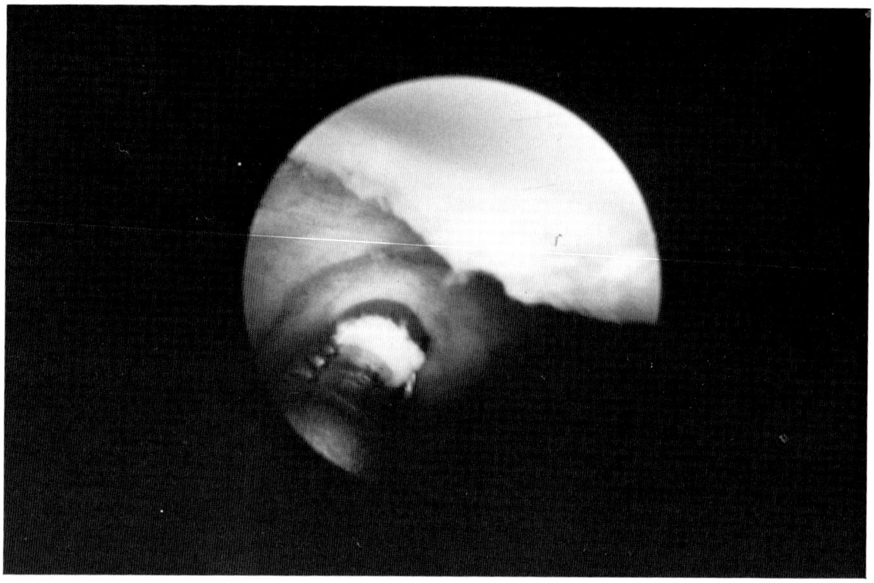

**Figure 1–6** The lesion after having been shaved. There are some doubts that this has any long-term beneficial effect.

## Lateral Retinacular Release

This can be done arthroscopically or through a very small, 1-cm arthrotomy incision. If the arthroscopist has the equipment to do this using an electrocautery, then the troublesome bleeding that sometimes follows this procedure can be avoided. It is technically more difficult and more time-consuming to do this procedure arthroscopically.

## Cutting Of Plica

This is a very popular procedure easily done and, like shaving the patella, is done far too often (Figure 1–7). It has been quite some time since I saw a patient in whom I thought the plica was responsible for the symptoms and whom symptoms were relieved by dividing this structure. It may be necessary to remove soft tissue structures including the plica in order to obtain an unobstructed view of the knee joint. There is certainly no harm in cutting the plica, but the biggest danger is that it may divert the surgeon's attention, and he may miss pathology elsewhere in the joint that is the real cause of the patient's complaints.

## Suture Of Meniscus

This is a procedure that is done with increasing frequency, both as an open procedure and arthroscopically. There is little doubt in anyone's mind now that preserving the meniscus is most important, and with techniques and new equipment, arthroscopic suture of the meniscus has become a fairly routine procedure in the hands of experienced arthroscopic surgeons. Arthroscopic suture has a special application to those tears located within the substance of the meniscus in the outer 25% of the body of the meniscus. These tears are most difficult to suture openly unless one removes the outer rim of the meniscus, which is something that should be avoided.

## Drilling Of Femoral Condyle

It is my belief that localized lesions, such as those seen in osteochondritis, that have separated should be replaced and pinned, if at all possible. Other lesions, such as those seen with chondral fractures, should be drilled down to bleeding bone. In most cases, I have removed the entire cortex in the base of the defect, which Ficat has recently referred to as spongialization. Some of these lesions are accessible to arthroscopic drilling. Those further back in the condyle are much more difficult to drill. My own preference in most cases is to do this through a very small arthrotomy incision (Figure 1–8), then the edges of the lesion can be cleanly and sharply defined and excised and the cortical bone can be removed. This can be done in much less time through a miniarthrotomy incision, and this is especially true when a large fat pad makes arthroscopic visualization difficult. Drilling down to cancellous bone results in some bleeding into the joint, and this of course makes placing other drill holes into the defect more difficult, if done arthroscopically.

## Abrasion Arthroplasty

Abrasion arthroplasty has become very popular in the past year or two, largely because it is performed with special sophisticated equipment, which seems to have an attraction for some orthopaedic surgeons. My own feeling is that this is an unsound procedure because it is usually performed in patients who have angular deformity and in whom the normal articular cartilage has broken down because of

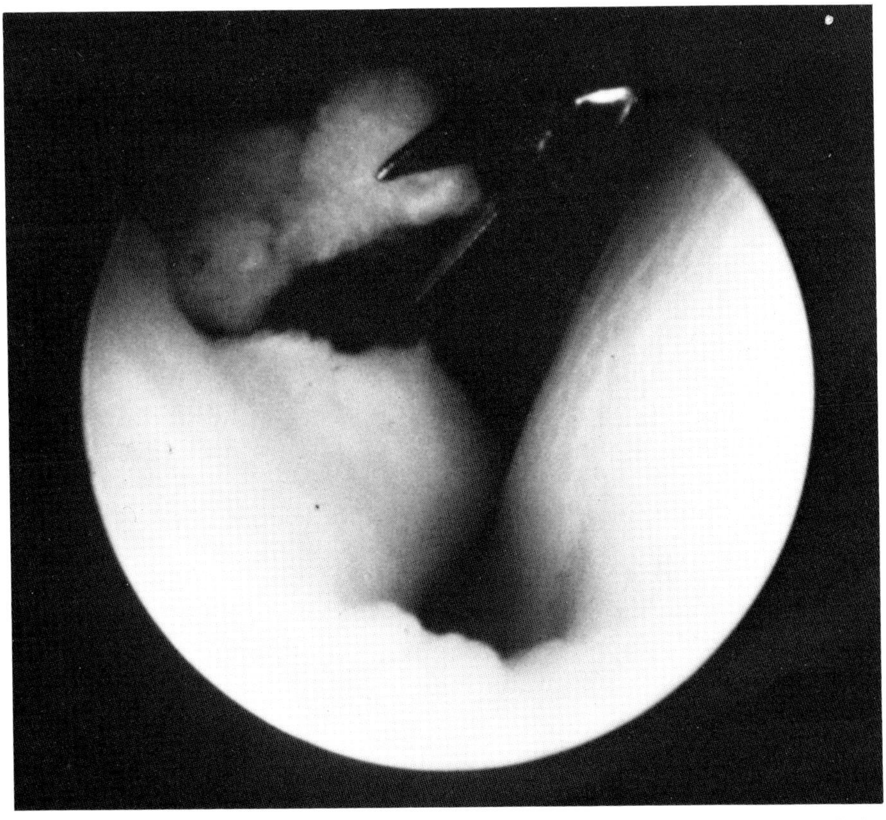

**Figure 1–7** A fairly good-sized medial plica that is being resected, although there is little reason to think that this has been producing symptoms.

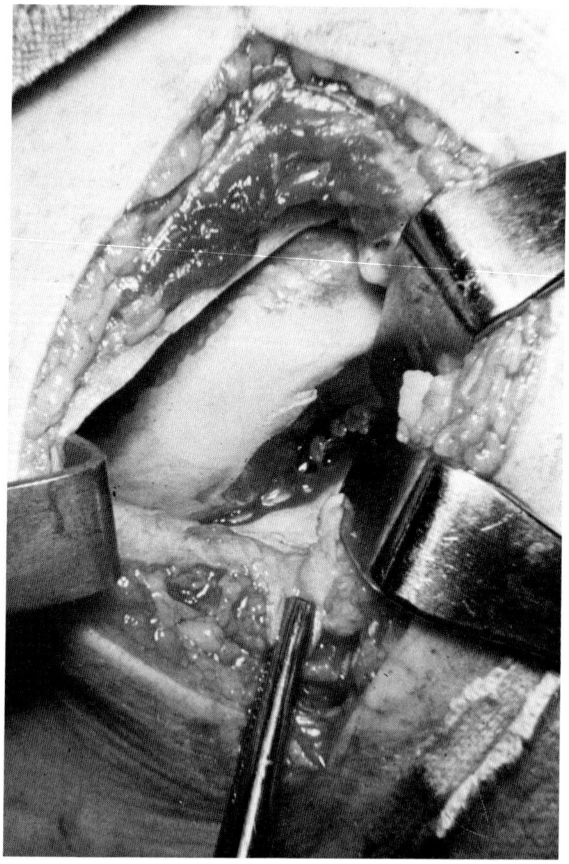

**Figure 1–8** Osteochondritic lesion of the medial femoral condyle which has been cored down to cancellous bone, a process that Ficat refers to as spongialization. It is much easier and better to perform this surgery through an arthrotomy incision. The scar in the skin is of secondary importance.

overload. It is unrealistic to think that the fibrocartilage resulting from the abrasion arthroplasty will survive for very long. Most of these patients need an osteotomy to realign the leg, not an abrasion arthroplasty.

### Future Developments

The frontier as far as arthroscopic surgery is concerned appears to be almost unlimited, and new procedures are constantly surfacing. One of these is a reconstruction of the cruciate ligament using a graft such as the semitendinosus, which is obtained by an open procedure and inserted by a closed arthroscopic procedure. Closed arthroscopic reconstruction of chronic recurrent dislocation of the shoulder is another such procedure. These operations are usually being done only by highly skilled, experienced arthroscopic surgeons, and whether or not such surgery will have any permanent place in the field of arthroscopic surgery is doubtful. Certainly, the results are not yet known.

## Arthroscopy Of Other Joints

There is scarcely any joint in the body that has not been investigated arthroscopically on at least a few occasions. Most of these efforts can be classified as a "triumph of technology over reason." The shoulder is the one joint other than the knee joint that is being arthroscoped with increasing frequency. It is a large joint, and it certainly lends itself to diagnostic arthroscopy (Figure 1–9), and even to some surgical procedures such as removal of the loose body. Currently, most of the interest centers on the glenoid labrum, excising it when it is loose or fragmented and occasionally inserting a staple to reattach it to the glenoid. This surgery is still in its infancy, and it is not known how successful it will be. Much of this surgery requires an anterior as well as a posterior approach to the shoulder, and already some complications have been reported with injury to the neurovascular structures in the front of the shoulder. These complications are similar to those reported in the knee joint where an attempt to do an arthroscopic menisccctomy through a posterior medial approach has resulted in damage to the popliteal vessels and even the loss of a limb.

## Summary

In summary, I think that there are three things that an arthroscopist should keep in mind. First, as a general rule, there is no urgency about scheduling an arthroscopy, except in acute trauma and rarely should the decision for arthroscopy be made on the patient's first visit. Second, diagnostic arthroscopy when used properly has been a great boom to orthopaedic surgery as well as to the patient, and with arthrography advanced to its present state, exploratory arthrotomies should be a thing of the past. Third, arthroscopic surgery, especially arthroscopic meniscectomy, is an exciting and highly satisfying procedure to both surgeon and patient alike: however, there is still a place for arthrotomy using a small incision after the patient's pathology has been pinpointed by a diagnostic arthroscopy. A well executed arthrotomy is superior to an arthroscopy poorly done.

The place of diagnostic arthroscopy has now become well-established in the field of orthopaedic surgery. It is my belief that arthroscopic surgery has yet to find its proper place in the armamentarium of the orthopedic surgeon.

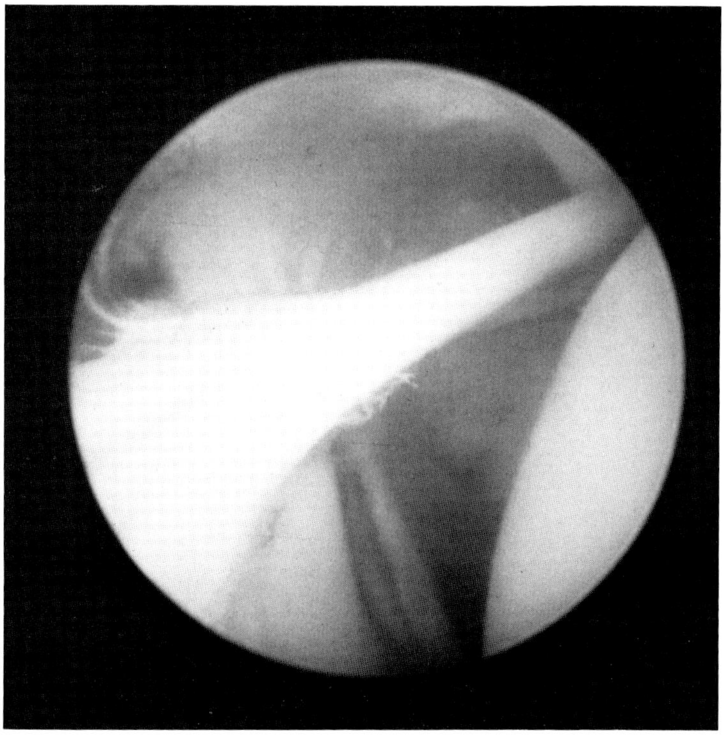

**Figure 1–9** View of the interior of the shoulder showing a tear of the glenoid labrum.

## *References*

1. Casscells S W. The place of arthroscopy and the diagnosis and treatment of internal derangement of the knee and analysis of 1,000 cases. Clin Orthop 151:135, 1980
2. Hamberg P P, Gillquist J, Lyshom J. A comparison between arthroscopic meniscectomy and modified open meniscectomy. J Bone Joint Surg [Br] 66:189, 1984
3. Joyce M J, Mankin H J. Caveat arthroscopos: Extra-articular lesions of bone simulating intra-articular pathology of the knee. J Bone Joint Surg [Am] 65:289, 1983
4. Keene J S, Dyreby J R. High tibial osteotomy in the treatment of osteoarthritis of the knee. The role of preoperative arthroscopy. J Bone Joint Surg [Am] 64:36, 1983
5. Noble J, Erat K. In defense of the meniscus. J Bone Joint Surg [Br] 62:7–11, 1980
6. Smillie I S. Diseases of the Knee Joint, p 84. Churchill Livingstone Ltd, Edinburgh, 1974
7. Watson-Jones Sir R. Fractures and Joint Injuries, pp 768–769. Williams & Wilkins, Baltimore, 1955.

# The Care of Arthroscopic Equipment

# 2

Anna Marie Cable

The care and maintenance of arthroscopic systems is a complex procedure. The nurse's role in the use and management of all arthroscopic equipment is essential to any surgeon who performs arthroscopic procedures.

The care of all arthroscopic instrumentation is of utmost importance in managing the inventory. The instrumentation is of precision quality and requires delicate handling. The total function of any one piece is dependent on proper care (1).

The arthroscope, sheath, trocars, and cannula systems should be stored and sterilized in a sterilization tray. All knives, probes, forceps, and scissors should also be stored in a tray that will ensure that the cutting edge of the instrument retains its sharpness (Figure 2–1). Instrument guards that are steam autoclavable protect the instruments well, and the same forceps can be assembled according to size on a rack on the sterile field (Figure 2–2). Instruments should not be dropped on one another. All metal-to-metal contact should be avoided.

Fiberoptic light cables should be stored separately in either a completely straight fashion or coiled to prevent fiber bundle breakage. Retrieval from the sterile field by the scrub or circulating nurse at the conclusion of the procedure is done with care that the cable does not fall or become damaged in any way. Careless handling will irreversibly damage the fibers and decrease optical transmission into the joint (2).

The light source itself is a very important piece of equipment. The medical electronics department in your institution must initially check the unit for electrical leakage and confirm that its voltage meets requirements for use in the operating room. A replacement bulb or bulbs should be stored near the source to provide for

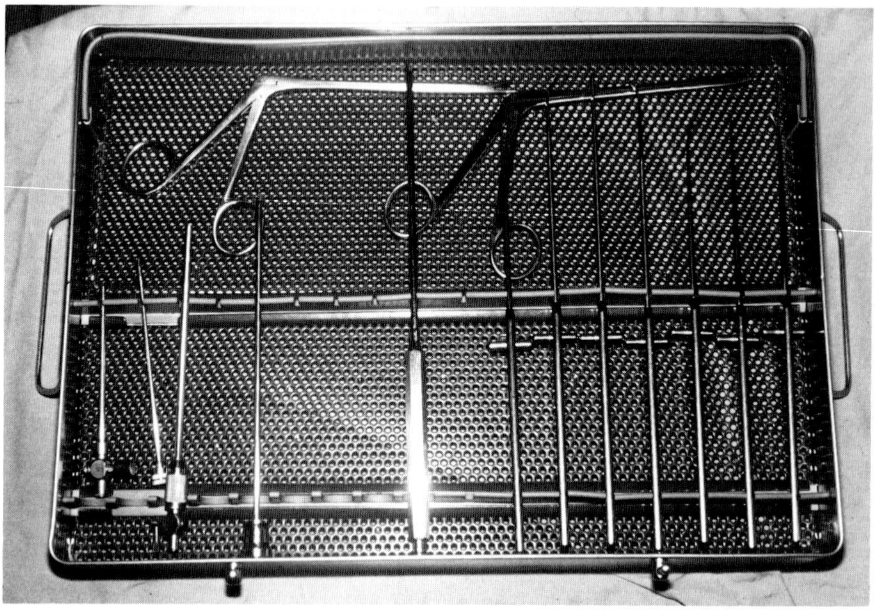

**Figure 2–1** Instrument sterilization tray.

changing of lamps when necessary. For increased lamp life, intensity must be decreased before the source is turned off. If your unit is equipped with a fan, allow it to run for several minutes before switching the power off.

General cleaning of arthroscopic instrumentation should be carried out with attention to every detail. Use a variety of soft brushes, pipe cleaners, or cotton swabs to clean sheaths and cannulas inside and out. A mild soap or detergent and

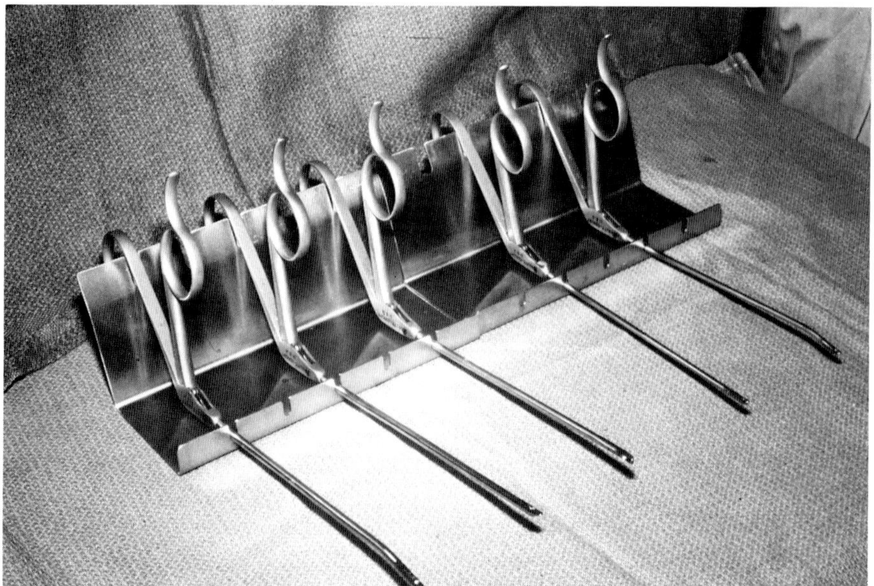

**Figure 2–2** Sterile forcep rack.

warm, distilled water will remove all debris remaining after a procedure. Air is used to blow out retained water particles before instruments are returned to storage trays.

Objective lenses and ocular windows on arthroscopes should be cleaned with alcohol swabs. Similar care should be given to the fiber ends of the light cable. Remove any adaptor for access (Figure 2–3). Residue must be removed to guarantee maximum light transmission.

Surgical instrument cleaner or lubricating oil should be routinely applied to stopcocks, locks, hinges, knob nuts, or other mechanical parts.

Instruments should not only be properly cleaned after each use, but examined for any defects. Optics can be checked extra-articularly by connecting the scope to the light cable and source and observing fine print or linen fibers for clarity. Also check the arthroscope with your eye for a crystal clear picture. Fogginess denotes a leak in the eyepiece, and a blocked view or "half moon" effect means that the fibers are broken or the ocular lens is dislodged. The light cable can be checked quickly by holding one end to a bright light and looking at the other end. (Figure 2–4). Black dots indicate broken fiberoptic fibers; so when it appears that more than one-third of the entire field is blackened, the cable should be replaced. Sharp cutting instruments must be checked for breaks or burrs. When damaged, these items should be sent to the manufacturer for repair or replacement. Backup instrumentation can be used during "down time."

Service by corporate representatives is very important to a surgeon or institution that must work with limited pieces of instrumentation or are unable to obtain loaners from the manufacturer during "down time." Most companies have a toll-free number to call for specific instructions on how to return items for repair or refurbishing. A representative can also be called locally, to assist in expediting such repairs.

Use the corporate representatives as resource persons. They can readily supply you with updated printed material or manuals regarding new or existing instruments or equipment. Become familiar with the representative so that you will feel comfortable if and when you should need to call him or her if a problem arises

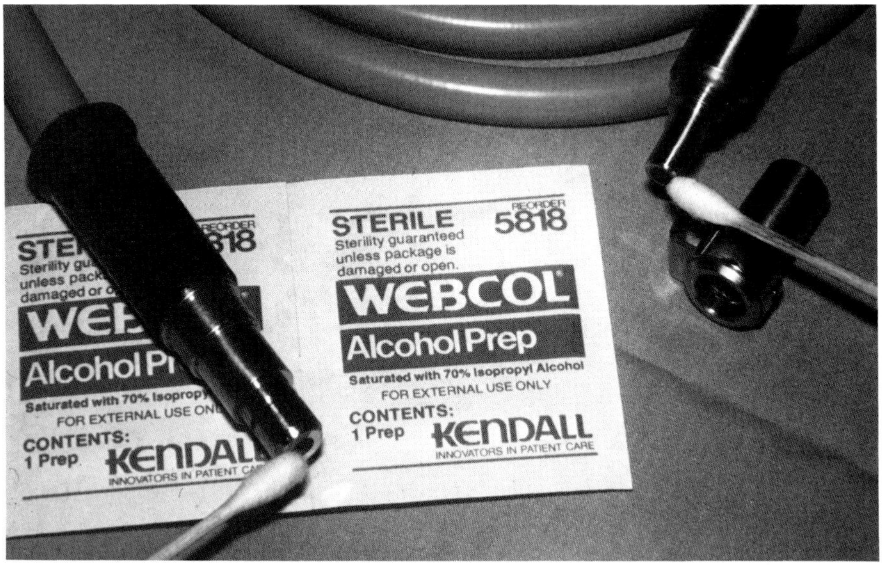


**Figure 2–3** Cleaning of light cable ends.

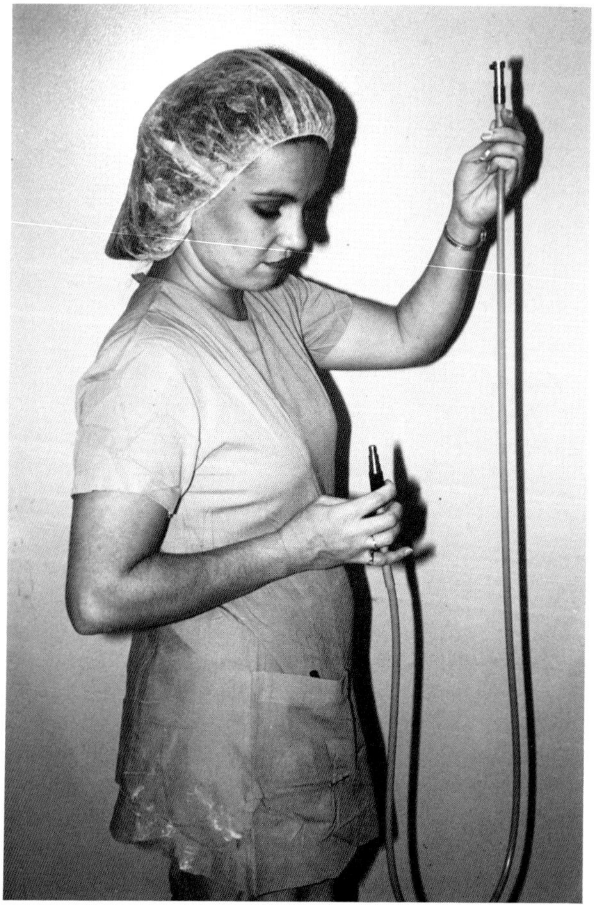

**Figure 2–4** Checking cable for broken fibers.

while using the product or if you would like to evaluate a new product on a trial basis. The industry is constantly eager to hear comments from those using its products in the operating room since this information can be valuable for future designs or modifications of products or instrumentation in the arthroscopic field.

The principles of sterilization and storage of instrumentation can be applied to maintaining the function and quality of all instrumentation to provide the arthroscopic surgeon with precision tools for the needs of each and every procedure.

By rule, each instrument is sterilized according to its manufacturer's instructions. Gas sterilization is the method of choice by most surgeons, but it has two drawbacks. The first is cost: gas sterilization is most expensive. The second drawback is that an institution's inventory may not permit gas sterilization of instrumentation for other than the first procedure of the day; thus subsequent procedures would rely upon sterilization by soaking in gluteraldehyde. Disinfection with 2% gluteraldehyde or activated dialdehyde solution is more economical but doesn't achieve complete sterilization because it fails to destroy spore-forming organisms and hepatitis virus in the recommended time (3). Operating room standards state that the use of ''double standards'' should not occur; thus if several arthroscope sets can be purchased, gas sterilization, which is the best method, could be done for all procedures.

Extended soak periods or water rinses may result in leakage into the system of fiber bundles in a telescope. All metal instrumentation and fiberoptic light cables can be steam sterilized. However, repeated steam sterilization does decrease the sharpness of cutting instruments (4). Therefore all cutting instruments should be examined carefully before and after use and repaired and replaced if necessary.

After a contaminated arthroscopy, decontamination is best carried out by gas sterilization in appropriately labeled bags. If the arthroscope is steam autoclavable, then decontamination can be done in the operating room's steam autoclave.

Safe storage of all instruments and equipment provides for longevity and less breakage overall. All sterile supplies should be in one area. A specific cupboard or case cart that accommodates supplies in labeled bins makes case preparation easy and readily accessible (Figure 2–5). A mobile case cart also is a table top surface for soak and rinse pans, and it can be moved easily from suite to suite.

Disposable drape packs or extremity sheets aid in the sterile draping of the affected extremity. Several suppliers are available. Single-use arthroscopy procedure trays can be custom made to include all supplies normally used for each arthroscopy. This practice helps avoid lost charges, aids in setup time, and is very cost-effective to the institution.

Intravenous poles should be accessible for irrigation fluid bags. The circulating nurse performs the sterile connection of inflow tubing to the bag as well as the connection of outflow suction tubing to a collection system equipped with a specimen collector. This is accomplished on the affected side of the patient. Then the light cable is connected to the light source, and the camera is either draped sterilely or connected to its console from the opposite side of the patient.

Surgical abrasion or cutting systems provide for intra-articular meniscal trimming, cutting, or shaving. Several systems are available that operate by either air power or battery. Adequate cleaning and lubrication where necessary help maintain these pieces in precision quality and function. Proper connections are a must for use.

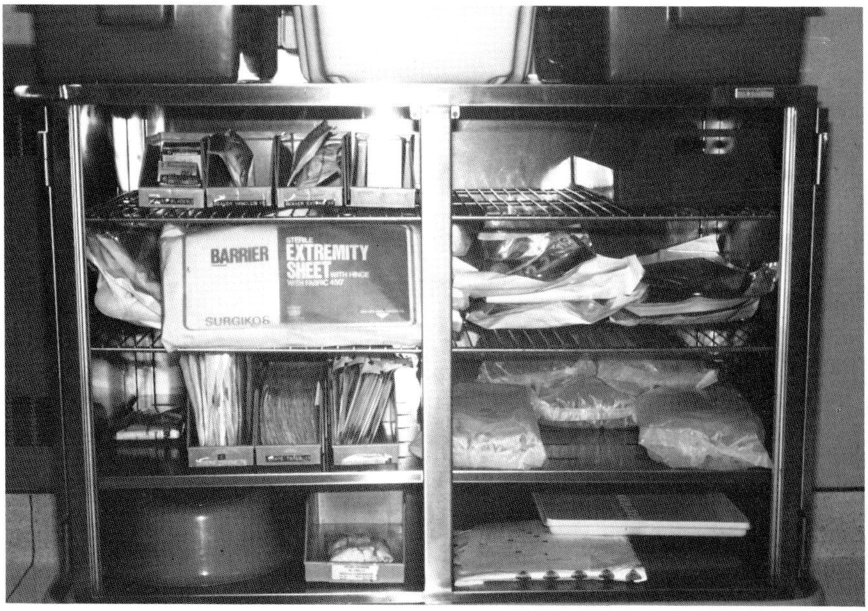


**Figure 2–5** Mobile storage case cart.

Arthroscopic leg holders are devices that stabilize the affected extremity and relieve the surgeon of the need to manipulate the leg during the procedure. Several models are available at varied costs. A well leg support, made of molded foam, protects the unaffected leg during surgery (Figure 2–6). Routine cleaning consists of soap and water, with new covers for the leg wraps for each patient.

"Everything has its place" is a necessary rule in the care and maintenance of expensive and delicate arthroscopic instruments and equipment.

Education of all personnel to the correct handling of all instrumentation is done by the nurse in charge of the equipment in conjunction with in-service education by sales representatives about new products in the operating room. Personnel should know instrument care in preparation for a case and between cases, as well as daily terminal care. One person should be responsible for all instruments and equipment. Surgeons can refer any complaints or suggestions to him or her and expect quick follow-through on a problem or topic. This person can become most familiar with new products and be instrumental in the preparation of budgetary appropriations for the continuing purchase of items. Stock inventory of all patient charge items must be maintained by this nurse. Repairs also can be handled by him or her or by a materials management person or unit manager equipped to rush a product to the manufacturer. Enough stress cannot be placed on the fact that the individual who maintains arthroscopic inventory is assuming a great responsibility to the patient, surgeon, operating room staff, and institution.

Video equipment is stored on a Surgicenter® table or in a mobile console. The monitor, camera console, videocassette recorder, and fiberoptic light source all fit nicely on a Surgicenter® table. Damp dusting of all surface areas must be done before the first procedure of the day. A mobile console that locks provides storage for all video equipment as well as instrumentation trays, cables, and the leg holder (Figure 2–7). The console can be adapted with hooks, handles, and cord storage brackets to aid its use.

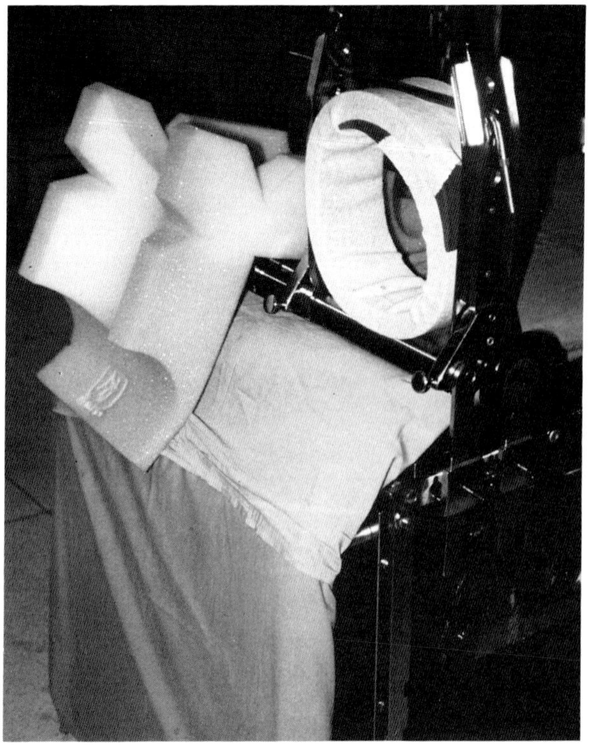

**Figure 2–6** Leg holder and well leg support.

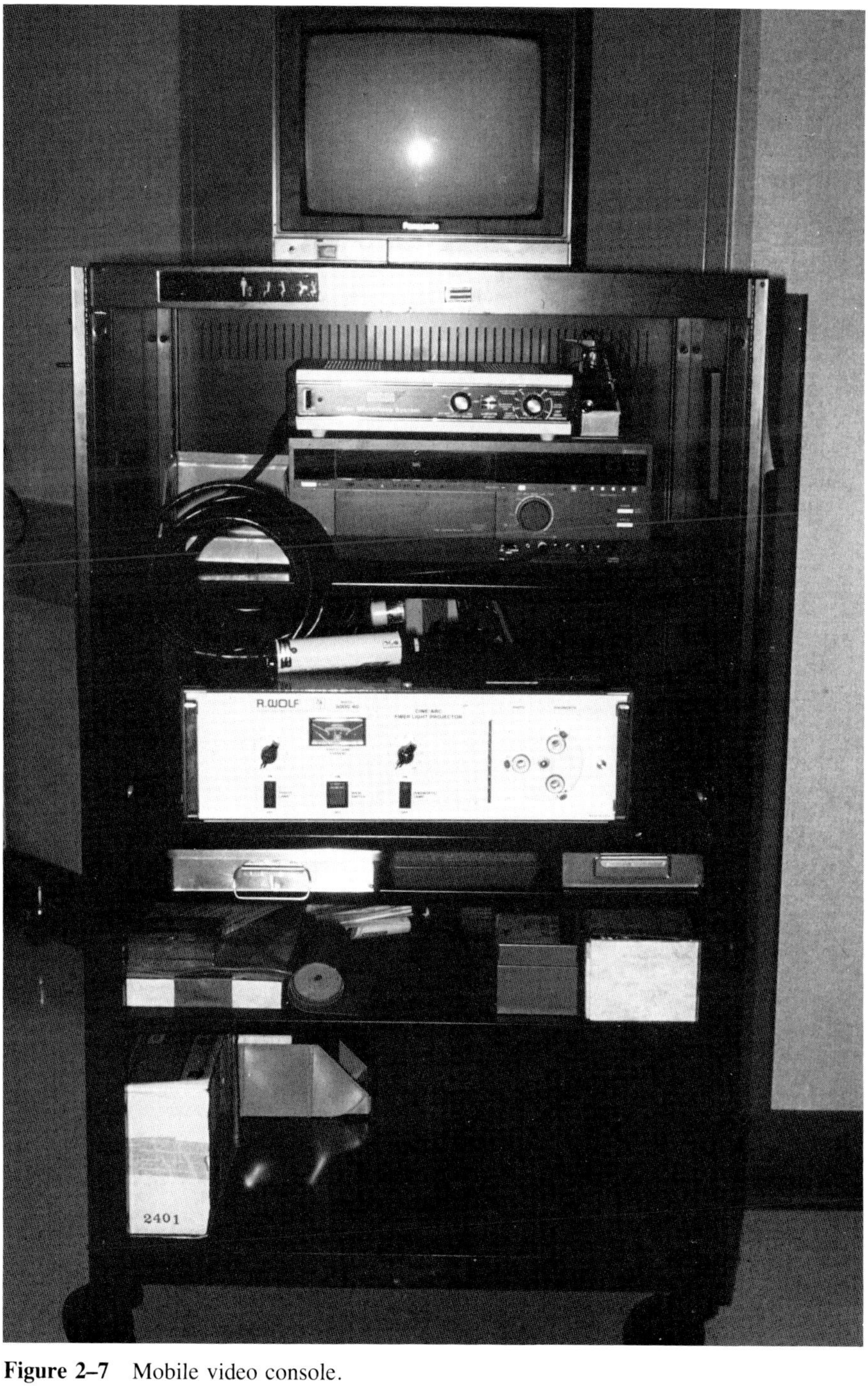


**Figure 2–7** Mobile video console.

The color monitor requires little care other than dust-free maintenance after the knobs or switches are set for optimal viewing color and clarity on the screen. The videocassette recorder requires proper care and maintenance for maximum functioning (5). Corresponding tapes should be available for each surgeon's use. A cleaning cassette tape can be used periodically to clean the sensitive video heads. Before recording a procedure, it is helpful to record several frames of the patient's information found on the chart's fact sheet or the patient's stamper plate. This aids the surgeon in correctly identifying each recording. The counter should also be monitored, and start and finish marks should be printed on the cassette cover.

Cameras are of two types. First, there are microvideo tube cameras that weigh 6–8 ounces and require microcouplers and sterile covers before use on an arthroscope. The medical photography department can assist in cleaning the lens and focusable microcoupler. The cable should be neatly coiled and stored free of tangles. It should never be disconnected from the console, except for servicing.

If this camera has a focus ring or control, make sure the camera is in optimal focus for each procedure. The diaphragm on the microcoupler must be opened before draping of the camera. Attaching the eyepiece to the coupler involves inserting it into the sterile cover and securely sealing the cover to the arthroscope with steristrips.

The controller panel on the camera console provides for color compensation according to the available light source. The color bars are used for determining hues.

The second type of camera, the solid-state video camera, is entirely soakable in glutaraldehyde. After a double distilled water rinse, a microfoam instrument wipe, used in cleaning the arthroscope, can clean the lens before it is wiped dry with a gauze sponge. Care in connecting the cable to the console is important, in that failure to align contact points can result in broken points and malfunction of the entire system. Make sure the camera is properly aligned and seated on the eyepiece of the arthroscope. The lens may need to be wiped dry if fogginess occurs and disrupts resolution on the monitor.

Corporate servicing on video equipment must be quick and efficient. Contact the service representative when a problem occurs that cannot be corrected by yourself or the medical photography department. If the equipment must be sent to a service center, make sure it is properly identified with a model and serial number and securely packaged in a shipping case.

Arthroscopy is a new and exciting form of surgery incorporating precision instrumentation and high-technology video recording. It is a very interesting and controversial field that will be discussed and improved upon for many years to come.

## *References*


1. McGinty J B, Berci G. Arthroscopy Guidelines. Karl Storz Endoscopy-America, Inc., Culver City, Ca. 1983
2. MacDonald E, Rigid endoscopes. AORN Journal 40:56–63, 1984
3. Johnson L, Schneider D, Austin M. Two percent glutaraldehyde: A disinfectant in arthroscopy and arthroscopic surgery. Bone Joint Surg [Am] 64:237–239, 1982
4. Stearns C. Preparation of arthroscopic instrumentation: The sterilization vs. disinfection controversy. Arthroscopy of the Knee: National Association of Orthopaedic Nurses, 24–29, 1983
5. Thayer J L, Jackson D W. Videoarthroscopy: What an orthopaedist should know about video equipment. Contemp Orthop 6:187–193, 1983

# Arthroscopic Treatment of Chondromalacia Patellae

# 3

John W. Ewing

## Anterior Knee Pain

A chapter in a textbook of arthroscopic surgical techniques covering arthroscopic patellar shaving for chondromalacia patellae would be inappropriate without at least a short discussion about the anterior knee pain syndrome.

There continues to be a general association of the term "chondromalacia patellae" with a clinical syndrome. This association is indeed unfortunate. Chrondromalacia patellae means simply softening of the articular surface of the patella. This particular entity of softening or even disruption of the patellar articular surface exists for the most part as a clinically silent or painless condition. The cause of chondromalacia patellae is unknown. It has been suggested that lack of compression may lead to cartilage softening (4), but other authors feel that too much compression is the etiology (7). Malalignment of the patella, i.e., lateral subluxation, has a high association with chondromalacia (3), but certainly not all subluxing patellae exhibit chondromalacic changes. Conversely, significant patellar chondromalacia is found in knees that, by any criteria, show no malalignment. Some authors have suggested that chondromalacia patellae is a normally anticipated event in the aging process (5), but necropsy studies in the elderly (2) and even arthroscopic observations of patellae in older patients would seem to dispute this contention. Suffice it to say that chondromalacia patellae is a commonly observed anatomical state that does not, in and of itself, always constitute a clinical syndrome. This is not to say, however, that chondromalacia cannot ever be the cause of anterior knee pain.

Anterior knee pain is one of the most frequent complaints presented to the orthopaedist. All too often we are confronted with the young patient, more frequently female than male, who presents with a complaint of significant parapatellar pain but has little or nothing in the way of physical findings or x-ray abnormalities to support a specific diagnosis. The list of conditions that constitute differential diagnosis includes parapatellar synovitis, bursitis, tendinitis, osteoarthritis, plica syndrome, osteochondritis dissecans, loose body, torn meniscus, excessive lateral pressure syndrome, recurrent dislocation of the patella, subluxing patella, unrecognized hip pathology, overpronation of the foot, soft tissue or bony neoplasm, and finally, chondromalacia. For the most part, the anterior knee pain syndrome is treated symptomatically once a sincere effort has been made to pinpoint a specific diagnosis. Rest from activities and anti-inflammatory drugs are used initially along with isometric quadriceps strengthening and hamstring-stretching exercises. Appropriate footwear modifications where indicated in runners is often very useful. The use of patellar and infrapatellar supports have also been valuable in my practice in managing these patients' painful knees.

When careful physical examination and x-ray evaluation including properly executed tangential views of the patella have not revealed a specific diagnosis, the tendency now is to turn to either arthrography or arthroscopy for help. The yield of positive results from arthrography is low in this instance and usually ambiguous. When a suggestion of a meniscal lesion is made, arthroscopy is then indicated to confirm the impression. If the patient's symptoms remain vague and no particular points of tenderness can be found, such as consistent tenderness over the medial shelf or significant pain on direct patellar compression, then the yield of significantly helpful information from arthroscopic examination is also very low. Continued conservative, symptomatic treatment along with an alteration of activity level on the patient's part are indicated in this syndrome rather than arthroscopic intervention.

Patellar malalignment syndromes including excessive lateral pressure syndrome are better diagnosed by standard noninvasive means rather than by arthroscopic techniques.

If, on the other hand, the physical examination reveals significant persistent pain on direct patellar compression, with or without true patellar crepitation, and the patient's symptoms have persisted for more than 3–6 months despite adequate conservative care, then arthroscopy is indicated to inspect the knee and in particular, the patellar surface. Patellar crepitation, which is a palpable sensation felt by the examiner by lightly resting the hand on the patella while the patient performs a deep knee bend, almost always indicates chondromalacia patella. The absence of crepitation, however, does not mean that the articular surface is normal. Care must be taken to avoid using crepitation as an indication for arthroscopic intervention. The vast majority of crepitant patellae are painless, and the patients who are led to seek attention for this peculiar symptom are best managed by a reassuring discussion that the crepitation they feel needs no specific care. Pain remains as the single indicator for arthroscopic intervention when chondromalacia patellae is suspected as the cause of the anterior pain syndrome.

## Technique

The arthroscopic patellar debridement is best carried out under general or spinal anesthesia. Local anesthesia can be used for this procedure at the surgeon's discretion. The procedure is easily done on an outpatient basis since postoperative discomfort is only moderate to minimal and managed nicely by oral analgesics and limited activities. Arthroscopic examination of all compartments of the knee is carried out through standard anterior approaches. If an unsuspected tear of either meniscus is found, it is treated by partial meniscectomy, and the patellar debridement is carried out at the same sitting. If, as is usually the case, the only mechanical abnormality found is disruption of the patellar articular surface, then the debridement is best carried out from the proximal approach. The use of a tourniquet is optional, as is the use of a thigh holder; we routinely employ both. The tourniquet is inflated prior to the placement of the thigh holder. The thigh holder is then placed over the inflated tourniquet to allow ample room for proximal approaches. The affected leg is placed in full extension following the arthroscopic exam. The heel of the affected leg is placed on a padded Mayo stand, and the opposite leg is allowed to flex to 90 degrees over the end of a flexed operating table (Figure 3–1). This allows for unimpeded use of either the medial or lateral proximal puncture site for either the television camera-equipped arthroscope or the operating instruments. The inflow cannula for knee distention is placed through the anterior lateral puncture site. The video monitor is placed at the foot of the table, and the surgeon and assistants are positioned at each side of the patient and work from above the

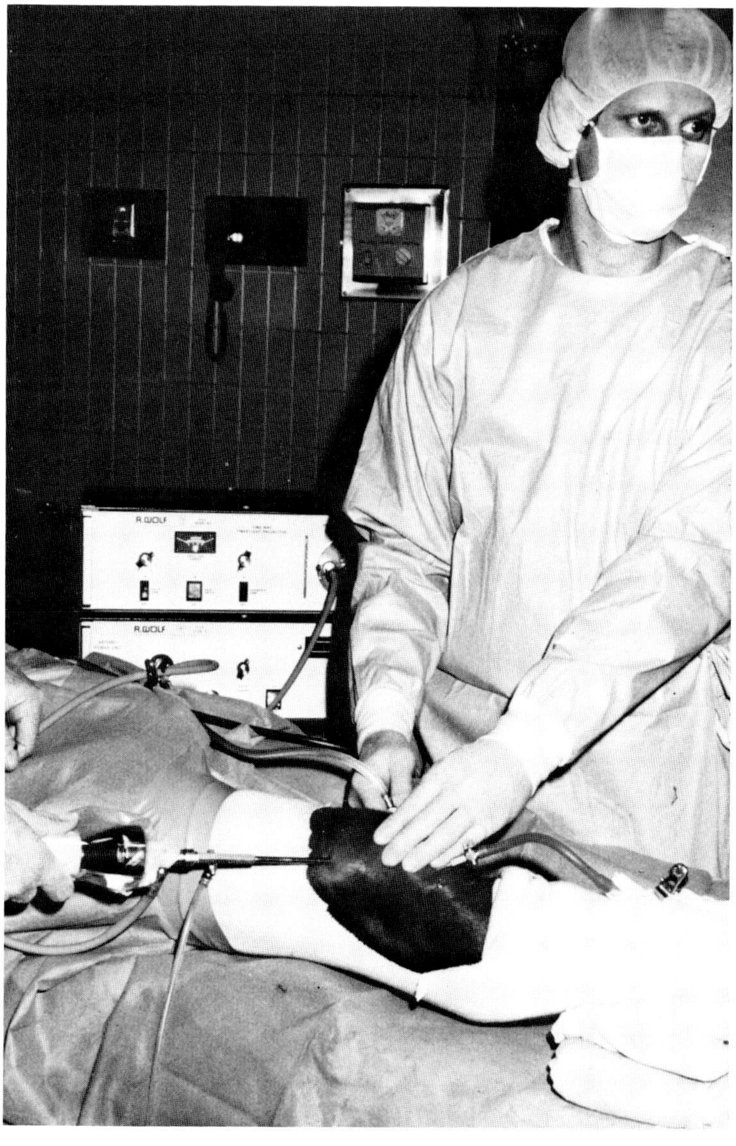

**Figure 3–1** Surgeon using the intra-articular shaver from the proximal approach, enabling the surgeon to operate in a bimanual fashion, which improves technique.

knee (Figure 3–2). With the knee adequately distended with either saline or Ringers lactate, the superolateral puncture is made on the line that extends proximally along the patellofemoral joint line approximately three finger breadths above the superior pole of the patella with the knee in full extension. A 4- to 5-mm arthroscope with 30 degrees fore-oblique lens affords an excellent view of the patellofemoral joint from this approach. The proximomedial portal is made selectively after first entering the knee superiorly and medially with an 18-gauge spinal needle. The optimum portal is one that allows the easiest access to the entire patellar surface, as determined by manipulation of the spinal needle. When this portal site has been determined, it is made with a number 11 surgical blade (Figure 3–3). This medial portal is usually one to two finger breadths above the superior pole of the patella in the extended knee along the medial patellofemoral joint line. Probing of the patellar surface is carried out through this medial portal using a standard 3-mm blunt probe. The chondromalacic nature of the patellar surface is then evaluated. A motorized cutting-suctioning device is then placed through the proximomedial portal, and the loose fibrillated articular cartilage is removed. On many occasions these are plate-like lesions of articular cartilage that are not attached to the deep zone of cartilage and are best removed by hand-held instruments. (Figures 3–4 to 3–6). The goal of the surgery is to remove all abnormally mobile articular cartilage and leave no undermined areas of poorly attached cartilage. In many instances there is a very obvious parapatellar synovitis. This synovial tissue is also removed at the time of surgery. If access to the lesional area of the patella is difficult from the medial portal, switching to the lateral portal for instruments and the medial for the arthroscope will often help. Accessory medial or lateral portals should be made without

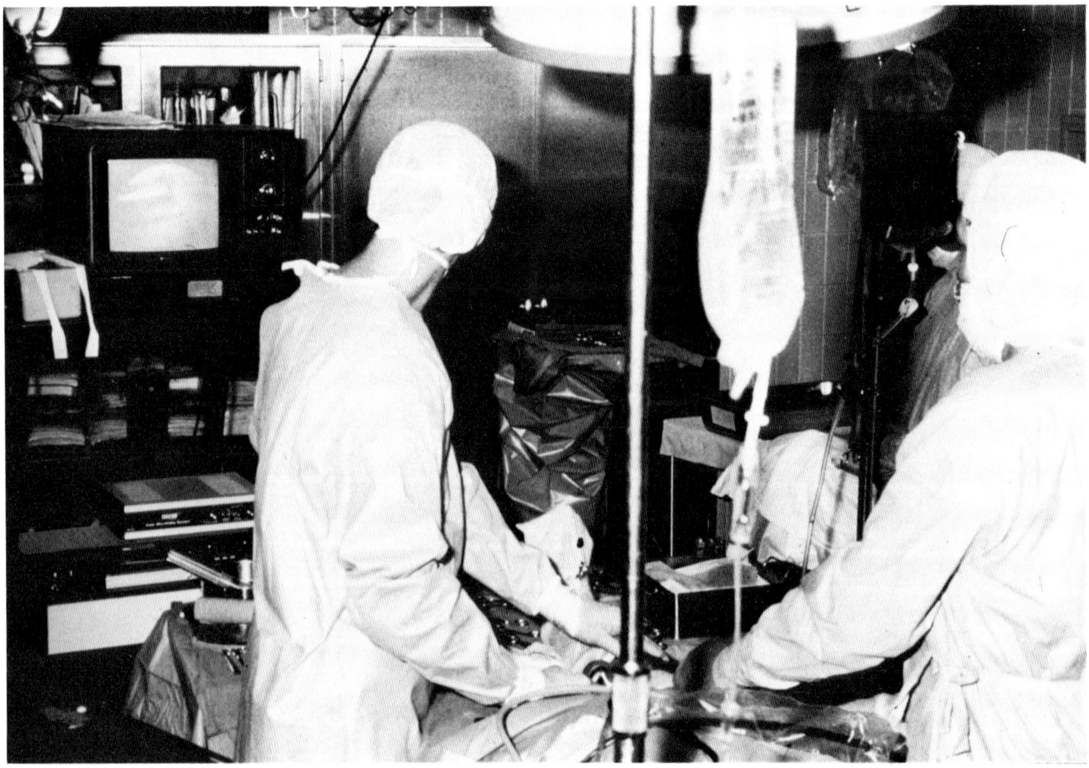

**Figure 3–2** Surgical setup. Note the monitor at the foot of the table for ease of viewing for the entire team.

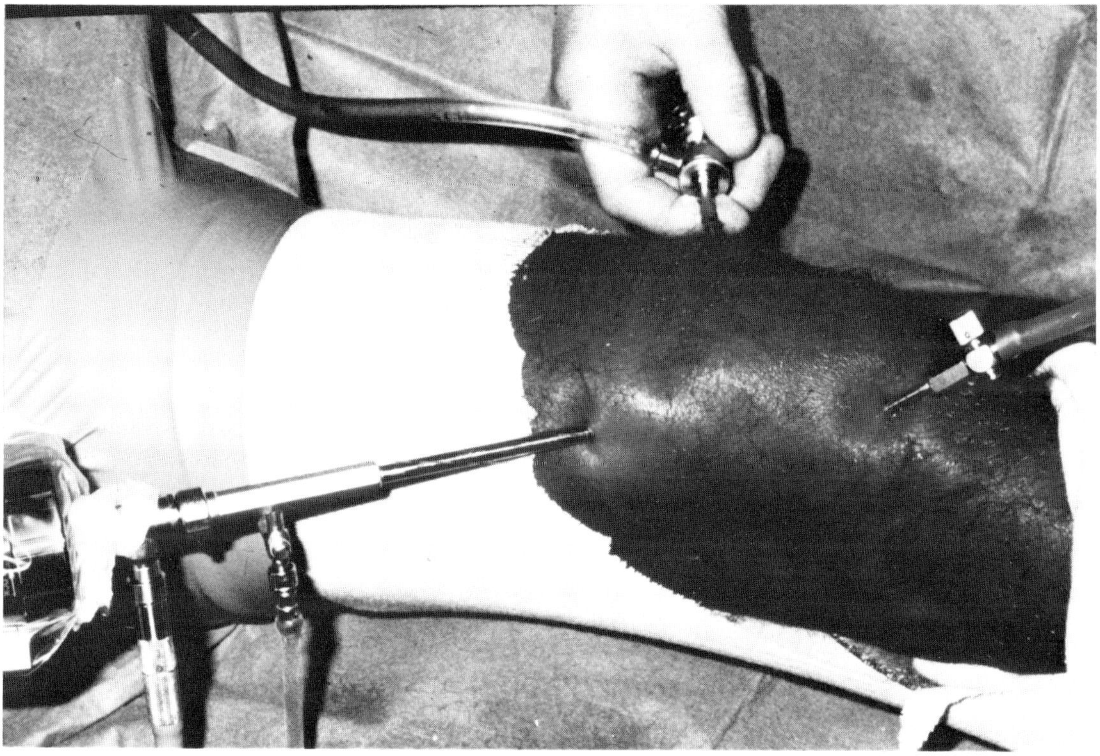

**Figure 3–3** A close-up view of the proximal approach for patellar surgery. The arthroscope is placed superolaterally, the intra-articular shaver is placed superomedially, and the inflow is in the anterolateral portal. (Note: The outflow is from the sidearm of the arthroscopic cannula.)

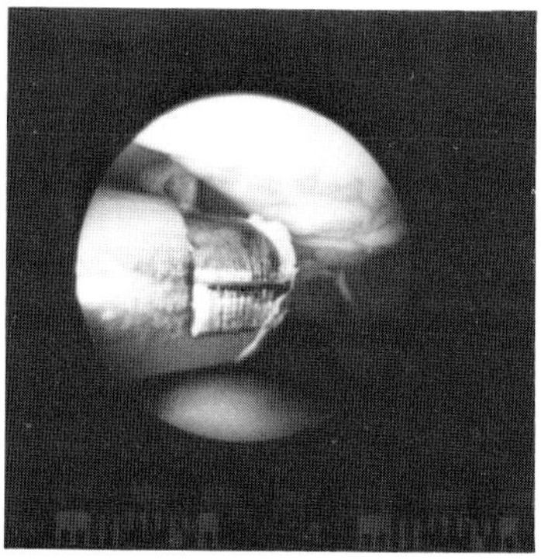

**Figure 3–4** The intra-articular shaver in action during the debridement of the grade III lesion of the patella.

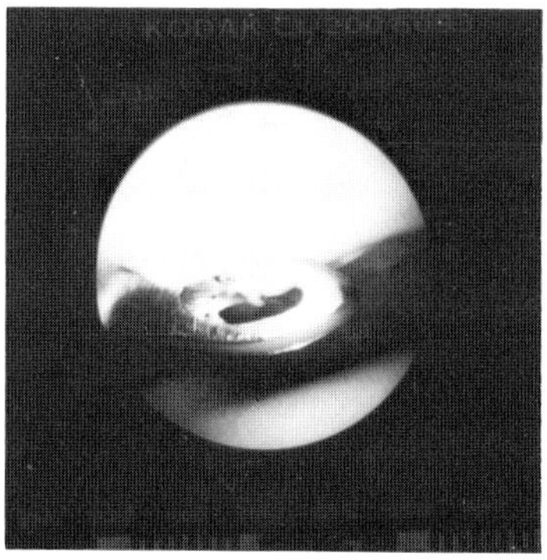

**Figure 3–5** The patellar trimmer while in use on a grade II lesion. This instrument is especially helpful as the fenestrations in the cutting jaws permit visualization of the area being trimmed. This permits more precise debridement and decreases surgical time.

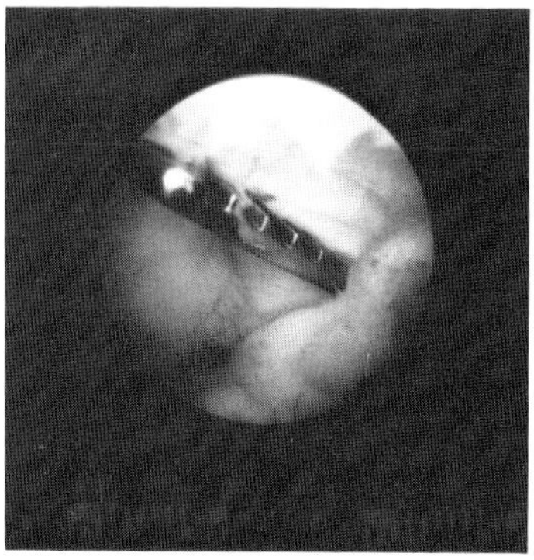

**Figure 3–6** The chondral rasp is used to smooth the surface as a final touch to the debridement. Its flat surface aids in creating a smoother articular surface with minimal loss of articular cartilage.

hesitation to improve the surgical exposure if it remains difficult to gain access. It is helpful to have an outflow established during the surgical procedure. We utilize flexible tubing attached to the sidearm of the arthroscopic cannula as an outflow (Figure 3–3). Final probing of the patellar surface is always done to ensure that there are no remaining undermined flaps of diseased articular cartilage. Finally, the knee is irrigated copiously and aspirated to remove all small fragments of cartilagenous debris and then is drained. A simple compressive bandage is applied to the leg, and the patient is allowed to return home following recovery from anesthesia. Crutch walking with weight bearing is advised, but most patients are fully weight bearing in 3 days. Unlimited activities are permitted when all signs of effusion are gone and full painless range of motion is present. Patients are usually able to participate in unlimited activities 4 weeks from surgery. The Outerbridge classification (7) has been used by this author to classify the degree of involvement.

Grade I changes exhibit only softening and swelling of the articular surface. In grade II chondromalacia, actual fragmentation and fissuring of the articular surface are noted in an area measuring ½ inch or less. Grade III is the same as Grade II, but it covers an area of erosion greater than ½ inch. In grade IV changes, there is an erosion down to and exposing subchondral bone.

Occasionally, one sees very superficial changes on the patellar surface without softening or fissuring. These changes do not constitute a pathological condition and should be ignored (Figures 3–7 and 3–8). Grade I changes are not subjected to surgical treatment, and grade II changes are removed only when they occur in the middle one-third of the patellar surface. It is quite common to see grade II changes on the surface of the very medial portion or odd facet of the patella (Figure 3–9). These lesions are likewise not felt to be a cause for patellofemoral pain and are left alone. In grade IV patellar disease, there is usually little to no remaining healthy articular cartilage on the patellar surface, which makes patellar debridement impractical. Thus the majority of the treatable patellar lesions fall into the grade III category, with only a few grade II lesions being added to this group (Figures 3–10 to 3–12).

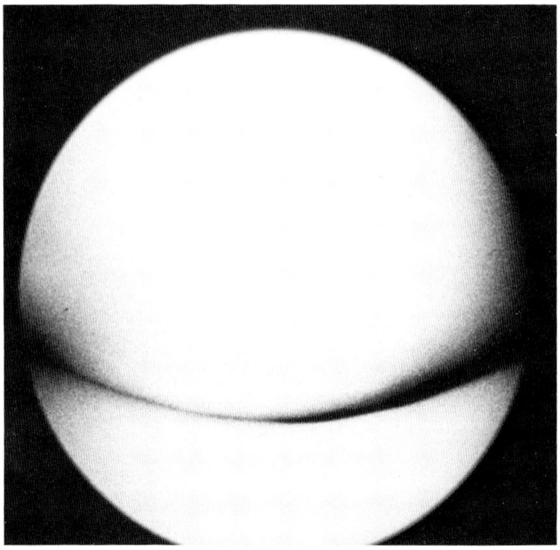

**Figure 3–7** A normal patella seen from the superolateral view.

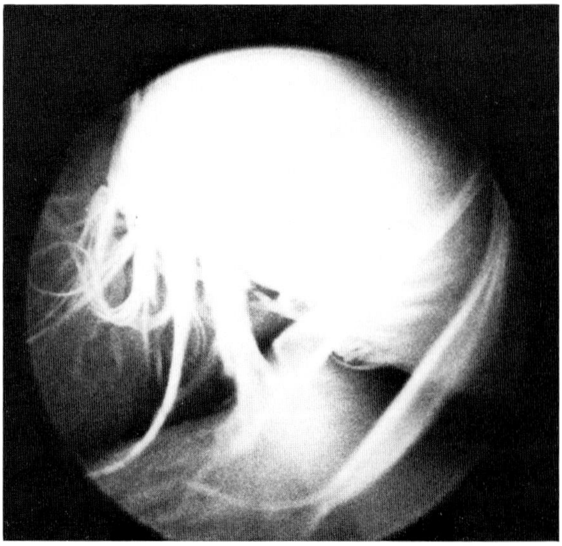

**Figure 3–8** Superficial "bacon strip" changes commonly seen near the superior pole of the patella and requiring no treatment.

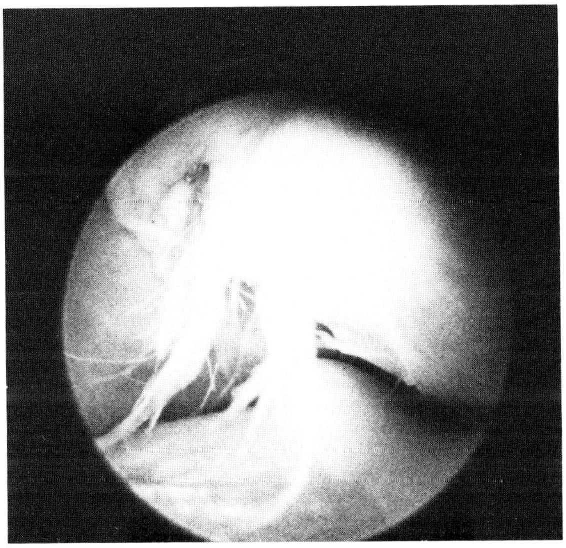

**Figure 3–9** The odd facet area of chondromalacia. Not considered pathologic and should be left alone.

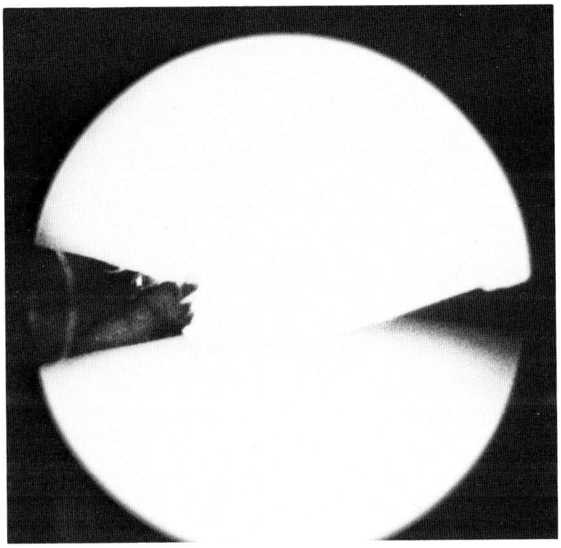

**Figure 3–10** A pathological grade II patellar lesion of the middle one-third of the patella.

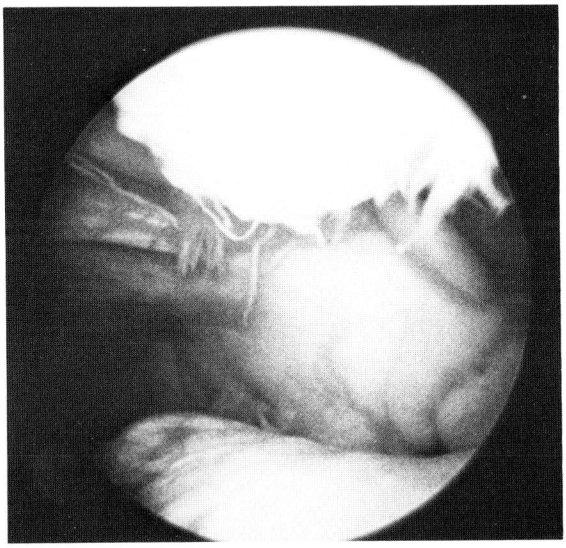

**Figure 3–11** A pathological grade III lesion somewhat "global" in location.

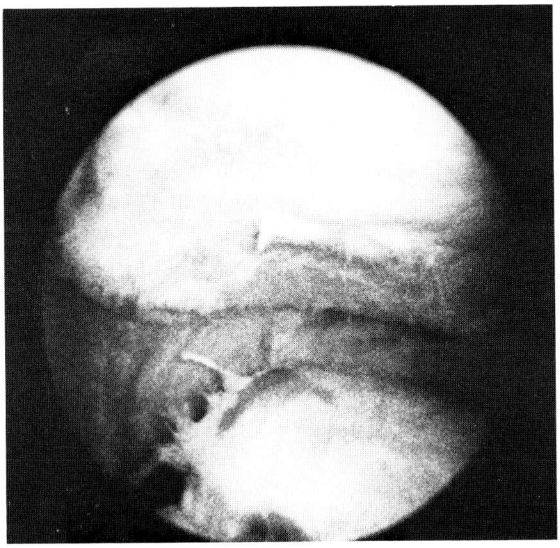

**Figure 3–12** Grade IV chondral lesion. Note the exposed subchondral bone.

# Results

In 1977 Dr. Lanny Johnson developed a motorized, cutting-suction device that provided a way to debride the patellar surface by means of arthroscopic control with minimal surgical trauma. Encouraged by reports of his early good results (6), we began to treat carefully selected cases of chronic anterior knee pain whose etiology seemed to be from chondromalacia patellae. In the initial phase, from 1977 to 1979, all cases were operated upon only after an initial diagnostic arthroscopy, performed some months prior to the patellar shaving. We found no patients

**Table 3–1** Phase I: Initial Patient Evaluation, 1981, by Gender

| | EXCELLENT | | GOOD | | FAIR | | POOR | |
|---|---|---|---|---|---|---|---|---|
| | No. | % | No. | % | No. | % | No. | % |
| All patients (n = 56) | 21 | 37.5 | 22 | 39.3 | 7 | 12.5 | 6 | 10.7 |
| Females (n = 39) | 11 | 28.2 | 19 | 48.7 | 5 | 12.8 | 4 | 10.3 |
| Males (n = 17) | 10 | 58.8 | 3 | 17.6 | 2 | 11.8 | 2 | 11.8 |

in the initial group whose pain was relieved by diagnostic arthroscopy alone. It was my intention to follow these patients closely for a long enough period of time to determine whether there was any relief of painful symptoms, and, if the relief was significant, whether it was only temporary. The initial patient evaluation was carried out in 1981. The second reevaluation of the patients in this continuing prospective analysis was carried out in the spring of 1984.

In the 1981 review, six patients were lost to follow-up. Fifty-two patients, 37 females and 15 males, in whom 56 patellar shavings were performed, were available for study. Their ages ranged from 16 to 64 years, with the average being 38 years; 27 of the 56 operations were done in patients over the age of 40. Right and left knees were done with equal frequency. The length of follow-up from the time of surgery ranged from 9 to 44 months, with an average of 24 months. The average duration of symptoms prior to surgical intervention was 3 years; only five patients were operated on after less than 6 months of disabling pain.

Results were categorized into four groups: "Excellent" meant that the knee was completely free from pain, with no functional limitations. "Good" meant that there had been a marked relief of pain and a decided improvement in functional capabilities. "Fair" indicated that although there had been some pain relief, the functional capacity of the patient had not been upgraded. And "Poor" indicated that there had been no change in the character of the syndrome. (No patients reported being worse following surgery.)

Seventy-seven percent of patients were in the excellent and good categories and were considered to have satisfactory results. Patients in the "fair" and "poor" groups were considered unsatisfactory. A similar grading system has been described by Bentley (1). Overall results and results by gender are shown in Table 3–1.

The differences between excellent and good, when compared by gender, are striking; nearly 60% of males achieved excellent results, while only 28% of females did.

Results were also analyzed by age (Table 3–2). It appeared from these data that older patients did better with isolated patellar shaving. The over-50 group yielded 84% satisfactory results, while the 40–50 age group yielded 85% satisfactory results.

**Table 3–2** Phase I: Initial Patient Evaluation, 1981, by Age

| RESULTS | 10–19 YEARS | 20–29 YEARS | 30–39 YEARS | 40–49 YEARS | >50 YEARS |
|---|---|---|---|---|---|
| Excellent | 2 | 5 | 5 | 5 | 4 |
| Good | 1 | 4 | 3 | 7 | 7 |
| Fair | 0 | 1 | 4 | 1 | 1 |
| Poor | 1 | 2 | 1 | 1 | 1 |
| Total | 4 | 12 | 13 | 14 | 13 |

**Table 3–3** Phase II: Reevaluation of Patients, 1984

| | EXCELLENT | GOOD | FAIR | POOR |
|---|---|---|---|---|
| No. of Patients | 23 | 23 | 3 | 2 |
| Percent | 45 | 45 | 6 | 4 |

This group of patients was evaluated for a second time in 1984, some 30 months after the initial evaluation. At this time we excluded any patients with less than 30 months follow-up from the time of surgery. Also eliminated from further follow-up were the 13 unsatisfactory cases found in the initial study. The six patients lost to follow-up in the original review were found and were evaluated in the second phase; however, four different patients included in the first phase were now lost. Six new cases with too short a follow-up time to be included in the original group now had at least 30 months postoperative time and were included in the second phase. We were thus left with a patient series of 51 knees in 47 patients for evaluation. Thirty-four of the patients (72%) were available for physical examination, and the remaining 13 patients were evaluated by questionnaire and telephone.

The duration of follow-up in the phase II study ranged from 30 to 72 months, with an average of 48 months. The age range was still 16–64 years, but the average age dropped slightly to 36 years. There were 30 females and 17 males in this second study group. Four patients had both knees operated. Of the original six patients lost to follow-up, five were satisfactory and one patient was an unsatisfactory result from the time of her original surgery. Using the same criteria to judge results as in the first study, we found 46 satisfactory and 5 unsatisfactory results (Table 3–3).

Four unsatisfactory results in phase II had been satisfactory in phase I. Thus the results had deteriorated somewhat. The fifth unsatisfactory result was in a patient added to the series following phase I. The other five patients added to the series as "new cases" were graded as satisfactory.

In the final analysis we were left with a total of 46 satisfactory results and 18 unsatisfactory. The overall percentage of success in this group was 71.8% (Table 3–4).

## Discussion

Chondromalacia patellae is for the most part a benign, painless disruption of the articular cartilage of the patellar surface. When no other reasonable diagnosis can be established to explain persistent disabling anterior knee pain, chondromalacia should be considered as the etiology. The exact mechanism of this pain in these patients is not clear since the condition remains asymptomatic in so many other patients. The small series of less than 70 patients presented in this chapter are part

**Table 3–4** Phase II: Overall Results

| SATISFACTORY | | UNSATISFACTORY | |
|---|---|---|---|
| No. | % | No. | % |
| 46 | 71.8 | 18 | 28.2 |

of a total series of more than 1300 arthroscopic surgical procedures performed by the author. Thus only 5% of the total surgical population in a busy arthroscopic practice represent patellar shaving.

The relative frequency of chondromalacia patellae, combined with the common complaint of anterior knee pain, therefore, tempts the orthopaedist to perform more arthroscopic procedures than are indicated. The ease with which the patella can be approached arthroscopically also creates a situation in which this procedure can be abused. It should be remembered that the poorest results were in the youngest patients and very few teenagers have been subjected to patellar shaving by this author for this reason.

While it would be preferable to have objective criteria to evaluate results of this surgical procedure, we have not been able to establish such criteria. In our evaluation in phase II, we used thigh girth measurements as well as cybex analysis, but we could not establish a relationship with either measured strength or atrophy and the final result. The weaker legs with atrophy were evenly distributed in both the satisfactory and unsatisfactory groups.

Arthroscopic patellar debridement of grade III chondromalacia patellae is a reasonable procedure with predictable long-term results when properly performed in the carefully selected patient with persistent anterior knee pain.

## *References*

1. Bentley G. Chondromalacia patella. J Bone Joint Surg [Am] 52:221, 1970
2. Cassells S W. Gross pathological changes in the knee joint of the aged individual—A study of 300 cases. Clin Orthop 132:225, 1978
3. Ewing J W, Kleinman R. Arthroscopic patellar shaving (with and without lateral release) found effective for chronic patello-femoral pain. Field of View (2):5, 1982
4. Goodfellow J W, Bullough P. The pattern of aging of the articular cartilage of the elbow joint. J Bone Joint Surg [Br] 49:175–181, 1967
5. Heine J. Arthritis deformans. Virchows Arch [Pathol Anat] 260:521, 1926
6. Johnson L L. diagnostic and Surgical Arthroscopy, 2nd ed, p 326. C V Mosby, St. Louis, 1981
7. Outerbridge R E. The etiology of chondromalacia patellae. J Bone Joint Surg [Br] 43:752–757, 1961

# Patellofemoral Problems and Malalignment

# 4

James M. Fox
Orrin H. Sherman
David Pevsner

The role of surgical lateral release of the patella needs to be placed in perspective by a thorough understanding of the anatomical structures involved, their deformities and pathology, the surgical opportunities and their resultant effect, and finally, the kind of rehabilitation program needed to return functional control to these structures. The goal of this chapter is to discuss these various entities in an attempt to understand the place of lateral release in the control of patellofemoral dysfunction.

## Anatomy of the Patellofemoral Joint

The patellofemoral joint consists of the trochlear groove of the femur and the patella with its lateral, medial, and odd facets (Figure 4–1). The patella is phylogenetically a sesamoid bone in the quadriceps tendon. Its dual purpose is 1) to protect the femoral articular surface and 2) by virtue of the fulcrum effect, to increase the efficiency of the quadriceps mechanism (46) and facilitate full knee extension (81).

Normal function of the patellofemoral joint is dependent upon adequate stabilization and guidance of the patella. The factors that influence this function are 1) dynamic structures (quadriceps mechanism), 2) static structures (lateral retinaculum), and 3) configuration of the patella and trochlear groove or sulcus.

The quadriceps tendon arises from four muscles: the vastus lateralis, vastus intermedius, rectus femoris, and vastus medialis. The inferior fibers of the vastus medialis run in an oblique direction from the adductor tubercle to the superior medial aspect of the patella, at a 65-degree angle (Figure 4–2). The vastus medialis

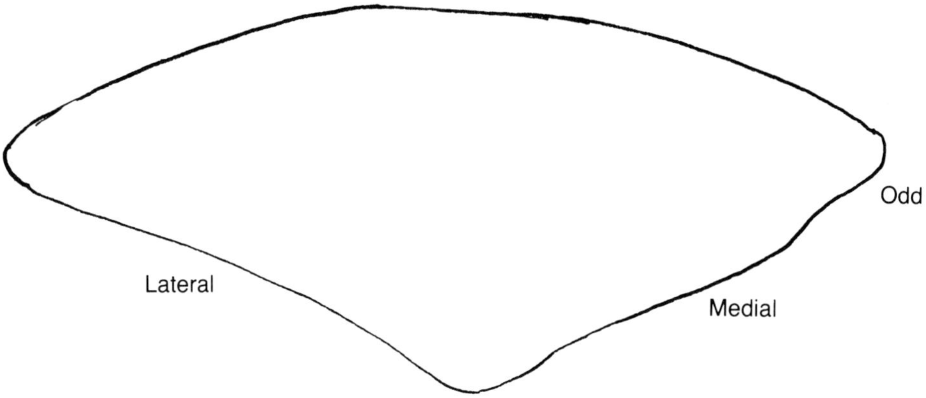


**Figure 4–1** Patellar facets.

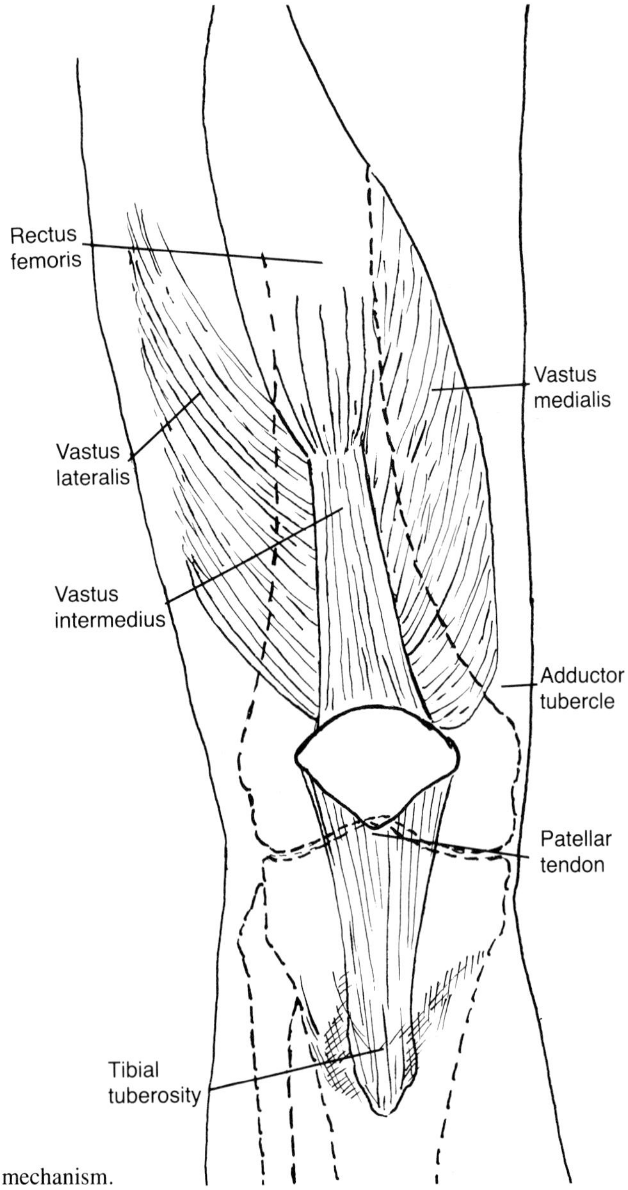


**Figure 4–2** Quadriceps mechanism.

obliquus (VMO) serves a patella-centering function (55). The quadriceps muscle has an axial deviation laterally of 10–15 degrees from the vertical. This is measured clinically as the Q angle. The vastus medialis obliquus counteracts the laterally deviating vector (K) resulting from the Q angle (Figure 4–3). This lateral vector is increased by a weakening of the VMO, an abnormally high insertion of the VMO on the patella, a stretched VMO and medial retinaculum secondary to dislocation, an injury to the VMO by a previous medial parapatellar incision, an unusually powerfully developed vastus lateralis, lateral retinacular tightness or fibrosis, congenital genu recurvatum with resultant laxity in the extensor mechanism, and patella alta where only vertically oriented fibers of the VMO are present.

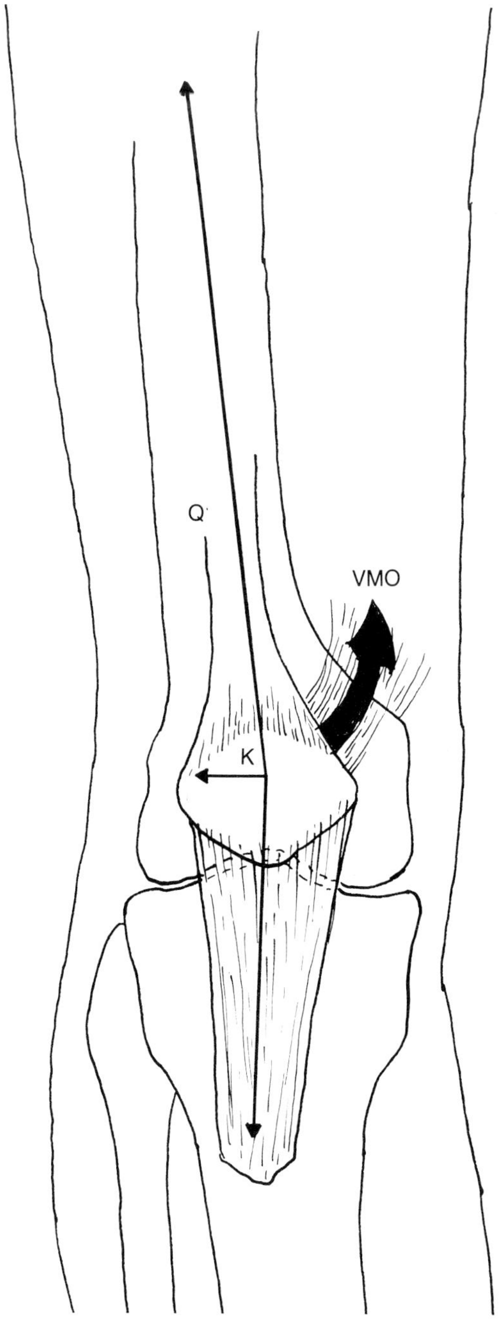


**Figure 4–3** Q angle vector K opposed by VMO.

The lateral retinacular structures can be divided into three layers. Superficially, at the superolateral border of the patella is the fibrous expansion of the vastus lateralis. These fibers are longitudinally oriented along the lateral border of the patella, merging distally with the patellar tendon. Interdigitating with this fibrous expansion of the vastus lateralis is the superficial oblique retinaculum. This structure originates from the iliotibial band (ITB) and merges into the anterior aspect of the patellar tendon. The ITB, as the distal expansion of the tensor fascia lata and gluteus maximus, inserts onto Gerdy's tubercle. Some fibers extend across Gerdy's tubercle to the tibial tuberosity.

Deep in this superficial layer is the deep transverse retinaculum. These fibers are deep in the superficial oblique retinaculum and run from the ITB to the patella. This structure ends at the level of the patellar tendon. The patellotibial ligament starts at the lower border of the deep transverse retinaculum. These fibers run from the distal patella obliquely and distally to insert in the coronary ligament of the lateral meniscus and proximal tibia. The transverse patellofemoral ligament runs from the lateral intermuscular septum and lateral epicondyle to the lateral patella at the proximal half. This is the epicondylopatellar ligament described by Kaplan (45).

The deepest layer, the capsulosynovial, is beneath the deep transverse retinaculum. This structure, although composed of two layers, the capsule and synovium, is adherent and essentially one layer at this point (Figure 4–4). The depth

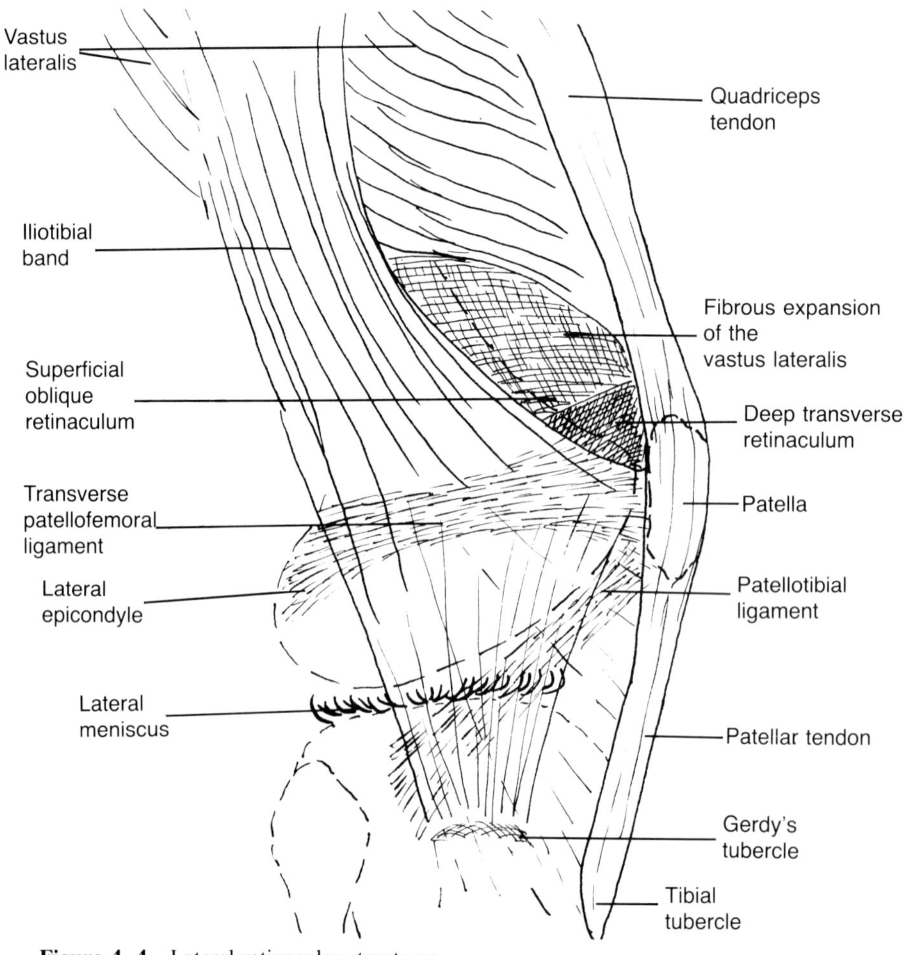


**Figure 4–4** Lateral retinacular structures.

of the femoral groove and the height of the lateral femoral condyle buttress the patella against lateral dislocations. The combination of a low profile of the femoral groove and a deficiency of the medial patellar facet can result in patellar instability. Wiberg (86) has described three types of patellae (Figure 4–5). Type I has equal medial and lateral facets. Type II has a more vertical and smaller medial facet and is the most common patellar configuration. Types I and II are the most stable, with equal distribution of forces over well-formed medial and lateral facets. Type III shows a more vertical and dysplastic medial facet and a greater tendency towards instability.

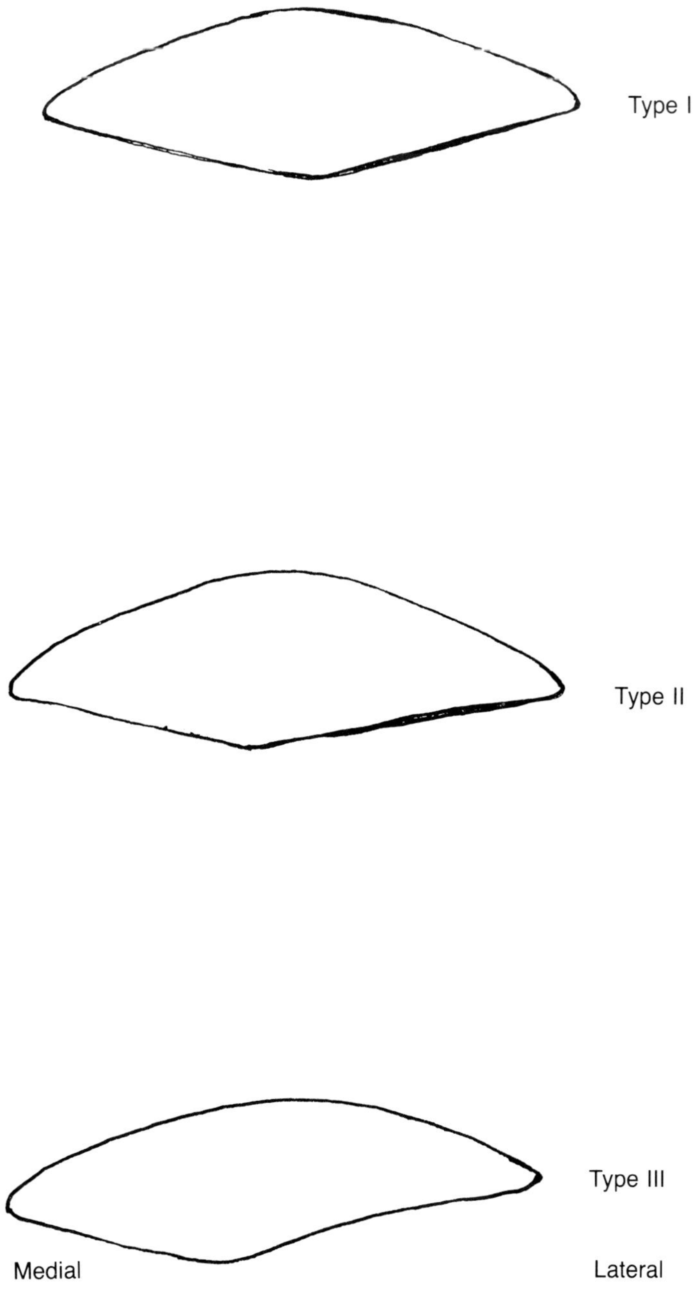


**Figure 4–5** Wiberg patellar types (86).

As the knee flexes and extends, the patella contacts the femoral groove at different points and with different forces. According to Aglietti et al. (1) and Goodfellow et al. (31), there is no contact at full extension. At 30 degrees of flexion, there is contact between the inferior articular surface of the patella and the upper femoral condyles. With initiation of flexion this contact is only between the lateral femoral condyle and lateral facet, but by 30 degrees of flexion, the contact is evenly distributed. At 60 degrees of flexion, the superior half of the patella and the femoral groove inferior to the 30-degree contact point are opposed with an increased contact area. At 90 degrees of flexion, the superior half of the patella and the femoral groove above the notch are in contact with an increased contact area. At 120 degrees of flexion, only the superior aspect of the patellar articular surface and the femoral groove adjacent to the notch are in contact. At 140 degrees of flexion, the odd facet of the patella comes into contact with the medial femoral condyle.

# Pathology

## Patellar Instability: Subluxation and Dislocation

The reported incidence of patellar subluxation or dislocation is 0.01–0.73%, with a recurrence rate of 0.01–0.03%. The female-to-male ratio is 2:1, with the more traumatic incidences occurring in males. Bilateral symptoms occur in one-third of the patients. The average age of occurrence in females is 15 years and in males is 16 years. A positive family history is present in 20–25% of the patients.

The mechanism of injury is usually one with the knee flexed and in valgus with the leg externally rotated. Quadriceps contraction during the push-off phase of a side-step cut subluxates or dislocates the patella laterally.

Several predisposing factors are associated with patellar instability. These are 1) weak VMO, 2) high insertion of VMO, 3) shallow femoral groove, 4) flat lateral femoral condyle, 5) patella alta with a flat patella, 6) generalized ligamentous laxity with recurvatum, 7) externally rotated tibias, 8) femoral anteversion, and 9) valgus knees.

The diagnosis of patellar dislocation is made by either observing a laterally dislocated patella or by a positive history of a reduction. Subluxation is not as easy to diagnose. The acute case may have a history similar to an acute dislocation but without the frank dislocation. Recurrent subluxation may be characterized by a "catching" sensation, "giving way," or medial knee pain.

Physical examination following a dislocation or subluxation may demonstrate lateral patellar tilt or "grasshopper eyes," as described by Hughston (42), when the patient is sitting with the knees flexed 90 degrees and viewed from above. A positive "apprehension sign" (15), medial retinacular tenderness, or an effusion may be present. Slocum et al. (75) made the diagnosis of patella alta by the presence of a small, high-riding patella associated with an enlarged fat pad and calf muscle.

Regarding x-ray views of the patellofemoral joint, it is the tangential and lateral positions that appear to be the most useful for evaluation. The tangential view of the flexed knee shows the intercondylar sulcus, patellar position in the sulcus, and the shape of the lateral femoral condyle. Each x-ray technique is basically a modification of the tangential view in order to develop criteria. A case requiring multiple x-ray positions is obviously quite a subtle situation. The subtleness and the difficulty in diagnosis arise from the dynamic quality of the relationship. An x-ray view shows only one point in time for the entire relationship that constitutes synchronous movement of the patellofemoral joint. With progressive flexion of the knee, the patella is being drawn into the sulcus by the flexed length of the patellar tendon, resisted by the dynamic forces of the quadriceps. The x-ray images recorded are not of the fluid movement of the joint but of a fixed point in time and space. Muscles are not contracting and their forces do not exist. All of the various x-ray techniques do assist in attempts to confirm the diagnosis, but in the borderline situation they can only be a source of additional inference.

One entity that is intimately related to patellofemoral dysfunction is lateral facet compression or, as described by Ficat et al. (21), excessive lateral pressure syndrome (ELPS). It is considered by Ficat to be a separate syndrome, but it should be regarded as part of a more generalized quadriceps mechanism malalignment. Pathomechanically, the syndrome results from a lateral shift of the equilibrium between the medial and lateral patellofemoral ligaments and retinaculum. This excessive lateral pull can be the result of hypertrophy or fibrosis of the lateral capsule or abnormal insertion from the iliotibial tract. An abnormal localized protrusion of the lateral facet of the trochlea femoris can also be involved (27). As a result of this lateral pull, the lateral facet undergoes hyperpressure while the medial facet is subjected to hypopressure (Figure 4–6).

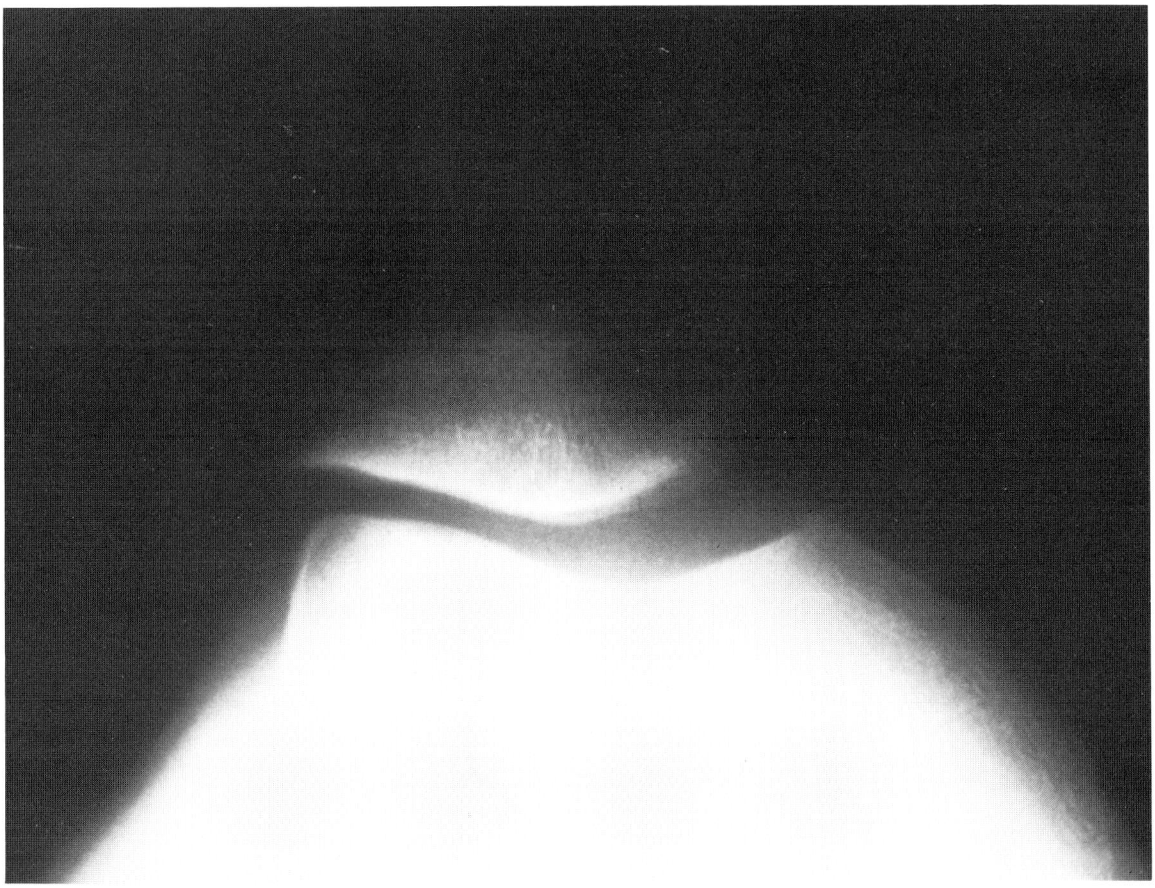

**Figure 4–6** Hyperpressure-hypopressure.

Chondromalacia of the lateral facet is a manifestation of ELPS and is most frequently located at the level of the critical zone lateral to the medial ridge (23). Infrequently, the chondromalacia centers on the lateral facet or extends the entire width of the lateral facet.

Ficat et al. (21) reviewed 115 knees that underwent lateral retinacular release for ELPS. There was an 80% good to excellent result at an average follow-up of 20 months.

## Traumatic Injuries

Traumatic lesions to the patellofemoral joint may be secondary to indirect or direct injury. Indirect trauma to the patellar articular surface is caused by direct application of force to the patella. The mechanism of injury is usually a fall on the knee, contusion from a hard object, or a dashboard injury. The patient usually complains of slight swelling and discomfort early on, followed by a quiescent period of several weeks or months with only mild symptoms. Later on, retropatellar pain develops with symptoms of chondromalacia.

Soto-Hall (78) described the pathological changes that occurred after acute trauma. Initially there was edema, then softening and fissuring, followed by fraying of the articular cartilage and in some cases, erosion to subchondral bone.

Donohue et al. (16) have shown experimentally the effects of indirect blunt trauma on adult canine articular cartilage. After impaction there were significant alterations in histological, biochemical, and ultrastructural characteristics without disruptions of the articular surface. The authors felt that this model of articular cartilage "contusion" may have been representative of the joint damage that is observed following indirect blunt trauma to the articular surface without radiographic evidence of fracture.

Direct trauma to the patellofemoral joint may result in an osteochondral fracture. The mechanism of injury is usually the repositioning of a dislocated patella rather than the dislocation itself. It may in part be due to strong quadriceps contraction at the time of repositioning, which can result in a tangential fracture of the medial facet of the patella or of the lateral femoral condyle. The incidence of osteochondral fracture following patellar dislocation is reported to be between 5% and 50% (66, 72).

The treatment for either type of traumatic lesion is dependent upon the location and size of the injury. In this situation we have had good results with arthroscopic removal of loose bodies, debridement of the lesion, or if the osteochondral fracture is large, repositioning it. This is then followed by a lateral release.

## Bipartite Patella with Stress Fracture

An uncommon congenital abnormality of the patellofemoral joint is a bipartite patella. The incidence is reported to be 2–3% (84). According to Smillie (76) the lesion is not necessarily bilateral nor symmetrical. The bipartite patella is usually asymptomatic, but occasionally movement in the synchondrosis between the primary patella and its attached anomalous part can result in pain. We have also seen stress fractures occurring in this synchondrosis with subsequent nonunion (Figure 4–7).

These patients complain of the gradual onset of pain associated with high levels of repetitive activity. Pain and tenderness are localized to the superolateral pole of the patella. A positive bone scan confirms the diagnosis (Figure 4–8). If symptoms are not relieved by conservative modalities, we have had good results with drilling across the synchondrosis under arthroscopic visualization.

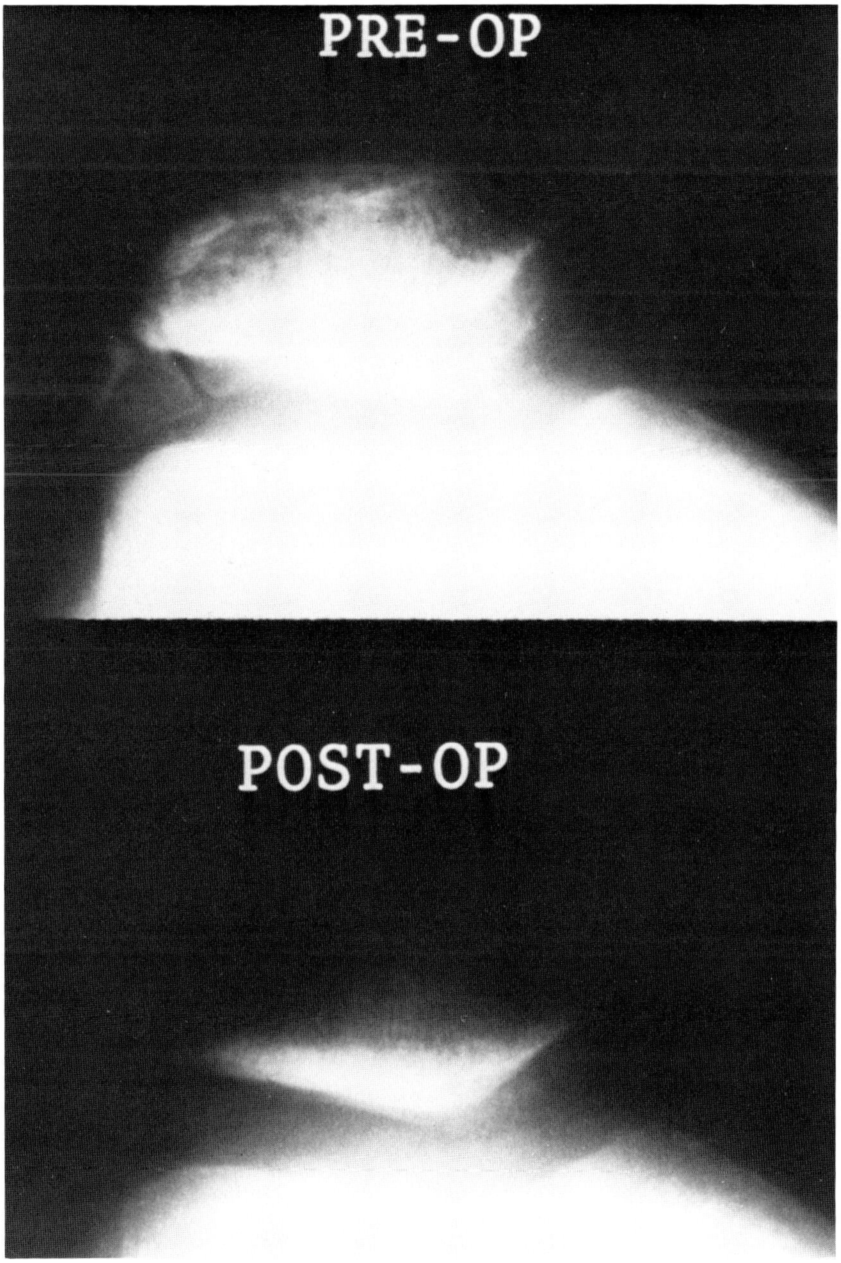


**Figure 4–7** Stress fracture in bipartite patella.

## Postoperative Fibrosis with Compression

Following an arthrotomy with a lateral capsular incision or a lateral release with insufficient postoperative mobilization, lateral capsular fibrosis may ensue. This can result in a strong lateral tether and subsequent ELPS. After performing an anterior cruciate ligament reconstruction, closure of the medial capsular incision may be difficult and under tension. This may also result in patellar compression. Larson et al. (54) performed a Z-plasty lengthening to deal with this compression, and we routinely employ this procedure in all our anterior cruciate ligament reconstructions. Secondary lateral capsular fibrosis and compression may require a lateral release.

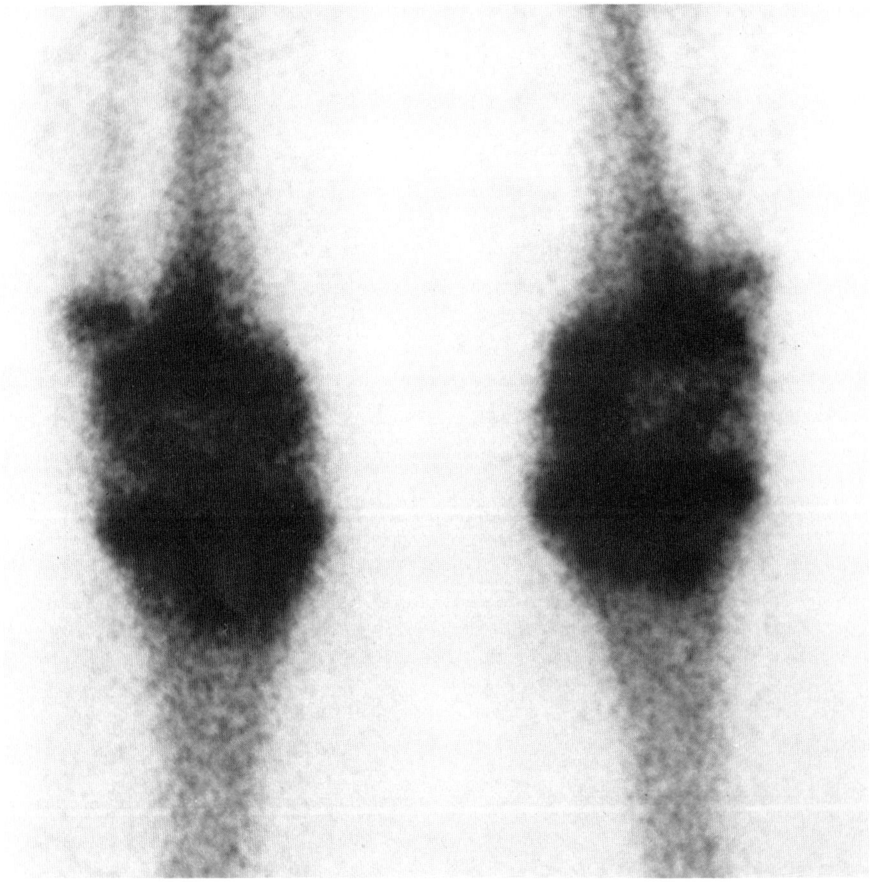

**Figure 4–8** Positive bone scan for bipartite patella with stress fracture.

## Patellofemoral Dysfunction Secondary to Change in Instant Center of Knee Motions

The mechanics of joint motion dictate that the instant center of knee motion be located along the line that is perpendicular to the joint surfaces at the point where they contact. In other words, if the knee joint is functioning normally, then the joint surfaces will roll and slide over one another. In the abnormal situation the joint surfaces will not slide and the instant center will be off this perpendicular line. This condition may occur when either a meniscus or ligamentous structure or both are not in their normal anatomical positions.

The menisci increase the congruency of the joint by increasing joint contact area and decreasing joint capsule stress (53). A torn meniscus will therefore require larger shifts of the tibia to produce the same shift of the contact point as in a normal knee. This shift will result in a change in the instant center of knee motion.

The cruciate ligaments can be thought of as those structures that limit the position of the instant center of the knee joint. If the point of contact of the knee is forced to shift from the anterior position to a more posterior position as a result of a torn anterior cruciate ligament, then the instant center of motion would similarly shift from a location along the perpendicular line from the anterior contact point to a position along the perpendicular line above the posterior contact point.

In the normal knee the relatively posterior placement of the contact point, and therefore the center of rotation, results in an increase in the moment arm of the quadriceps mechanism and a decrease in the functional load on the patellofemoral joint. When the load is moved anteriorly as a result of a meniscal tear or ligamentous damage, the instant center shifts posteriorly as a result of a shift of the contact point. Consequently, the hamstrings develop a greater moment arm and there is a change in the functional load on the patellofemoral joint.

## Medial Synovial Shelf

The plica synovialis mediopatellaris or "medial synovial shelf" represents the persistence of an embryonic synovial septum in an adult knee, and is present in 20–55% of all knees. It is a three-dimensional synovial fold that runs from the medial wall of the knee joint just proximal to the patella, obliquely and distally to its insertion in the anterior fat pad. Because of its location, it may bowstring during flexion and make contact with the medial femoral condyle and/or the medial facet of the patella.

The "shelf" may become inflamed and thickened during strenuous activity or as a result of blunt trauma to the front of the knee. Patients will complain of pain along the shelf, which can be mistaken for medial retinacular pain or meniscal symptoms. Patients may also describe a snapping with flexion and extension as the shelf bowstrings over the medial femoral condyle. Often, the thickened structure can be palpated as a tender band.

Treatment is initially conservative. If this fails, arthroscopic resection of the medial synovial shelf can yield good to excellent results in greater than 90% of the patients (25). Histologically, the resected tissue reveals chronic fibrosis, mucoid degeneration, and chronic inflammation.

## Reflex Sympathetic Dystrophy

Protracted knee or patellar pain can follow minor trauma or surgery. When symptoms persist and overshadow all therapeutic intervention, reflex sympathetic dystrophy should be given a high index of suspicion. Originally described as Sudeck's atrophy or shoulder-hand syndrome, this sympathetic nerve disturbance can be observed in the knee.

The constellation of symptoms that make a diagnosis are 1) causalgia, which is a burning pain that may be associated with hyperesthesia; 2) stiffness secondary to edema, capsular thickening, and muscle atrophy; 3) vascular changes such as skin discoloration, cold skin temperature, and hair loss; 4) x-ray changes such as marked decalcification, which is most severe or restricted to the patella; and 5) positive bone scan with marked increase in uptake (Figure 4–9).

Once the diagnosis has been made, therapy is a formidable challenge. Physical therapy, transcutaneous electrical nerve stimulation (TENS), and sympathetic ganglion blocks have been used with variable results.

## Osteochondritis Dissecans

Osteochondritis dissecans has been described as a condition of uncertain etiology, characterized by the separation of a subchondral fragment of bone from the convex articular surface of a joint. The patella is infrequently involved, but when it is, a loose fragment may sometimes separate, usually in the region of the central ridge or inferior pole. Although a history of causative trauma is usually lacking, Edwards and Bentley (19) felt that repetitive shearing stress on the patellar surface was an important etiological factor. He found that in four of five patients, symptoms began after flexing the knee under load, and three showed patellar subluxation on tangential radiographs.

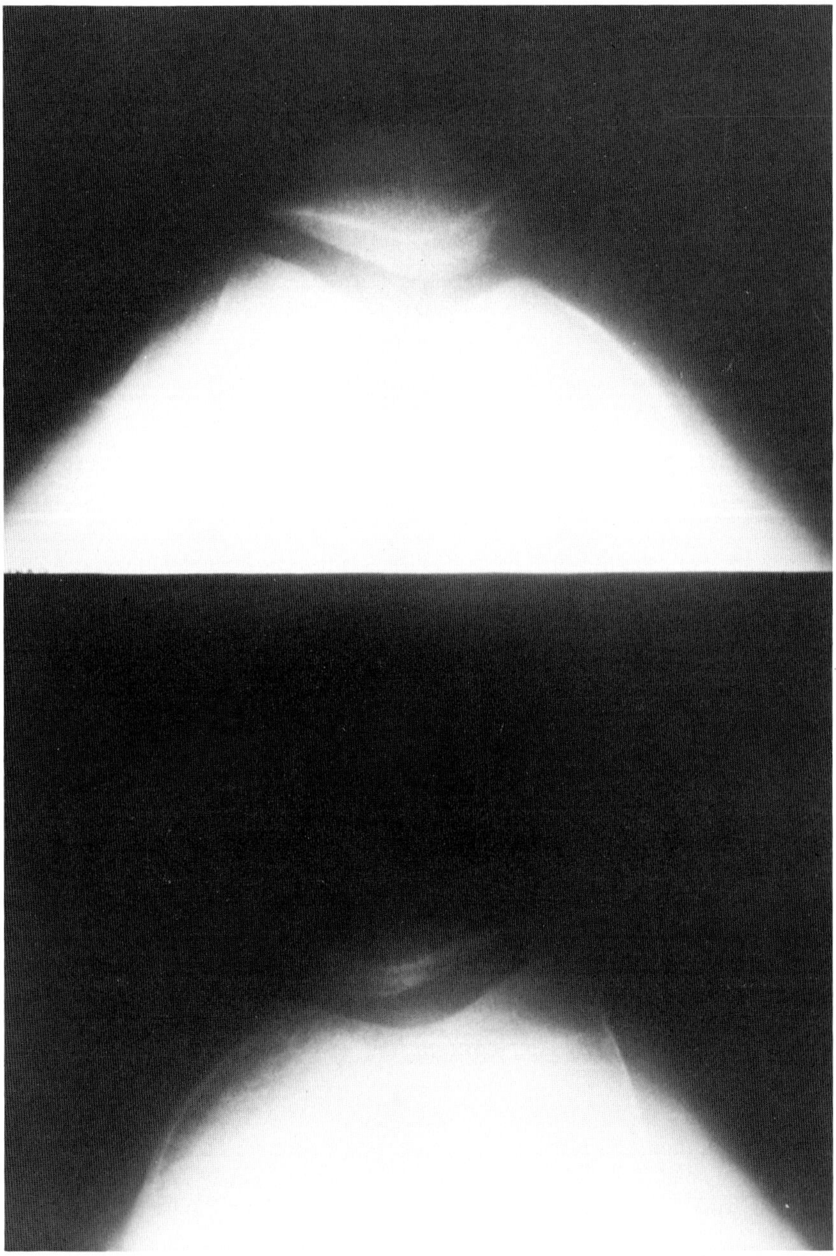

A

**Figure 4–9** Sympathetic dystrophy. **A** X-rays show marked change.

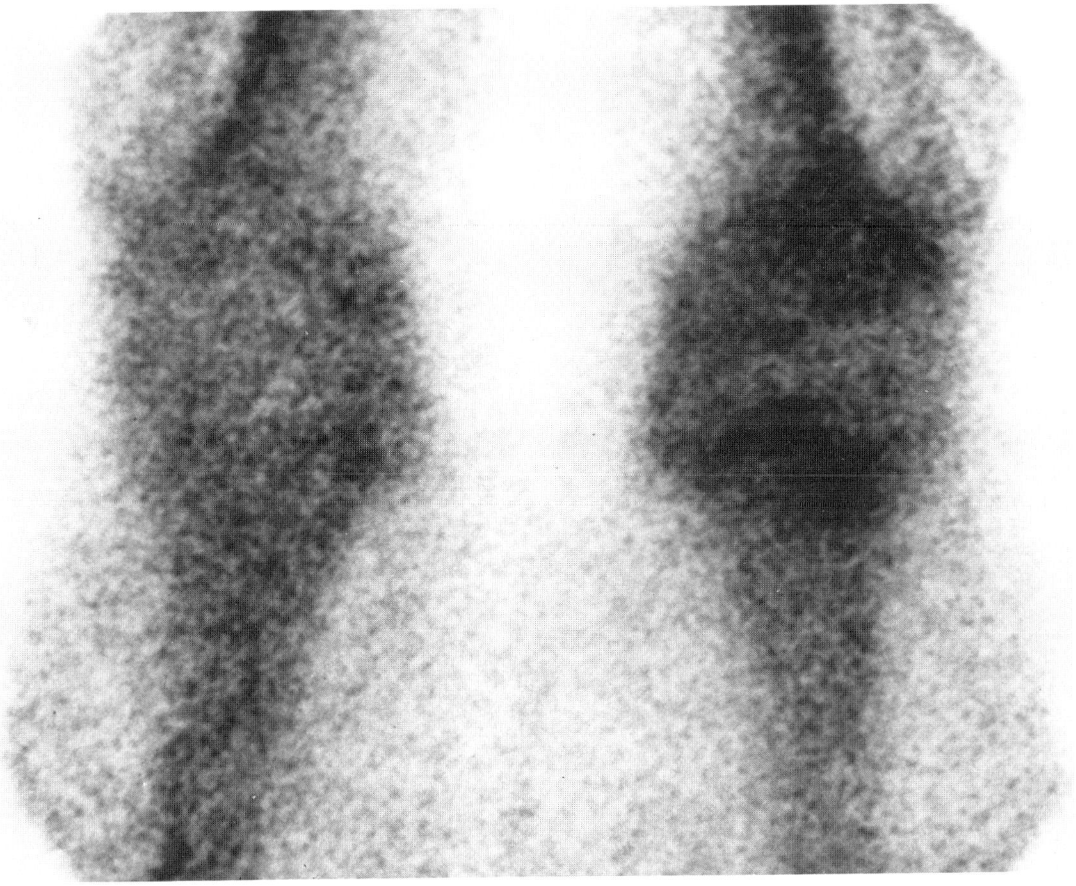

B

**Figure 4–9** (*cont.*) **B** bone scan.

Complaints are generally mild until the osteochondritis fragments partially or completely separate. Symptoms may then either be those typical of a patellofemoral disorder or secondary to the loose body formation. Treatment is directed at removal of the partially detached fragment of loose body.

## Surgical Procedures

The application of surgical procedures for the patellofemoral joint can be questioned. As we have emphasized, this is an extremely dynamic functioning relationship, and not only the application, but the degree of application, of surgical procedures is difficult to determine by strict criteria. The patellofemoral relationships can be likened to those of the glenohumeral joint, which is also controlled with muscular function and limited passive anatomical restraints. Therefore, altering the active restraints can be a confusing aspect for the surgeon. How much something should be loosened or tightened must be correlated to the entire arc of movement and also to the inhibition of movement that occurs in the anesthetized state. (The glenohumeral joint is a very forgiving joint, whereas the patellofemoral joint is a very unforgiving one with a long memory and at times can even carry a grudge.)

In those entities that are related to dysfunctional tightness of this joint, in particular lateral facet compression, stress fractures of the lateral facet of the patella, contracture of the lateral patellofemoral ligament secondary to trauma, and arthrofibrosis from previous trauma or "surgical trauma," the application of lateral release is an accepted efficacious procedure. However, the role of lateral release in patellofemoral instability is not as clear-cut. As previously noted, the patellofemoral mechanism is a very finely tuned one, and there may be multiple causes of instability, either simple or complex.

Surgical procedures for patellar instability can be divided into 1) proximal realignments, 2) bony procedures, 3) distal realignments, and 4) patellectomy.

Proximal realignments historically began with Huebscher (41) in 1850. In this type of operation, the medial side of the capsule was scraped and scarified in order to bring about a contraction. Later on, Bevan (6) described a medial reefing using the vastus medialis. These medial reefings proved inadequate, so attempts at correction were made by means of a fascial transplant (18).

With the tethering of the patella medially, an open space resulted sometimes at the site of the lateral incision. This was filled in by a transplant removed from the medial side (14). An alternative method was to transplant a strip of medial capsule, fascia, and the vastus medialis over the superior pole of the patella into the gap on the lateral side (51). Free fascial transplants have also been utilized. A strip of fascia lata or peroneal tendon was fastened to the patella and the medial femoral condyle (29). Or, the fascial strip removed from the lateral side was run subcutaneously over the patella and fixed to the medial femoral condyle (48).

More recently, proximal realignments have been described employing a quadricepsplasty. Robbins and Ulin (71) obtained a 94% good-to-excellent result with no recurrences. Madigan et al. (56) utilized a lateral and distal transfer of the VMO plus a lateral release in one-half of the patients. He only achieved a 58% good to excellent result with a 26% recurrence rate. A predisposing factor for failure was genu valgum of greater than 15 degrees. Crosby and Insall (12), using a proximal fascial sling, obtained 75% good to excellent results with a 25% recurrence rate. There was no x-ray evidence of osteoarthritis at follow-up. Complications associated with proximal realignment are increased patellofemoral compression, limitation of flexion, and patellar rotation.

Bony procedures to prevent the patella from slipping laterally have included using osteotomes to elevate the lateral femoral condyle (2) and to place a bone block from the patella into the lateral femoral condyle (20).

Distal realignment utilizing the pes tendon has yielded satisfactory results with no recurrences (4, 87). The tendons function as a "physiological sling." Galeazzi (28) first reported using the semitendonosis. The problem with the technique was that the repair was essentially longitudinal. Others (3, 52) have modified this procedure, either by changing the direction of pull or by combining it with other forms of distal realignments. Overall, the success rate of this procedure has been 70–85% good to excellent results except in cases with preoperative ligamentous laxity or symptoms present for greater than 2 years (33). Unfortunately, with this procedure the complication rate has been excessively high.

A procedure employing the transfer of the patellar tendon was reported by Roux (73). This involved a lateral release, medial repair, and a complete transfer of the patellar tendon medially, leaving the inferior periosteum intact. Goldthwait (30) only transferred the lateral one-half of the patellar tendon in his realignments.

Hauser (37) reported a procedure that transferred the patellar tendon and tibial tubercle distally and medially. He did establish criteria for a successful operation for patellar instability: 1) prevention of recurrence, 2) patient security, 3) full functional capacity of the knee, 4) normal appearance of the knee, 5) minimal risk to the patient, and 6) short convalescence. Since Hauser's original description, many variations have been described, especially in fixation of the tibial tubercle transfer (11, 13, 17, 24, 27, 32, 34, 35, 40, 44, 57, 60, 79, 82). The results have all been satisfactory with respect to prevention of recurrence.

Complications associated with tibial tubercle transfers have been unacceptably frequent. Osteoarthritis following the procedure has been reported to be as high as 100% (12, 61). The reasons given by the authors for such poor results are delay in performing the operation and insufficient correction of patella alta. Overall complication rates are as high as 49% (9, 77). Patella baja (7) and compartment syndromes secondary to damage to the anterior tibial recurrent vessels (83) have been reported. If the procedure is done in children prior to epiphyseal closure, recurvatum is a frequent complication (40). This is a result of the epiphysiodesis that occurs if removal of the block of tibial tubercle damages the proximal tibial epiphysis and if the cavity is filled by a piece of bone taken from a new bed.

Proximal and distal realignments combined have been used for patellar instability (43, 75). A tibial tubercle transfer of the patellar tendon is only used in those who are skeletally mature. Loss of motion requiring manipulation has been a problem (38).

## Lateral Retinacular Release

Lateral retinacular release has frequently been done during a realignment procedure, but as an isolated procedure, it is relatively recent. Initially, a lateral release was done as an open procedure (10, 21, 62, 64, 88), one of the benefits being the ability to visualize and secure hemostasis. A percutaneous lateral release has also been popular (8, 36, 67). This is either done through an arthroscopy incision or through a separate puncture. A common problem with this technique has been postoperative hemarthrosis.

Arthroscopic lateral retinacular release enables the procedure to be done under direct visualization (59, 63) but still does not adequately prevent hemarthrosis. The advent of electrosurgical lateral release appears to meet the needs of achieving hemostasis (65). In a review of 214 cases of electrosurgical lateral release done by us, the hemarthrosis rate was 1.4%. The results of isolated lateral retinacular release done as an open, percutancous, or arthroscopic procedure have yielded 75–80% good to excellent results, a number that compares favorably to formal realignment procedures.

Patellectomy has also been used to treat patellar instability and at times it has been called "the best operation for recurrent dislocations" (58). A quadricepsplasty is necessary to realign the abnormal pull of the quadriceps if success is to be achieved (61, 85). A common complication of this procedure is the persistent extensor lag (40).

**Role of Electrosurgery** Isolated lateral release has been utilized for instability of the patellofemoral joint either as an open procedure, including such things as Z-plasty, and as a subcutaneous procedure (open and closed). Arthroscopically controlled lateral release is credited to Drs. John McGinty and Robert Metcalf who introduced the arthroscopic method. In all of these procedures, a major complication is one of hemarthroses. The lateral retinacular and capsular aspect of the patellofemoral joint has a rich blood supply and a frequency of postoperative hemarthrosis varying between 10% to 30%. In an attempt to alleviate the problems of hemarthrosis, suction drainage, compressive pads, and immobilization dressings have been employed. The problem with hemarthrosis is the irritation of the joint, secondary to the hemosiderin deposits; distention of the joint; and resultant pain and inhibition of movement (Figure 4–10).

The ideal surgical procedure would involve immediate hemostasis to allow for rapid movement of the joint; protecting this area from recurrent binding down with fibrose tissue; maintaining the articular surface nourishment through active range-of-motion exercises; and continued strengthening of the quadriceps. The principle of lateral release is to release a deforming structure that is tending to tether or pull the patella laterally with the flexion movement, and with this release, to allow the medial restrictive forces, in particular the vastus medialis obliquus musculature, to maintain control as the patella passes through into the femoral groove and trochlear notch.

In March of 1981 we began working with electrosurgical apparatus to obtain immediate hemostasis. This was performed with arthroscopic techniques previously demonstrated by Dr. Lanny Johnson, with visualization via the arthroscope from the medial aspect of the joint and direct inspection of the division of the lateral patellofemoral ligament and lateral capsule.

The use of electrosurgery dates back to the early twentieth century, but it is Drs. Harvey Cushing and W. T. Bovie who have received credit for the true clinical application in modern day surgery. Delivery generators, solid-state transistorized equipment, have made available relatively safe ''nonaggressive'' sources of energy.

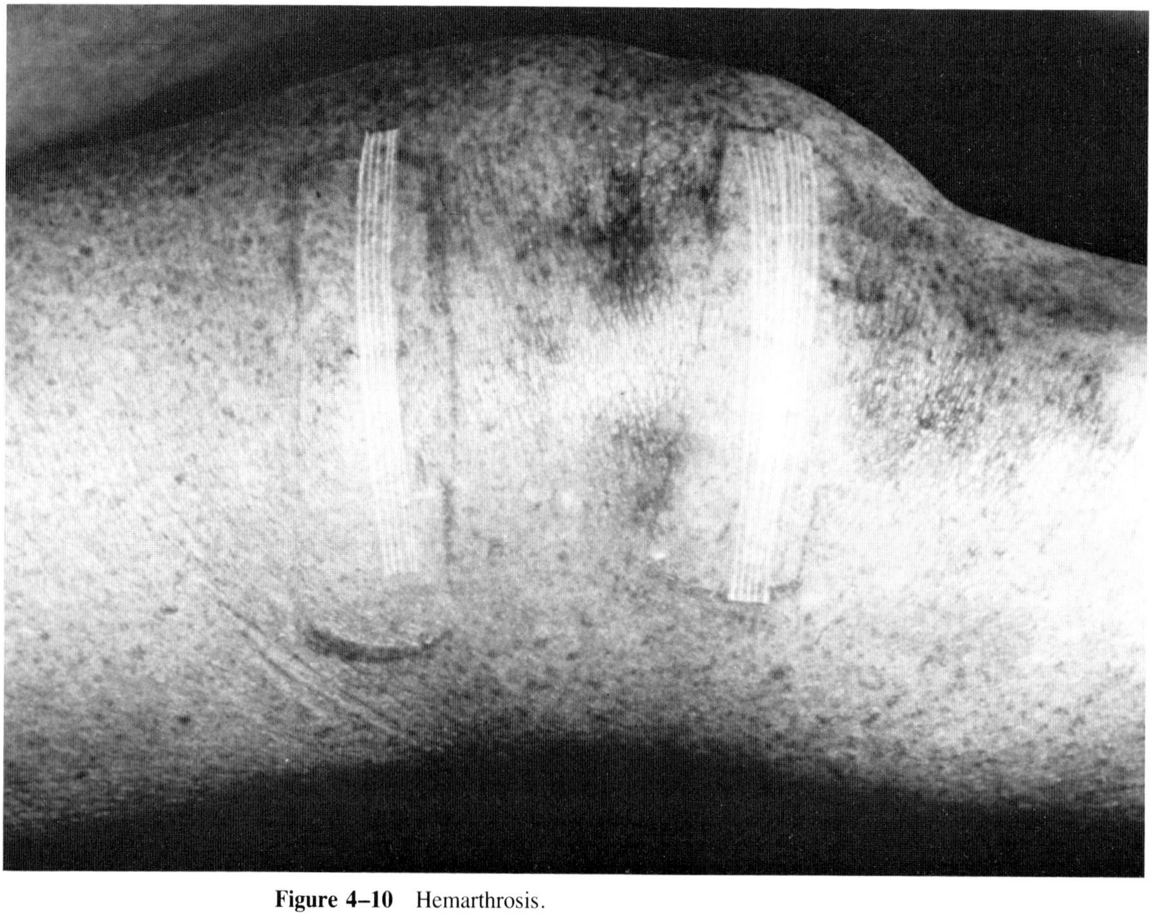

**Figure 4–10** Hemarthrosis.

With continued efforts at development, in conjunction with commercial support, a delivery system was formulated to include specially designed electro-tips, insulated to allow for concentration of the electrofrequency wave at the cutting tip. As experience was gained, rapid cutting and coagulation could be obtained in a sequential manner, and confidence was gained in the effectiveness of the system.

**Surgical Technique** After completion of a diagnostic arthroscopic procedure by an anterolateral portal, with secondary portals used depending upon the need to investigate associated positions, the arthroscope is transferred to a medial portal, and the electrosurgical device is inserted through the standard anterolateral portal. Irrigation fluid is changed to a nonconductive fluid. The release is performed with the generator setting initially at approximately 30 watts of power (we would recommend a digital readout generator for confirmation). Power settings are decreased or increased as necessary. It is important to use the lowest power setting that is effective as all the cutting is performed by hydrolysis of the cells and desiccation. Therefore, a minimal power setting will cause the least amount of trauma.

Release is begun proximally and carried superiorly with division of the internal synovial and then the capsular layer. Prior to the release, a spinal needle is placed at the superolateral pole of the patella to serve as a geographic landmark for orientation (Figure 4–11). The tourniquet is placed on the upper thigh but not inflated unless a large arterial bleeder is encountered that cannot be controlled initially. If the tourniquet inflation is necessary, deflation is done as soon as he-

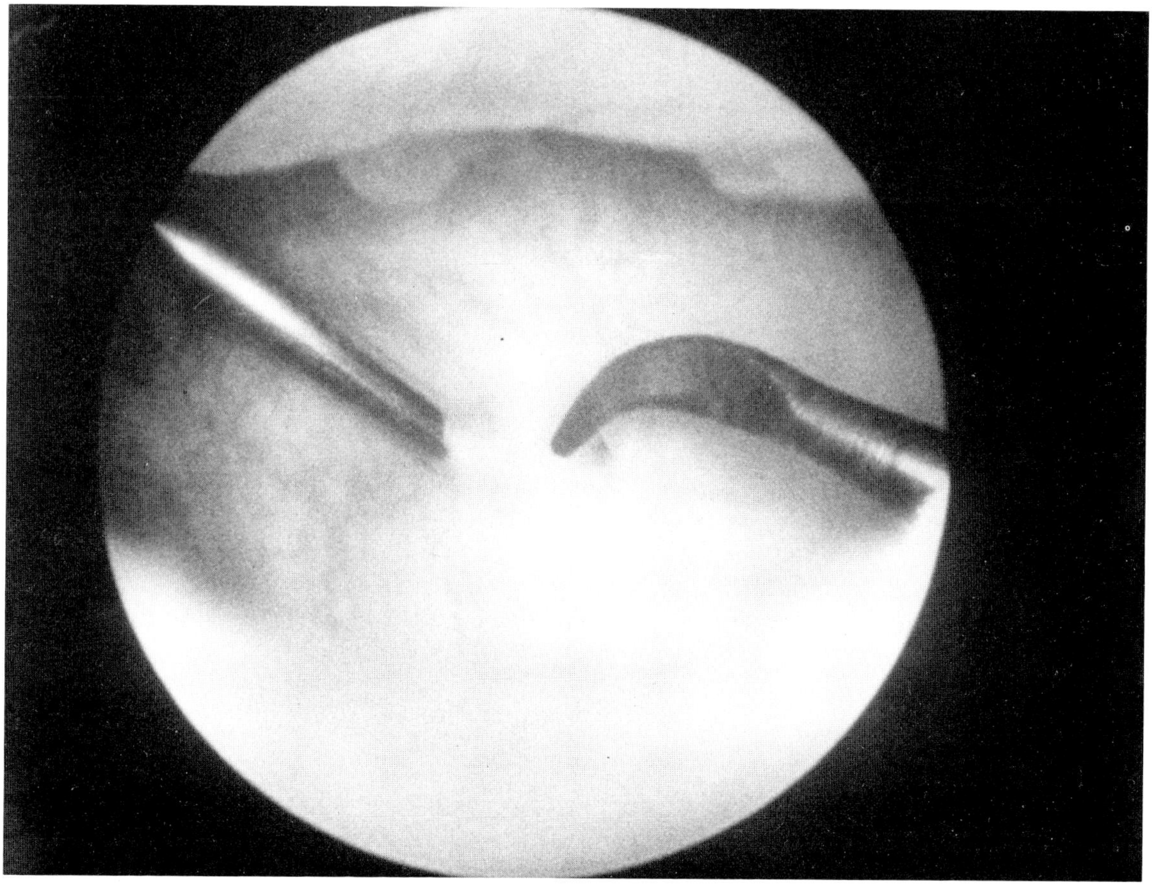

**Figure 4–11** Spinal needle placement and cutting-coagulating tip.

mostasis is obtained. This allows for direct visualization of vasculature as it is encountered. An alternative method is to inflate the tourniquet through the procedure, deflate it at the end, and then confirm hemostasis. The problem with this latter technique is that the occasional arterial or venous structure that was not coagulated initially causes rapid bleeding, and should this occur from numerous structures, the bleeding sources are obscured, making coagulation much more difficult. Also, infiltration with local anesthetic along the lateral capsular area increases the electrolyte contact, therefore increasing the resistance of the tissue and diminishing the effectiveness of the electrosurgical apparatus. For that reason infiltration with local anesthetic is contraindicated. After completion of the release to the desired proximal area, the knee is once again irrigated with the standard arthroscopic fluid and then thoroughly suctioned. Irrigation fluid is then discontinued, the knee is drained of any extraneous fluid, and the lateral aspect of the patella is palpated and everted to make sure that there are no further restrictive bands. If adequate release has been obtained, the patella can be everted 60–90 degrees to confirm its mobility. Surgical incisions are closed with adhesive tapes, and sterile padding is applied over the incisions and held in place with elastic support stocking, previously measured for the patient. In the postoperative phase, the patient is encouraged to maintain his isometric exercise program and active flexion of the knee joint.

Recently, this procedure has been performed on an outpatient basis, with the patients admitted the morning of surgery and discharged approximately 3–5 hours after their surgery. They are ambulated with crutches for external support and bear weight at whatever level comfortable. Patients continue with their crutches until adequate muscle control has been obtained and they are safe in standard ambulation. If the patient, in his daily routine, is faced with repetitive stair climbing, we encourage the continued use of crutches until further power in flexion maneuvers has been obtained. The patient is maintained in his isometric exercise program, and active flexion maneuvers are encouraged. At the 1-week postoperative visit, 90% of the patients have obtained 90-degree flexion, and within 2 weeks 100% of the patients have obtained 90-degree flexion.

The application of electrosurgery in orthopaedic surgery is beyond the scope of this chapter. But careful attention to and familiarity with all the principles is essential. This includes knowledge about radio frequencies, generator types available, grounding of return electrodes, use of fluid-sealed pencils, and numerous other factors related to this energy source.

One of the aspects that can be discussed is the choice of a nonconductive fluid, which is dependent upon availability and cost. To date, the procedures conducted in our office have utilized sterile water. This is obviously a nonconductive fluid but does cause reactive changes within the joint and a reactive synovitis and associated cartilage irritation. This apparently does have some relationship to dose exposure, and therefore, it is our recommendation that the use of sterile water be limited to only that point in the surgical procedure that involves the use of electrosurgery. This will diminish the frequency of any type of reactive synovitis. Although this is self limiting, this restriction is the prudent course.

As previously stated, the power setting should be limited to the lowest setting that still effectively produces energy. Comparing the cutting of meniscal tissue with a scalpel versus an electrosurgical apparatus demonstrates minimal difference in damage to the cell structures. However, the most limited force and destruction possible is the most prudent surgical technique.

Lastly, the specific surgical technique is one of "throwing the wave" before the electrode. This effect of electrosurgery, with activation of the energy source prior to touching the tissue, allows the operator to effect a cutting mode approximately 1 mm from the tip of the electrode and does not even require touching the tissue per se. This produces a much sharper, finer cutting line and diminishes the chance of tissue carbonization. This technique, with some practice, is easy to achieve and its effectiveness will become obvious to the surgeon. It is easily transposed to open surgical procedures and is a worthwhile technique to practice.

## Functional Rehabilitation Following Subcutaneous Lateral Release

### Acute Phase (Week 1)

The immediate postoperative period following subcutaneous lateral release presents the rehabilitation team with the first of many dilemmas encountered during the patient's recovery. After any trauma, control of the body's inflammatory response to the injury is paramount. Limiting the amount of inflammatory exudate has been shown to be directly correlated with early improvement in function, especially in the knee (39, 80).

Following subcutaneous lateral release it is especially important to ensure that rest and immobilization are used judiciously. Sherman et al. (74) demonstrated that a major finding among those with poor results after subcutaneous lateral release was a significant loss in range of motion (ROM). Thus, even in the acute phase, normal function is promoted by early motion and facilitory techniques to prevent "quadriceps dissociation" (5).

The first priority in any patient with knee problems is to achieve volitional control of the vastus medialis (VM) muscle (70). We have found that after facilitation of the VM has been initiated, patients are better able to establish or reestablish normal kinesthetic awareness of the limb and thus improve their ROM and gait. This fact combined with the need for early motion in the acute phase following subcutaneous lateral release require that inflammation be aggressively controlled at the site of the release during the acute phase. Compression wraps, cryotherapy, high-voltage galvanic electrical stimulation, and anti-inflammatory medication can all be used to control any local swelling at the site of the release (74).

Although facilitation of the VM is the first task necessary for progress to the subacute stages, it will not occur in the presence of pain due to reflex inhibition (5). Therefore, aggressive exercises or ambulation with pain are to be avoided during the acute phase. Crutches are often used by patients during the first week, although some patients will require the use of support for ambulation for 2–3 weeks after surgery, depending upon their ability to stabilize the patella dynamically during gait. TENS, functional electrical stimulation, and/or biofeedback can all be used to help control the patient's pain and assist the physical therapist in facilitating the individual's musculature (74). Special capsular mobilization techniques along with connective tissue massage in the subacute stage are especially important for restoration of distal and medial physiological joint play, prevention of adhesions in the suprapatellar pouch, and rescarring of the release itself (47) (Figure 4–12).

### Subacute Phase (Weeks 2–3)

As the inflammatory period following subcutaneous lateral release passes, it is important to guide the initial repair process about the site of the release, while preventing the deleterious effects of immobilization. From the first to third weeks

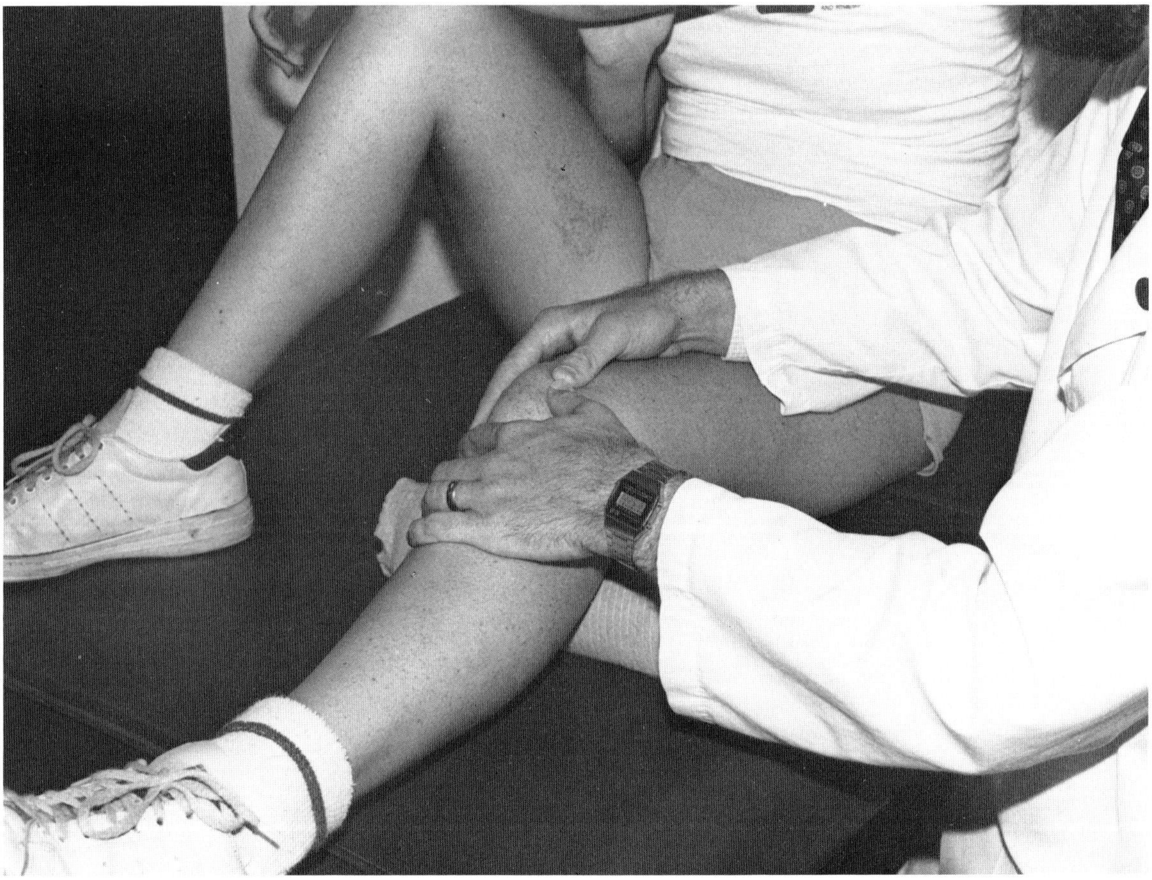

**Figure 4–12** Capsular mobilization.

following surgery, greater emphasis can be given to strengthening of the VM if volitional control has been established, with less concern for exacerbating the inflammatory process.

Techniques for quadriceps strengthening are initially limited to submaximal isometric exercises at terminal extension (70). Maximal contractions are used as soon as the patient is able to perform them without pain. Every patient must recover or acquire the ability to control the VM volitionally and contract it maximally without pain, or else progress to more complex motor skills requiring coordinated multimuscle responses will be impossible. Facilitory techniques such as those mentioned above are almost always continued in patients who have undergone subcutaneous lateral release, as the release itself is such an inhibitory influence on the musculature. Tone and control of the VM, then, is used as the primary clinical indicator of both patellar stabilization and of the readiness of the neuromotor system to begin training for more complex motor patterns.

Although the wound dressings are generally discarded at 48 hours postoperatively, a light wrap is often helpful in controlling swelling and in providing some static support for the patellofemoral joint. Aggressive anti-inflammatory measures must be continued as well. We have repeatedly found ice to be helpful, whereas modalities such as ultrasound and diathermy are avoided during this fragile period of anabolic fibroblastic activity (69). Continued protection from full weight bearing on an unprepared joint may also be required. However, it may be necessary to use a more intensive push on ROM than would otherwise be used with other types of surgical patients, even at the cost of some exacerbation in pain, swelling, and muscular inhibition, to avoid early maturation of a scar over the site of the release.

## Functional Rehabilitation Phase (3 Weeks to Completion)

After control of the VM is established and the repair process is well underway, functional integration of all of the components of complex movements can be begun. Many physical therapists choose to utilize the various methods of proprioceptive neuromuscular facilitation (PNF) (49) to promote these responses. Use of these techniques for strengthening can help ensure that the patient will not slip into previously learned patterns of substitution at any time during the strengthening process.

We have chosen, however, to initially further our strength training by continuing to use the same techniques of isometric contraction that the patient has already become familiar with and which he or she can duplicate at home. Resistance to the quadriceps muscle is delivered at the foot, preferably using an apparatus such as a quadriceps boot or sandbag. The patient is then asked to flex the hip (the classic straight-leg raise), but great care is also taken to ensure that he or she simultaneously maintains a maximum contraction of the VM, with complete knee extension (Figure 4–13). Short-arc exercises are next employed with similar attention to proper recruitment of the VM (74).

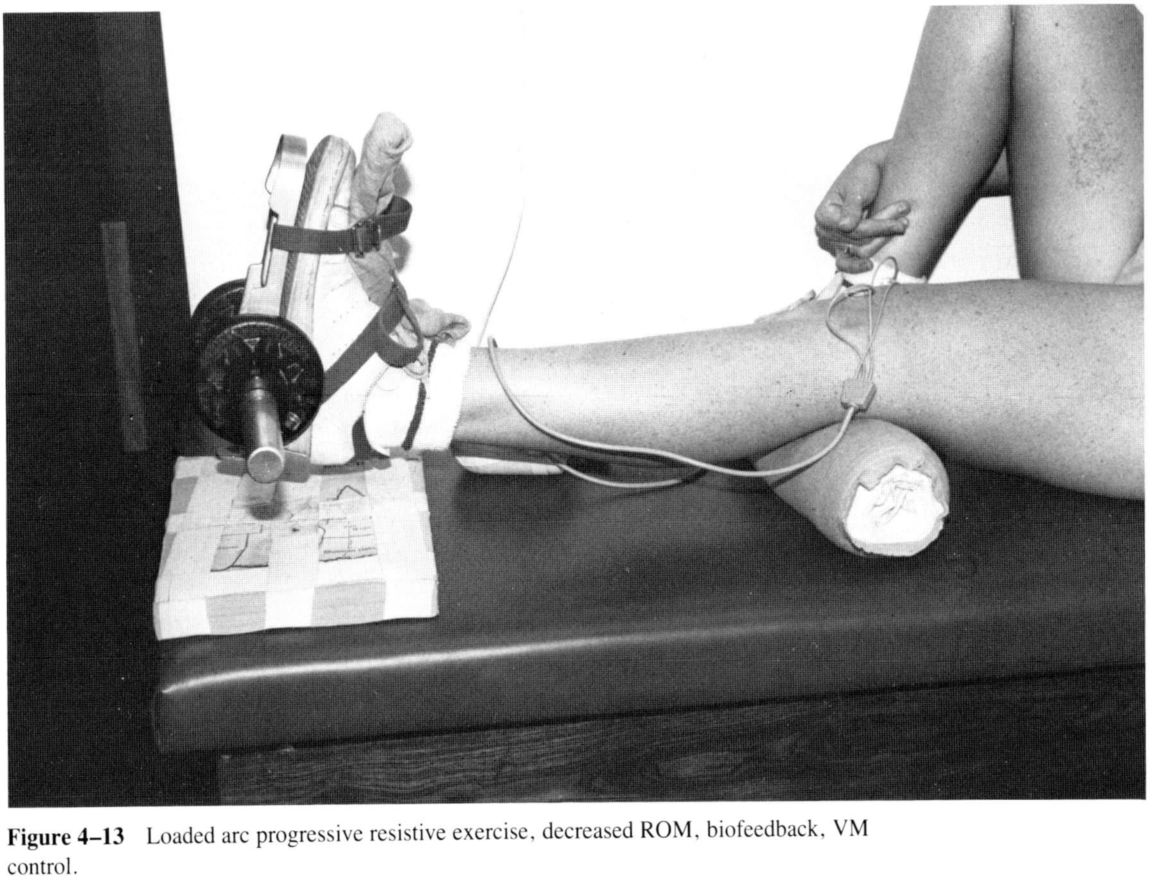

**Figure 4–13** Loaded arc progressive resistive exercise, decreased ROM, biofeedback, VM control.

When an adequate baseline level of strength for the VM has been achieved by the methods above, training through the rest of the ROM is begun via high-speed isokinetic exercise. The isokinetic bicycle ergometer has been our mode of choice. Isolating resisted knee extension from a sitting position causes very high retropatellar compressive forces, regardless of how the resistance is applied (22, 26, 68, 74). Use of the isokinetic bicycle ergometer can help minimize these forces. It is also a more functional motor activity, which can help make the patient's transition to VM control during movement much easier.

Toward the end of the rehabilitation process, strengthening exercises must shift to an eccentric emphasis. Eccentric quadriceps contractions are an integral part of most recreational activities. A balanced and coordinated release of the VM and the remaining quadriceps is especially difficult for patients following subcutaneous lateral release. In addition, eccentric strength training can also create high forces across the patella. We have found that exercises that allow for simultaneous hip and knee flexion during movement to be the best methods. Again, great care must be taken to avoid muscular substitution patterns that keep the VM from properly centering the patella as tension is released.

As progress is made with strength training, either with PNF or with more traditional types of progressive resistive exercise (PRE), the patient may be slowly and carefully advanced along a continuum of functional activities consistent with his degree of power and coordination. Beginning with unassisted walking using normalized motor function, the individual may progress through swimming, distance and/or hill walking on the treadmill, cycling at home, and running (74).

Constant postural reeducation and staged agility drills will be required at every stage of the activity continuum. Each patient must be closely monitored in the clinic, so that faulty body mechanics can be corrected. Supplemental training of other areas, such as the cardiovascular system, may be necessary, with appropriate screening in conjunction with the patient's primary physician.

Flexibility exercises are extremely important to conclude the rehabilitation process successfully. The hamstring and hip flexors are notoriously inflexible. Since flexibility is a composite of elasticity of the connective tissue components of the musculature, as well as a reflection of the level of residual tone, techniques of neuromuscular inhibition will be required (49, 50). Flexion of the knee should be pursued with the hip in extension so that the lateral capsular attachments near the release are stretched through the rectus femoris. Transverse friction massage may also be required over the release to obtain optimal scar formation near the release site (47) (Figure 4–14).

Since connective tissue repair will continue for well over a year, pain following subcutaneous lateral release may persist for some time (69). Since pain is such a potent inhibitor of normal patellofemoral function, it is not unusual for the rehabilitation of these patients to take many months. Formal physical therapy generally requires 12–16 weeks, although it is not unusual for patients who are particularly deficient in motor function to require much longer to complete their rehabilitation. Finally, residual degenerative changes of the articular surfaces may continually inhibit normal motor responses. Patients with significant joint disease often must continue to perform the basic isolated exercises for the VM indefinitely, in order to participate in rigorous activities.

In conclusion, successful rehabilitation after subcutaneous lateral release requires an approach that promotes patellofemoral function and integrates it with the remainder of the locomotor system. Experience has shown that spontaneous recovery of normal extensor mechanism function is quite rare. The difficulty of restoring normal patellar mechanics following subcutaneous lateral release is often complicated by a lack of fundamental motor skills in these patients. Thus gains in

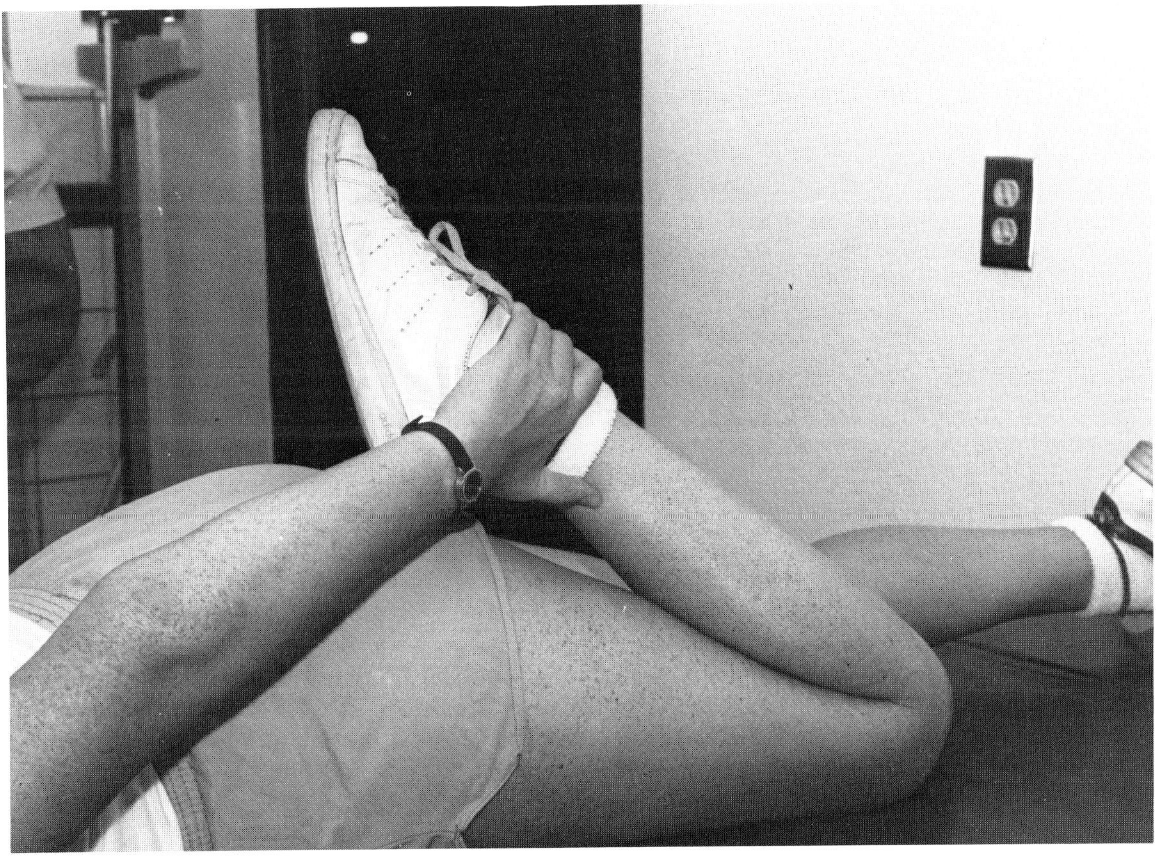

**Figure 4–14** Stretch SLR, prone position, hip extended.

strength and proprioceptive awareness throughout the ROM are attempted only after careful local preparation of the knee musculature with the types of PRE described above. Later improvement is sought using routines that demand normal motor patterns and that most closely approximate those of the patient's normal activities of daily living. Seventy-five percent of those patients utilizing this approach have achieved satisfactory results after subcutaneous lateral release (74).

## Summary

There are various questions the treating physician must answer prior to the application of lateral release. The first question that must be answered is "When is surgery indicated?" This is dependent upon the patient's response to conservative modalities, such as rehabilitation of the extensor mechanism for patellofemoral instability. In our experience, approximately 80–90% of patients with this diagnosis initially do respond to aggressive rehabilitation and strengthening programs. Those entities such as contraction of the lateral patellofemoral ligament, mobilization techniques, contrairritation, stretching, and patellofemoral enhancement procedures do play a role.

The second question that needs to be addressed is "In which patients can isolated lateral release can be applied?" In our experience, lateral release is, without question, definitely indicated in those patients with contraction of the lateral patellofemoral ligament, including such specific entities as the lateral facet compression syndrome or ELPS, as described by Ficat and Hungerford, and for those patients with arthrofibrosis and associated contracture. As for patellofemoral instability, we have found that it is the procedure of primary choice to release a deforming structure and thus allow further rehabilitation of the controlling forces. It appears to be the first rung on the surgical ladder of care. An isolated lateral release by arthroscopic control for visual division of the deforming structure and attempt at further rehabilitation is the primary surgical procedure. There remains a group of approximately 25% of patients whose symptoms are not adequately controlled over a long period of time, and for them more aggressive realignment procedures may become necessary. This may expose a certain percentage of patients to a secondary surgical procedure; however, the advantage of avoiding the major trauma associated with proximal and distal realignments appears to be well worth it.

The third question that any physician must answer is ''What method should be used to perform lateral release?'' Immediate hemostasis, early ROM, and the resultant advantageous rehabilitative techniques seem to indicate the application of electrosurgical modalities. The use of electrosurgical techniques in our arthroscopic procedures, in particular for lateral release, has been a definite step forward and has significantly diminished the frequency of hemarthrosis in our practice and the resultant morbidity to the patient population.

A caveat must be made regarding the technique of electrosurgery. Surgeons must familiarize themselves with various generators, and they must familiarize themselves and their staff with all the aspects of electrosurgical technique. Recently, publications have appeared that should help to disseminate this knowledge.

## *References*

1. Aglietti P, Insall J, Walker P. A new patellar prosthesis. Clin Orthop 107:175, 1975
2. Albee F. Orthopedic and Reconstructive Surgery, Industrial and Civilian, pp 624–630. WB Saunders, Philadelphia, 1919
3. Baker R, Carroll N. The semitendonosis tenodesis for recurrent dislocation of the patella. J Bone Joint Surg [Br] 54:103–108, 1972
4. Baksp D. Restoration of dynamic stability of the patella by pes anserinus transposition—A new approach. J Bone Joint Surg [Br] 63:399–403, 1981
5. Beck J, Wildermuth B. The female athlete's knee. Clinics in Sports Medicine (to be published)
6. Bevan A. Dislocation of the patella. Surg Clin North Am 4:929–935, 1920
7. Blazina ME, Fox JM, Jurgutis JG, Carlson GJ, Patella Baja (In Rera). A technical consideration in tibial tubercle transfer. Presented at post-graduate course on knees, AAOS, San Francisco, California, 1974.
8. Chen S, Ramanathan E. The treatment of patellar instability by lateral release. J Bone Joint Surg [Br] 66:344–349, 1984
9. Chrisman O, Snook G, Wilson T. A long-term prospective study of the Hauser and Roux-Goldthwait procedure for recurrent patellar dislocation. Clin Orthop 144:27–30, 1979
10. Coder L, Larson R. Z-plasty lateral retinacular release for the treatment of patellar compression syndrome. Clin Orthop 144:110–114, 1979
11. Cox JS. An evaluation of the Elmslie-Trillat procedure for management of patellar dislocations and subluxations: A preliminary report. Am J Sports Med 4:72–77, 1976
12. Crosby E, Insall J. Recurring dislocation of the patella—Relation of treatment of osteoarthritis. J Bone Joint Surg [Am] 58:9–13, 1976
13. DeCesare W. Late results of Hauser procedure for recurrent dislocation of the patella. Clin Orthop 140:137–144, 1979
14. Dickson J. Recurrent dislocation of the patella. Surg Clin North Am 16:997–1000, 1936
15. Dimon J. Apprehension test for subluxation of patella. Clin Orthop 103:39, 1974

16. Donohue J, Buss D, Oegema T, Thompson R. The effects of indirect blunt trauma on adult canine articular cartilage. J Bone Joint Surg [Am] 65:948–957, 1983
17. Dougherty J, Wirth C, Akbarnia B. Management of patellar subluxation—A modification of Hauser's technique. Clin Orthop 115:204–208, 1976
18. Edmonson A, Crenshaw A. (eds) Campbells' Operative Orthopedics, 6th ed. CV Mosby, St. Louis, 1980
19. Edwards D, Bentley G. Osteochondritis dissecans patellae. J Bone Joint Surg [Br] 59:58–63, 1977
20. Estor E, Estor H. La luxation recidivante de la rotule. Revue d'Orthopédie et de Chirurgie de l'Appareil Moteur 20:330–335, 1933
21. Ficat R, Ficat C, Bailleux A. Syndrome d'hyperpression externe de la rotule (SHPE). Rev Chir Orthop 61:39–59, 1975
22. Ficat R, Hungerford D. Disorders of the Patellofemoral Joint. Williams & Wilkins, Baltimore, 1977
23. Ficat R, Phillippe J, Hungerford D. Chondromalacia patellae: A system of classification. Clin Orthop 144:55–62, 1979
24. Fielding J, Liebler W. Tibial tubercle transfer: A long range follow-up study. Clin Orthop 144:31–35, 1979
25. Fox J, Blazina M, Del Pizzo W, et al. The synovial shelf syndrome. Paper presented at the Annual Meeting of the American Academy of Orthopaedic Surgeons, San Francisco, 1979
26. Frankel V, Nordin M. Basic Biomechanics of the Skeletal System. Lea & Febiger, Philadelphia, 1980
27. Fulkerson J. Anteromedialization of the tibial tuberosity for patellofemoral malalignment. Clin Orthop 177:176–181, 1983
28. Galeazzi R. Nouve applicazioni del trapianto musculore e tendineo. Clinica Ortopedica del l'Istituto Rachitici, Milano, pp 315–323, 1921
29. Gallie W, LeMesurier A. Habitual dislocation of the patella. J Bone Joint Surg 22:575–582, 1924
30. Goldthwait J. Slipping or recurring dislocation of the patella with the report of 11 cases. Boston Med Surg J 150:164–174, 1904
31. Goodfellow J, Hungerford D, Sindel M. Patellofemoral joint mechanics and pathology. I. Functional anatomy of the patellofemoral joint. J Bone Joint Surg [Br] 58:287, 1976
32. Grana W, O'Donoghue D. Patellar tendon transfer by the slot-block method for recurrent subluxation and dislocation of the patella. J Bone Joint Surg [Am] 59:736–741, 1977
33. Hall J, Micheli L, McMarama G. Semitendonosis tenodesis for recurrent subluxation or dislocation of the patella. Clin Orthop 144:31–35, 1979
34. Hampson W, Hill B. Late results of transfer of the tibial tubercle for recurrent dislocation of the patella. J Bone Joint Surg [Br] 57:209–213, 1975
35. Harrison, M. The results of a realignment operation for recurrent dislocation of the patella. J Bone Joint Surg [Br] 37:559–567, 1955
36. Harwin S, Stern R. Subcutaneous lateral retinacular release for chondromalacia of the patella. A preliminary report. Clin Orthop 156:207–210, 1981
37. Hauser E. Total tendon transplant for slipping patella—A new operation for recurrent dislocation of the patella. Gynecol and Obstet Invest 66:199–213, 1938
38. Henry J, Craven P. Surgical treatment of patellar instability: Indications and results. Am J Sports Med 9:82–85, 1981
39. Hettinga D. Normal joint structures and their reaction to injury. J Orthop Sports Phys Ther 1:16–21, 1979
40. Heywood A. Recurrent dislocation of the patella—A study of its pathology and treatment in one hundred six knees. J Bone Joint Surg [Br] 43:508–517, 1961
41. Huebscher C. Ueber Operationen bei habitueller Luxation des Kniescheibe. Z Orthop Chir 24:1–22, 1909
42. Hughston J. Subluxation of the patella. J Bone Joint Surg [Am] 50:1003–1026, 1968
43. Hughston J, Walsh W. Proximal and distal reconstruction of the extensor mechanism for patellar subluxation. Clin Orthop 144:36–42, 1979

44. Jones J, Francis K, Mahoney J. Recurrent dislocating patella in a long-term follow-up study. Clin Orthop 20:230–240, 1961
45. Kaplan E. Some aspects of functional anatomy of the human knee. Clin Orthop 23:18–29, 1962
46. Kaufer H. Mechanical function of the patella. J Bone Joint Surg [Am] 53:1551–1560, 1971
47. Kessler R, Hertling D. Management of Common Musculoskeletal Disorders. Harper & Row, Philadelphia, 1983
48. Klapp R. Die Operationen on der unteren Extremitaeten. In: Bier A, Braun H, Kuemmell H (eds) Chirurgische Operationslehre, vol 5, pp 330–662, Berlin, 1920
49. Knott M, Voss E. Proprioceptive Neuromuscular Facilitation. Harper & Row, Philadelphia, 1968
50. Korr I. The facilitated segment. In: Proceeding of the Third International Conference of the International Federation of Manipulative Therapists, Vail, Co, pp 143–146, 1977
51. Kroguis A. Zur operativen Behandlung der habituellen Luxation der Kniescheibe. Zentralbl Chir 31:254–257, 1904
52. Kummel B, Crutchlow W. Stabilization of the subluxating patella by semitendonis transfer to the lateral third of the infrapatellar tendon. Am J Sports Med 5:194–202, 1977
53. Kurosawa H, Fukobayoshi T, Nakajima H. Load bearing mode of the knee joint: Physical behavior of the knee joint with or without menisci. Clin Orthop 149:283, 1980
54. Larson R, Cabaud H, Slocum D, et al. The patellar compression syndrome: Surgical treatment by lateral retinacular release. Clin Orthop 134:158–167, 1978
55. Lieb F, Perry J. Quadriceps function an anatomical and mechanical study using amputated limbs. J Bone Joint Surg [Am] 50:1535, 1968
56. Madigan R, Wissinger H, Donaldson W. Preliminary experience with a method of quadricepsplasty in recurrent subluxation of the patella. J Bone Joint Surg [Am] 57:601–607, 1975
57. McCarroll H, Schwartzmann J. Lateral dislocation of the patella—Correction by simultaneous transplantation of the tibial tubercle and semitendonosis. J Bone Joint Surg 28:446–452, 1945
58. McFarland B. Excision of patella for dislocation. J Bone Joint Surg [Br] 30:158–159, 1948
59. McGinty J, McCarthy, JC. Endoscopic lateral retinacular release. A preliminary report. Clin Orthop 158:120–125, 1981
60. McKeever D. Transplantation of the tibial tubercle. J Bone Joint Surg [Am] 33:478–479, 1951
61. McNab I. Recurrent dislocation of the patella. J Bone Joint Surg [Am] 34:957–976, 1952
62. Merchant A, Mercer N. Lateral release of the patella. A preliminary report. Clin Orthop 103:40–45, 1974
63. Metcalf R. An arthroscopic method for lateral release of the subluxating or dislocating patella. Clin Orthop 167:9–18, 1982
64. Micheli L, Stanitsky C. Lateral patellar retinacular release. Am J Sports Med 9:330–336, 1981
65. Miller G, Dickason J, Fox J, et. al. The use of electrosurgery for arthroscopic subcutaneous lateral release. Orthopedics 5:309–314, 1982
66. O'Donoghue D. Treatment of acute dislocations of the patella. In: American Academy of Orthopaedic Surgeons (ed) Symposium on the Athlete's Knee, Surgical Repair and Reconstructions, pp 36–49. CV Mosby, St. Louis, 1980
67. Osborne A, Fulford P. Lateral release for chondromalacia patellae. J Bone Joint Surg [Br] 64:202–205, 1982
68. Outerbridge R, Dunlop J. The problem of chondromalacia patella. Clin Orthop 110:177–196, 1975
69. Peacock E, Van Winkle W. Wound Repair. WB Saunders, Philadelphia, 1976
70. Pevsner D, Johnson J, Blazina M. The patellofemoral joint and its implication in the rehabilitation of the knee. Phys Ther 59:869–874, 1979

71. Robbins H, Ulin R. A procedure for recurrent dislocation of the patella. Bull Hosp Joint Dis 34:148–155, 1973
72. Rorabeck C, Bobechko W. Acute dislocation of the patella with osteochondral fracture. A review of 18 cases. J Bone Joint Surg [Br] 58:237–240, 1976
73. Roux C. Luxation habituelle de la rotule: traitemente operatoire. Revue de Chirurgie 8:682–689, 1888
74. Sherman O, Fox J, Sperling H, et al. Patellar instability: Arthroscopic treatment by electrosurgical subcutaneous lateral release. Paper presented at the 10th Annual Meeting of the American Orthopaedic Society for Sports Medicine, Anaheim, CA, 1984
75. Slocum D, James S, Larson R. Surgical treatment of the dislocating patella in athletes. Paper presented at the Annual Meeting of the American Orthopaedic Association, Hot Springs, VA, 1973
76. Smillie I. Injuries of the Knee Joint, 2nd ed. Williams & Wilkins, Baltimore, 1951
77. Sorell C. Recurrent dislocation of patella—Considerations on present methods of treatment—Long-term follow-up study. Bull Hosp Joint Dis 25:94–125, 1964
78. Soto-Hall R. Traumatic degeneration of the articular cartilage of the patella. J Bone Joint Surg 27:426–431, 1945
79. Southwick W, Becker G, Albright J. Dovetail patellar tendon transfer for recurrent dislocating patella. JAMA 204:117–121, 1968
80. Stratford P. Electromyography of the quadriceps femoris muscle in subjects with normal knees and acutely effused knees. Phys Ther 62:279–283, 1982
81. Sutton F, Thompson C, Lipke J, Kettelkamp D. The effect of patellectomy on knee function. J Bone Joint Surg [Am] 58:537–540, 1976
82. Trillat A, Dejour H, Covelte A. Diagnostic et traitemente de subluxation recidivante de la rotule. Rev Chir Orthop 50:813–824, 1964
83. Wall J. Compartment syndrome as a complication of the Hauser procedure. J Bone Joint Surg [Am] 61:185–191, 1979
84. Weaver J. Bipartite patella as a cause of disability in the athlete. Am J Sports Med 5:137–143, 1977
85. West F, Soto-Hall R. Recurrent dislocation of the patella in the adult—End results of patellectomy with quadricepsplasty. J Bone Joint Surg [Am] 40:386–393, 1958
86. Wiberg G. Roentgenographic and anatomic studies on the femoropatellar joint with special reference to chondromalacia patella. Acta Orthop Scand 12:319, 1941
87. Wilber N. Recurrent lateral dislocation of the patella: Preliminary results of pes anserinus transfer. South Med J 67:531–533, 1974
88. Willner P. Recurrent dislocation of the patella. Clin Orthop 69:213–215, 1970

# Articular Cartilage and Its Relationship to Meniscal Lesions

# 5

S. Ward Casscells

In dealing with problems either inside or outside of the knee joint, it is important to recognize that the fate of the knee joint depends upon the integrity of the articular cartilage. This should be kept in mind when undertaking or planning any surgical procedure. It is also necessary to have some understanding of the pathophysiology of this important tissue as well as an understanding of the function of other tissues within the confines of the knee joint, especially the meniscus. The cruciate ligaments, of course, are also important, but this paper does not discuss the care of these ligaments in the overall treatment of knee injuries.

Although MacConaill (9) in 1932 and Fairbanks (6) in 1948 wrote on the important role that the meniscus plays in the function of the knee joint, this advice was largely ignored. Just a few years ago, orthopaedists were taught that a tight knee is a good knee and that to achieve this it may be necessary to remove the meniscus while doing a repair of the ligamentous structures. Now the tragic consequences of total meniscectomy are well known. The purpose of this paper is to emphasize that it is important to consider what is best for the articular cartilage when some surgical procedure is contemplated.

There is some confusion in the literature about the ability of the articular cartilage of the knee to withstand the rigors of a normal lifespan (1, 7, 12). In none of these previously reported series is there any clinical information about previous trauma to the joint surfaces or whether there is malalignment of the leg, both of which are important. My own impression, based on clinical observation, as well as a large series of cadaver knees (2), leads me to believe that the articular cartilage is capable of remaining intact throughout a normal lifespan of 70 years or more. This clinical observation is supported by the work of some investigators such as Ekholm (4), who in 1951 stated, "Even in unfavorable circumstances, articular surfaces are very resistant to wear and tear, and it is possible under physiological conditions that there is so little loss of surface tissue in a healthy adult joint that no multiplication of cartilage cells need occur to sustain cartilage." In 1969 Meachim (11) noted "surprisingly little evidence of a generalized aging change in properties of human cartilage 30 to 40 years of age." He also stated that "in middle and later years of adult life, there is no evidence of generalized change with age." If this is true, then what causes articular cartilage to break down in the absence of trauma and in the absence of diseases, such as rheumatoid arthritis, that specifically attack the cartilage? Although there are no statistics, there seems to be little doubt that overload of the cartilage is responsible. Clement Sledge (personal communication) has estimated the weight-bearing tolerance of articular cartilage as approximately 20–25 kg/cm$^2$. Weightman (16) has determined the weight-bearing tolerance to be 285 lb per square inch, which is comparable to Sledge's figures. With this knowledge as a background, this paper will explore why the articular cartilage breaks down, what is apt to accelerate this breakdown, and what role the torn or intact meniscus plays in this process.

## Alignment

Alignment is one factor that influences to a considerable degree the fate and survivability of the articular cartilage. Normally, the three joints of the lower extremity are mechanically aligned so that a plumbline dropped from the center of the femoral head passes through the center of the knee and the center of the ankle joints. Anatomically, there is an angle of approximately 6 degrees between the long axis of the femur and that of the tibia. It is not known how much malalignment or deviation from this angle of 6 degrees the articular cartilage will tolerate, and there are no statistics on the incidence of unicompartmental degenerative arthritis in patients with bowlegs or knock-knees. I have seen many 55- or 60-year-old patients with no history of trauma who have considerable medial compartment degenerative changes, with an anatomic angle of 0 degrees, and others with lateral compartment disease in whom the angle was 12 degrees valgus.

These are patients who have had no known trauma and no meniscectomy. On the basis of my own clinical experience with absolutely no data to back it up, I am under the impression that variations of as little as 5 or 6 degrees from the anatomic angle will result in degenerative arthritis by the time the patient is 55 or 60 years of age, if not sooner. In addition, almost all of these patients at this stage of their disease have some degenerative changes in the posterior horns of the respective menisci. Unfortunately, the meniscus has often been considered the cause of the problem rather than the result of it. What these patients need is not a meniscectomy, but an osteotomy to realign the leg, and the sooner it is done, the better the result.

## Trauma

Punched out defects in the articular surface of the knee joint, especially on the femoral side, are quite commonly seen following trauma. There may or may not be a concomitant tear of the meniscus. If there is a meniscal tear that necessitates meniscectomy, especially a total meniscectomy, and if in addition this patient has malalignment, the prognosis for survival of the articular cartilage is extremely poor.

It is my impression that a single punched out lesion in the femoral condyle may remain stable for many years if the patient has no malalignment and a normal meniscus. This may be true to a lesser extent if the patient is young and an active basketball or football player.

It is of utmost importance to the clinician to understand the relationship or lack of relationship of the torn meniscus to the articular cartilage so that he might be better able to treat his patients effectively. Despite the opinions of Watson-Jones (15), Smillie (13), Helfet (8), and other lesser known orthopaedic surgeons, there is no data, to my knowledge, that supports the theory that a torn meniscus poses any *significant* threat to the integrity of the articular cartilage. Minor superficial lesions probably do not break down to the point where they can be termed degenerative arthritis if the leg is normally aligned. This is my opinion and also that of long-time cartilage observers such as Mankin (10), Thompson (14), and Sledge (personal communication). Unfortunately, there is little or no clinical data in the literature on this general topic. My own data, based on a study of a large number of cadaver knees as well as clinical experience at arthroscopy and arthrotomy, have convinced me that the torn meniscus poses no serious threat to the articular cartilage (3). This is also the opinion of Fahme and colleagues (5), who stated that they found "little evidence that degenerative meniscal tears cause osteoarthritis or vice versa."

Researchers who work on animal models in laboratories and who submit their results to statistical analysis are quick to criticize clinical impressions such as those that have just been expressed because they are "unproven and anecdotal." It is likely that some clinical problems will never be resolved scientifically, such as the relationship between a torn meniscus and degenerative arthritis. Since this relationship has never been established either scientifically or clinically, it should not be necessary to disprove something that has never been proven. However, in the minds of many surgeons, this seems to be the case. Clinicians often cannot wait for a scientific solution to all their clinical problems, and they "must go with the available evidence." The available evidence suggests that the torn meniscus is not a "great threat to the knee joint with destructive power" as Smillie (13) has stated, nor should we "remove a meniscus because of the danger of leaving an unseen tear in the posterior horn," as advocated by Watson-Jones.

On the basis of our present knowledge, the following are suggestions on how to deal with a tear or suspected tear of the meniscus. All or part of the meniscus should be salvaged, whenever possible, by suture or limited partial meniscectomy. Increasing experience and knowledge has shown that many more meniscal tears can be treated by suture, either openly or arthroscopically. This includes some tears within the substance of the meniscus. Although his work has not been published, Charles Henning has had as much or more experience with arthroscopic suture than almost anyone else and has had a high degree of success in suturing menisci that were previously thought to be unsuturable (personal communication). Bucket-handle tears, for instance, often can be repaired by scarifying the adjacent soft tissue to produce bleeding; in a high percentage of cases, the tear will heal. There is nothing to be lost by trying.

Tears of the meniscus that have the potential for locking the joint and causing functional disability should be excised at least partially. Included in this category are flap tears which have the potential for causing functional disability, as the flap itself, usually has no weight-bearing function. Other tears such as the simple horizontal cleavage tear, which has no potential for locking the joint, need not be resected; I have many patients who have been treated in this conservative fashion. These patients, of course, can get into future trouble, especially if they are athletes, and further surgery may be required. Again, there is no harm in delay, and as this meniscus is capable of bearing weight, it should be preserved. In addition, excessive contouring and trimming of the meniscus is unnecessary and unwise as it further reduces the weight-bearing function of the meniscus.

Another situation that arises is a small tear, under a centimeter in diameter, that does not lend itself to suture or in which a suture is thought to be unnecessary. Or sometimes there is a tear that is only suspected but cannot be clearly demonstrated. These patients, I feel, should not have any surgery on the meniscus. Regarding meniscectomy in these patients, my own philosophy is "when in doubt, don't." I have never been disappointed when I have followed this guideline, but I have been embarrassed when I have not followed my own advice and removed a meniscus that, I realized too late, should not have been excised.

## *References*

1. Bennett GA, Waine H, Bauer W. Changes in the Knee Joint at Various Ages. Commonwealth Fund, Boston, 1942
2. Casscells SW. Gross pathologic changes in the knee joint of the aged individual. Clin Orthop 132:225–232, 1978
3. Casscells SW. The torn or degenerated meniscus and its relationship to degeneration of the weight-bearing areas of the femur and tibia. Clin Orthop 132:196–200, 1978
4. Ekholm R. Relationship between articular changes and function. Acta Orthop Scand 21:81, 1951
5. Fahme NRM, Williams EA, Noble J. Meniscal pathology and osteoarthritis of the knee. J Bone Joint Surg [Br] 65:24–29, 1983.
6. Fairbank TJ. Knee joint changes after meniscectomy. J Bone Joint Surg [Br] 30:664, 1948
7. Heine J. Arthritis deformans. Virchows Arch [Pathol Anat] 260:521, 1926
8. Helfet AJ. Managements of internal derangements of the knee, p 46. JB Lippincott, Philadelphia, 1963
9. MacConaill MA. The function of intra-articular fibrocartilages with special reference to the knee and inferior radio-ulnar joints. Irish Journal of Anatomy 66:210–227, 1932
10. Mankin HJ. Response of articular cartilage to mechanical injury. J Bone Joint Surg [Am] 64:460–465, 1982
11. Meachim G. Age changes in articular cartilage. Clin Orthop 64:33, 1969
12. Owre A. Chondromalacia of the patella. Acta Chir Scand [Suppl] 77:41, 1936
13. Smillie IS. Injuries of the Knee Joint, p 84. Churchill Livingstone, Edinburgh, 1946
14. Thompson RC. Surface injury to articular cartilage. Clin Orthop 107:239–248, 1975
15. Watson-Jones Sir R. Fractures and Joint Injuries, p 768–769. Williams & Wilkins, Baltimore, 1955
16. Weightman BO. Adult Articular Cartilage, p 225, Grune & Stratton, New York, 1972

# Arthroscopic Management of Osteochondritis Dissecans

# 6

James F. Guhl

The regenerated interest in the use of the arthroscope within the orthopaedic community in the 1960s, along with the development of the tungsten bulb, was instrumental in changing the approach to problems of the knee. Fiberoptics entered the picture a few years later, and simultaneously operative arthroscopy was introduced. This resulted in better diagnostic evaluation of osteochondritis dissecans as well as the surgical treatment for this problem with the arthroscope.

This author began evaluation and treatment of osteochondritis dissecans by this method in 1975. Over the past decade various aspects of this treatment and the results thereof at different stages were presented in courses and later published. A complete analysis of the results of this author's series is presented in this update.

In addition to a review of arthroscopic techniques, other methods affecting the approach to the treatment of osteochondritis dissecans will be considered. Recently, many surgeons have been using the arthroscopic approach advocated by the author in treating this entity. Valuable information has been obtained from some of these surgeons by personal communication. It seems appropriate to reevaluate conservative treatment as well as update the methods by which these lesions are treated by open techniques versus the arthroscopic approach and to emphasize newer methods recently introduced. The uses of scintiradiography and electrical stimulation are being worked out by others and are rapidly being accepted in the total treatment plan of osteochondritis. However, before enlarging on these points, it seems best to briefly review the methods used in the past.

Originally, restricted activity by either cast or an immobilizer, depending upon the attitude or activity level of the patient, was advocated in patients below the age of 12 years. This was reflected in the literature by Green (4), Green and

Banks (5), Helfet (9), and Campbell and Ranawat (2). In the age group between 12 and 15 years, intact lesions that showed delayed union by conservative methods were opened and drilled. The success rate of conservative treatment dropped as age increased, and it did not seem reasonable to pursue such treatment for intact lesions in patients over 15 years of age. Lesions that showed a partial separation on x-ray were best considered for drilling, fixing, and/or grafting. In 1970 Smillie (13) reported fixation of these fragments with small nails that were later removed. This, however, resulted in two operations. Aichroth (1) reported equally good results by excising loose or separated fragments and curetting the base. Scott and Stevenson (12), and Lindholm and Pylkkanen (10) reported bone peg fixation by arthrotomy. Lipscomb et al. (11) reported a small series of cases treated by curetting the base of the lesions, or the crater, filling them with cancellous bone, and fixing the fragments with Kirshner wires that were later removed.

With this experience in mind, and with the development of arthroscopic techniques, methods were developed for the treatment of osteochondritis dissecans by "closed surgery." The advantages were significant despite early criticism. Surgical trauma was lessened, scars were reduced, hospital stay and total rehabilitation time were decreased, and pain was reduced. The introduction of arthroscopy resulted in better evaluation of the lesion prior to treatment than was possible by x-ray alone. As time passed and techniques became refined, more accurate surgery seemed possible. Repeat procedures were better accepted by the patient, if necessary. Evaluation (and treatment) under local anesthesia became possible when healing was in question. Total treatment time was reduced by repeating procedures arthroscopically at an earlier date if delayed union was suspected or recognized.

During the past several years, less time was spent in cast immobilization. Earlier motion was subsequently provided by the use of hinged casts. The total approach in the treatment of osteochondritis dissecans became more promising, with reduced muscle atrophy, retained motion, and certainly reduced psychological impact on the patient.

Several reports on this treatment were then published. The first was a preliminary report in *Orthopedic Clinics of North America* in 1979 (6), at which time 23 cases were reviewed. In 1982 *Clinical Orthopedics and Related Research* carried a report on a total of 50 cases in detail (7). The combined results of another 22 cases added to this series were discussed in 1984 in *Orthopedics* (8). In this chapter the cases have been further reviewed and updated. Recently, new instruments and improved techniques, such as the use of the cannulated cancellous bone screw for fixation, have been added. Jigs designed for the repair and reconstruction of anterior cruciate ligaments were adapted to the treatment of osteochondritis dissecans to make pin fixation and bone grafting technically much easier. Bone grafts were employed more frequently, especially in younger patients in their early teens, as seen later in this update.

## Evaluation and Classification

### X-Ray

Routine x-rays, that is anteroposterior, lateral, and tunnel of both knees and left wrist and hand films for age, are ordered in addition to certain special views of value. Magnification views are helpful, especially in young patients. The bone scan is used to differentiate anomalies of ossification from osteochondritis dissecans in borderline cases. In patients older than 15 years, tomograms are important for further comparison, especially when grafting, by comparing pertinent cuts.

The following classification has been developed to define the amount of weight-bearing area to be treated: Lesions of the medial femoral condyle are central, centrolateral, and inferocentral (Figure 6–1). In the lateral femoral condyle, lesions are usually inferocentral, large, and more posterior (Figure 6–2). These have, in general, a poorer prognosis.

## Arthroscopy

The technique used for evaluation in meniscus surgery, that is probing, should also be employed before embarking on this type of surgery. In addition, the use of light dimming and methylene blue dye brings out further characteristics of the lesion. Viewing the lesion with an oblique scope from a tangential angle also may provide more information.

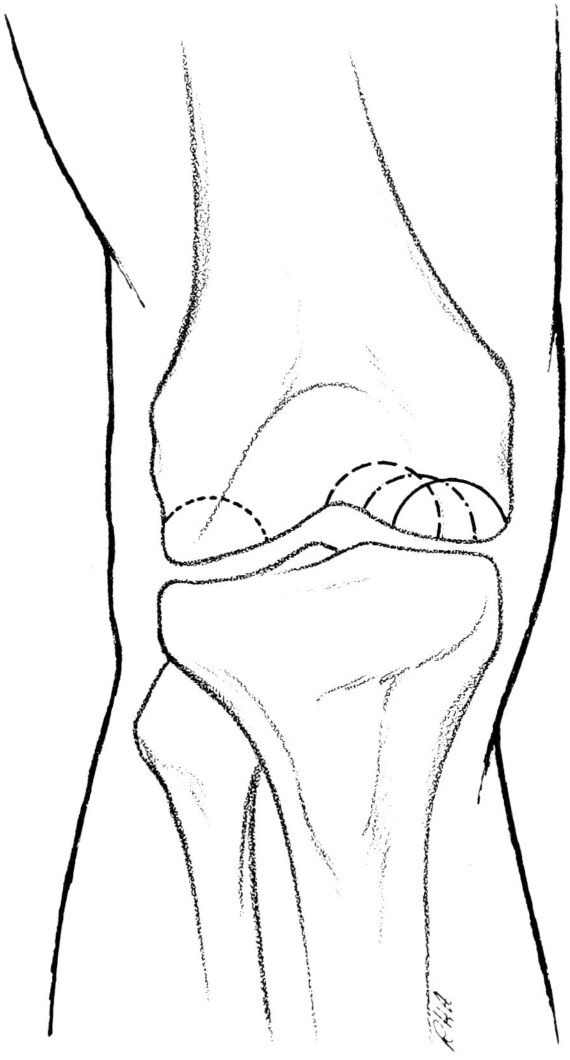

**Figure 6–1** Diagram showing x-ray classifications of lesions of the medial femoral condyle (right knee).

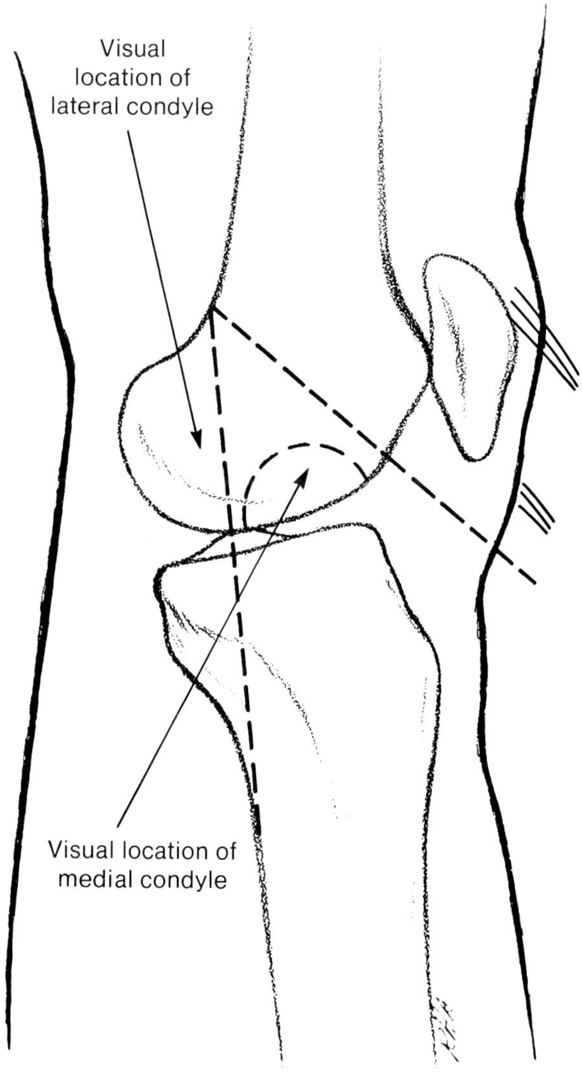


**Figure 6–2** Diagram for lesions of the lateral femoral condyle, compared to those in the medial femoral condyle, as seen on the lateral view. The lesion of the lateral femoral condyle is shown by a solid line. These are usually far posterior.

Lesions of osteochondritis dissecans are classified arthroscopically as follows: intact, early separation, partially detached, and craters with loose bodies either salvagable or unsalvagable. Intact lesions treated arthroscopically are those that are up to 3–4 cm in diameter with no break in the articular cartilage (Figure 6–3). They may be soft when probed and are usually slightly raised or depressed. Separated lesions are movable to a minimal degree when probed and have a break in the articular cartilage, usually of the lower third. Fibrous tissue usually protrudes in this area. Partially detached lesions can be displaced out of the crater but are usually held by a hinge of articular cartilage superiorly. There is a good amount of fibrous tissue between the lesion and crater in most cases. Craters are often filled with rough, fibrous tissue that is quite abrasive to the adjacent articular cartilage of the tibial plateau. The goal in reconstructing such defects is to develop a more acceptable fibrocartilagenous tissue (Figure 6–4). A large loose body that has completely detached fairly recently can often be replaced by arthroscopic or open methods, grafted, and/or fixed to form a more acceptable opposing surface.

# Arthroscopic Surgery

## Indications

In patients under 12 years of age, physiologically conservative treatment appears best. This consists of restricted activity or in some cases non-weight bearing with crutches. Cast immobilization is used less frequently than in the past, but

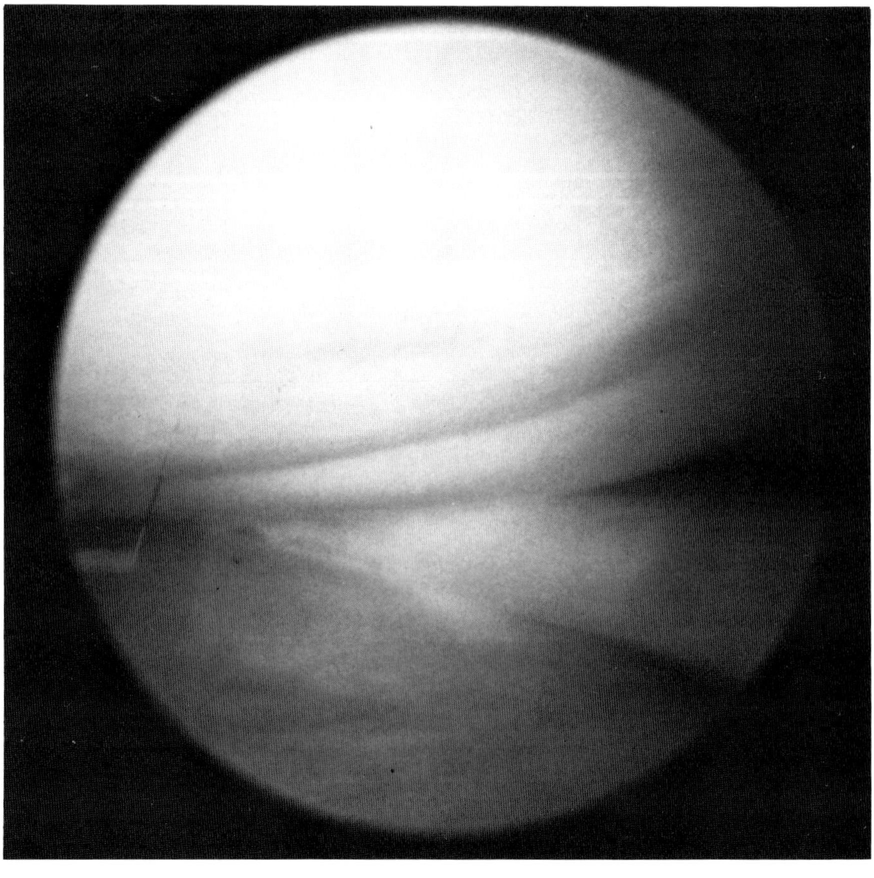

**Figure 6–3** Arthroscopic view of a typical intact lesion (right knee).

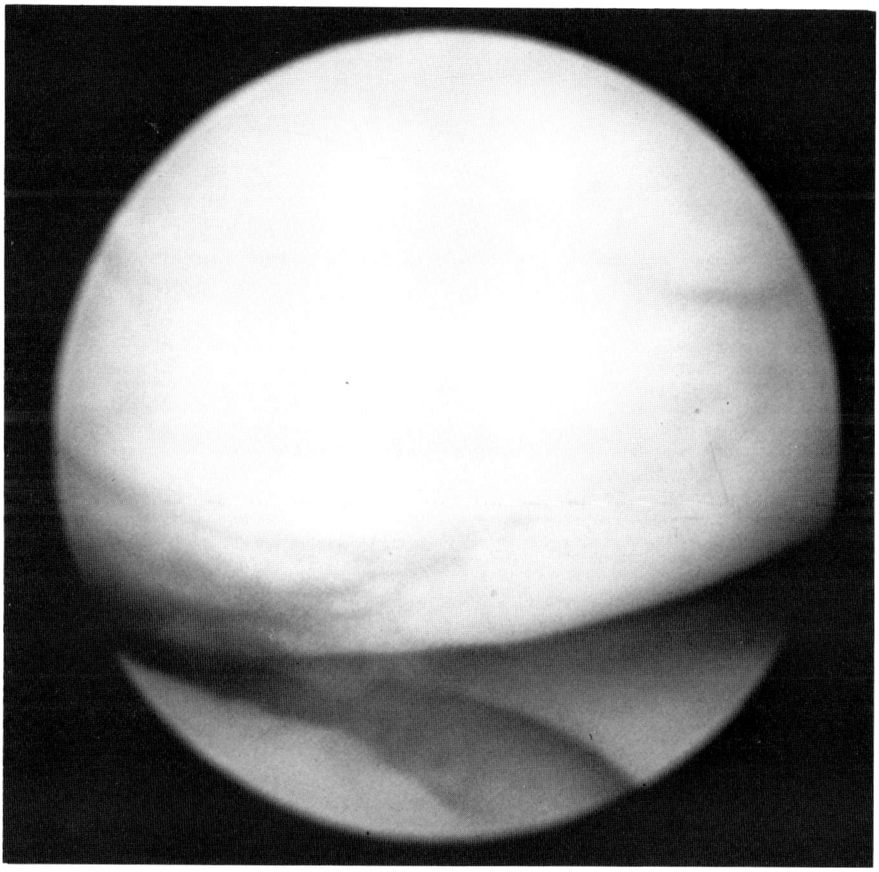

**Figure 6–4** Arthroscopic view of fibrocartilagenous tissue as it has replaced hyaline cartilage in filling a large defect (right knee).

since children at that age cannot always be trusted, it is still used at times, when necessary, in this author's experience. Cahill (personal communication) has used scintiradiography for follow-up at 6-week intervals in those patients he treats conservatively, until they are fully mature. When the scan shows decreased activity, healing is said to take place. Surgery is indicated in those patients where the lesion remains active.

This author would tend to prefer arthroscopic drilling versus conservative treatment in this age group over 12 years because there is an extremely low risk with this surgical treatment as compared with the hassle and the possibility of prolonged care by this conservative method, should it fail and ultimately require surgery. Also, experience has shown in my series in this age group that there has been a very high rate of healing by arthroscopic drilling. Also, several cases that were originally treated conservatively by others and subsequently referred to me were then drilled since they failed to heal by the former method.

The indications, therefore, for arthroscopic treatment are as follows: In patients 12 to 14 or 15 years of age, drilling arthroscopically is recommended for intact lesions. In older patients large lesions that are intact often must be grafted in addition to this. Lesions that show early separation are debrided at the border, drilled, and fixed accordingly with screws or pins if indicated. Partially detached lesions are debrided of fibrous tissue at the base of the lesion, and the crater is then reduced, grafted, and/or pinned. Grafts are used in the last two categories if the patient has reached maturity, when epiphyseal closure has occurred. Completely detached lesions can be salvaged, fixed, or grafted arthroscopically on occasion. Old craters are reconstructed and loose bodies are removed.

Open surgery should be done in large detached lesions (4 or 5 cm) that may require two or three grafts for fixation. Lesions with two or more salvageable loose fragments that can be fixed or grafted are best treated by open techniques. An arthrotomy is used occasionally for large lesions with hard sclerotic bases. Occasionally, lesions of the lateral femoral condyle, which are usually located far posterior, are difficult to treat arthroscopically and require open surgery as the only choice.

Henning (personal communication) has reviewed a fairly large series treated by electrical stimulation. This may be cumbersome and time consuming, and until further cases are reported, I would prefer to reserve this method for salvage cases. An example would be a large lesion that was grafted and now is undergoing a delayed union.

## Techniques

Arthroscopic surgical techniques, as of this date, are applicable in about 85% of the lesions of osteochondritis dissecans encountered in patients over 12 years of age. Other methods, as mentioned, are presently used for the remaining lesions according to the indications discussed. Classification must be considered by establishing the condition, size, and amount of weight-bearing area of each lesion to determine the method of arthroscopic treatment. The surgery is done under general anesthesia in an operating room or day-surgery center using sterile techniques.

**Drilling** Intact lesions are drilled with an 0.062 mm plain Kirshner wire by triangulation with the arthroscope (Figure 6–5). To begin the procedure the joint is distended with saline. The wire is best passed through a Needlescope cannula or a similar, small-diameter sheath to avoid involving soft tissue. The Needlescope obturator is at first lined up with the arthroscope and aimed for the center of the lesion. Drill holes are made here and other appropriate places within the borders of the lesion. The scope and wire are interchanged from the inferomedial to the inferolateral approach to keep the direction of drilling perpendicular to the cartilage surface. The weight-bearing area is avoided, if possible. However, it appears that no significant damage is done by using smooth wires of this size. Often the slits in the cartilage close after the wire is removed and can barely be seen a few moments later. Six to 10 holes are drilled to a depth of freshly bleeding bone, as noted when the tourniquet is deflated (see Figures 6–6 to 6–8).

**Pinning** Pinning was originally done with partially threaded wires, with the distal 3 inches having a raised thread. These are commercially available. Smooth or threaded pins can be used. The former should then be inserted at different angles to hold the lesion. Threaded wires are more difficult to insert and remove. More recently, Lanny Johnson (personal communication) developed a cannulated cancellous screw that could be inserted arthroscopically over a previously placed Kirshner wire (Figure 6–9). However, arthroscopy will be required for its removal.

The pins or wires are inserted from the inferolateral approach for lesions of the medial femoral condyle and aimed toward the condyle's posterosuperior flare for easier removal later. The scope is in the inferomedial portal (Figure 6–10). The wires are then withdrawn from the condyle, from above, until they disappear beneath the skin and are passed into the joint (Figure 6–11). The joint is then

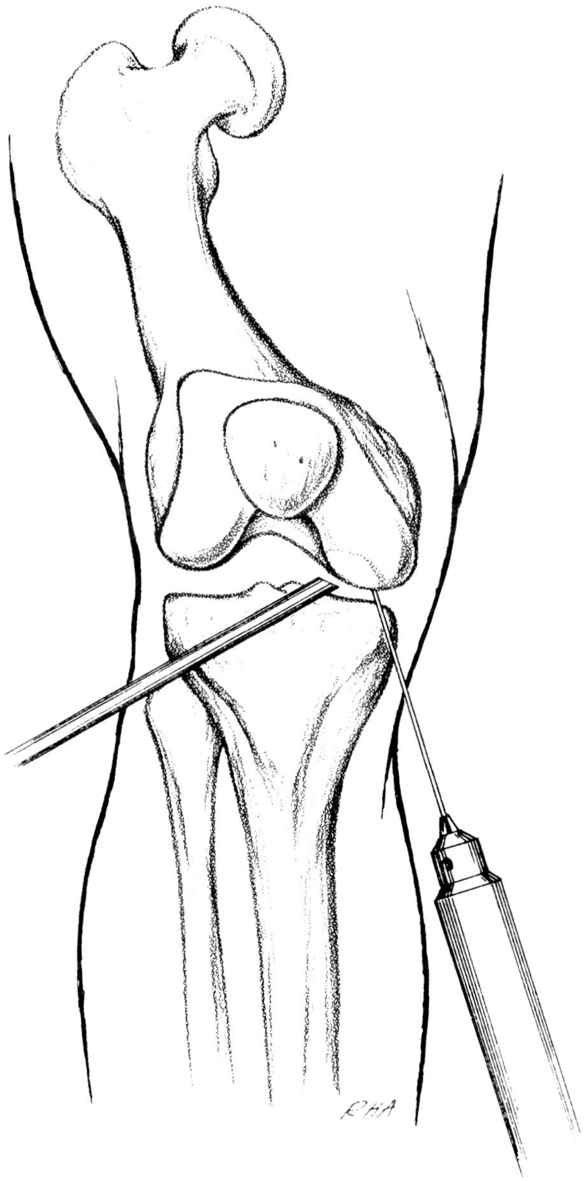

**Figure 6–5** Diagram showing the technique of drilling.

redistended and the scope reinserted in the inferolateral portal. The remaining centimeter of the wire is withdrawn until the end is flush or slightly below the articular cartilage (Figure 6–12). The proximal ends are cut beneath the skin of the proximal portion of the medial condyle and removed under local anesthesia in 4–6 weeks.

Another method that may prove to be easier and is presently under development is insertion of the wires with the use of jigs. There are many jigs under development at this time for arthroscopic anterior cruciate reconstruction (Figure 6–13). The principle of all of the jigs is the same: there is a point within the joint and a second point outside the joint that can be accurately lined up to determine the exact path of the wire (Figures 6–14 and 6–15). This can also be used for accurate placement of pins or reamers when grafting bone, thus making that procedure easier and more accurately and rapidly accomplished.

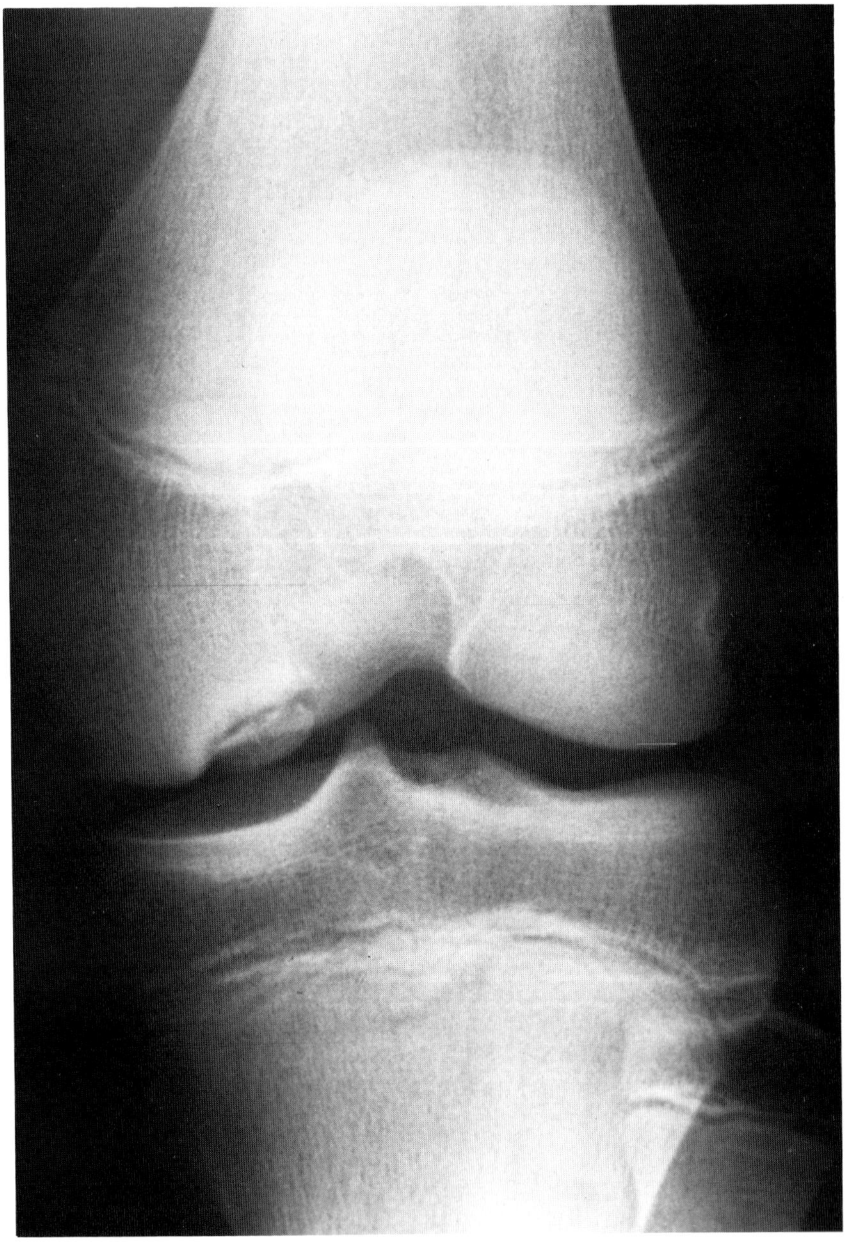

**Figure 6–6** X-ray of an intact lesion (left knee).

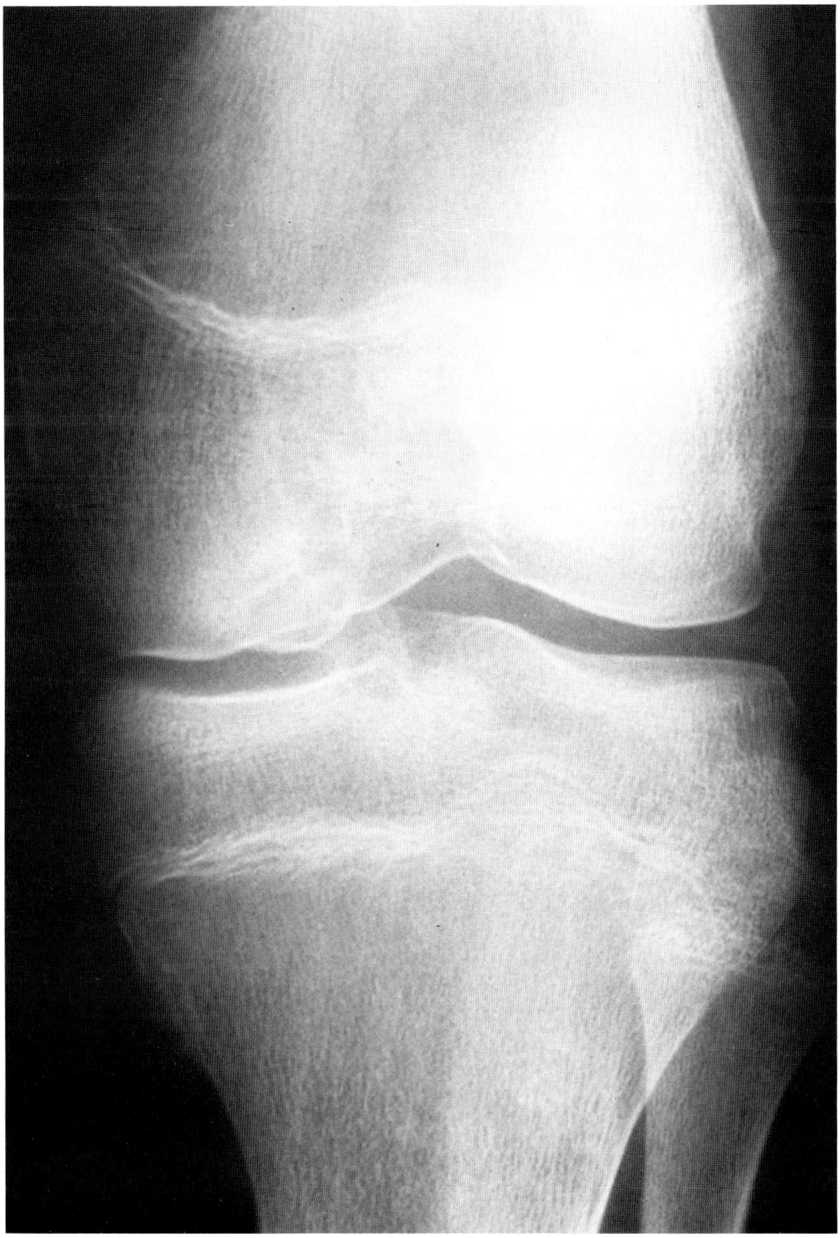

**Figure 6–7** X-ray showing healing of the intact lesion shown in Figure 6–6 8 weeks after arthroscopic drilling (left knee).

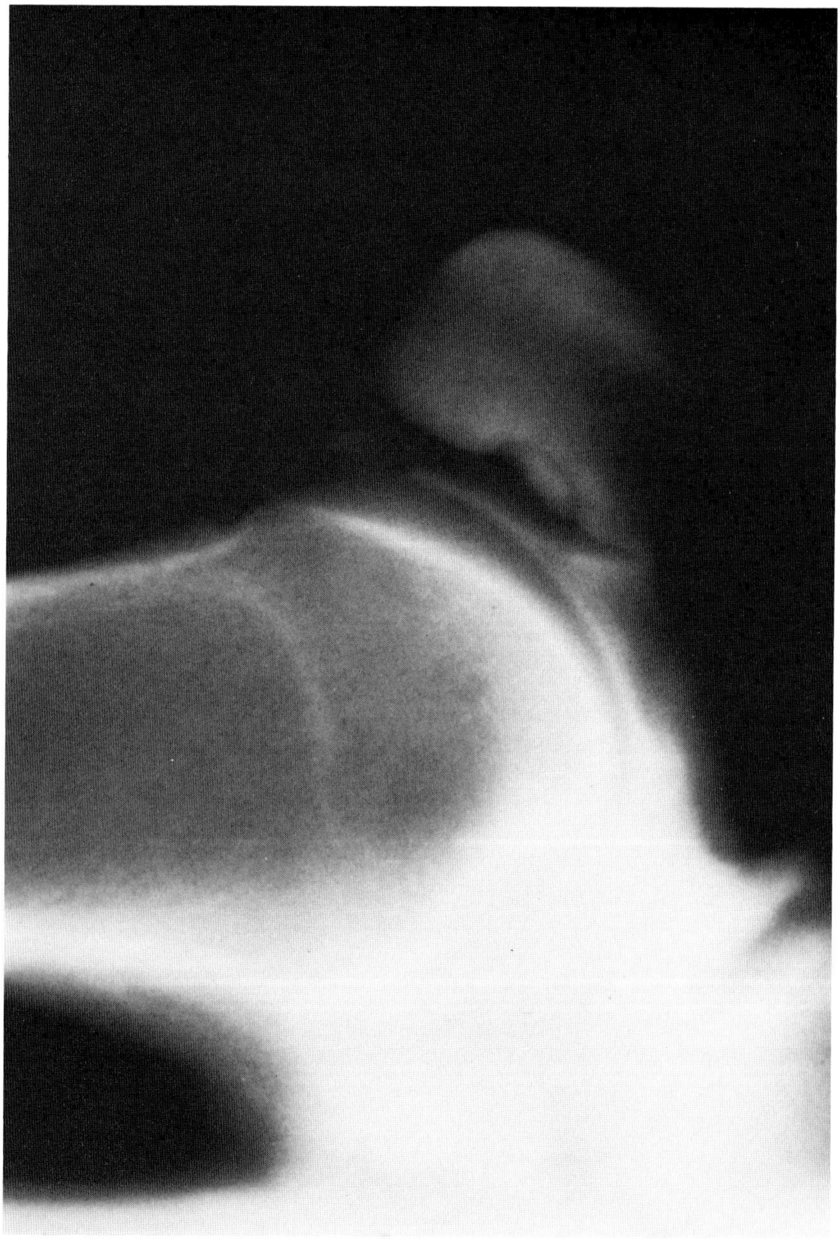

**Figure 6–8** Symptomatic patella lesion. Recommended treatment: lateral release and drill if the lesion is intact, or excise and debride or abrade if the lesion is partially separated or detached (right knee). (Courtesy of James Smith, M.D., Seattle, Washington)

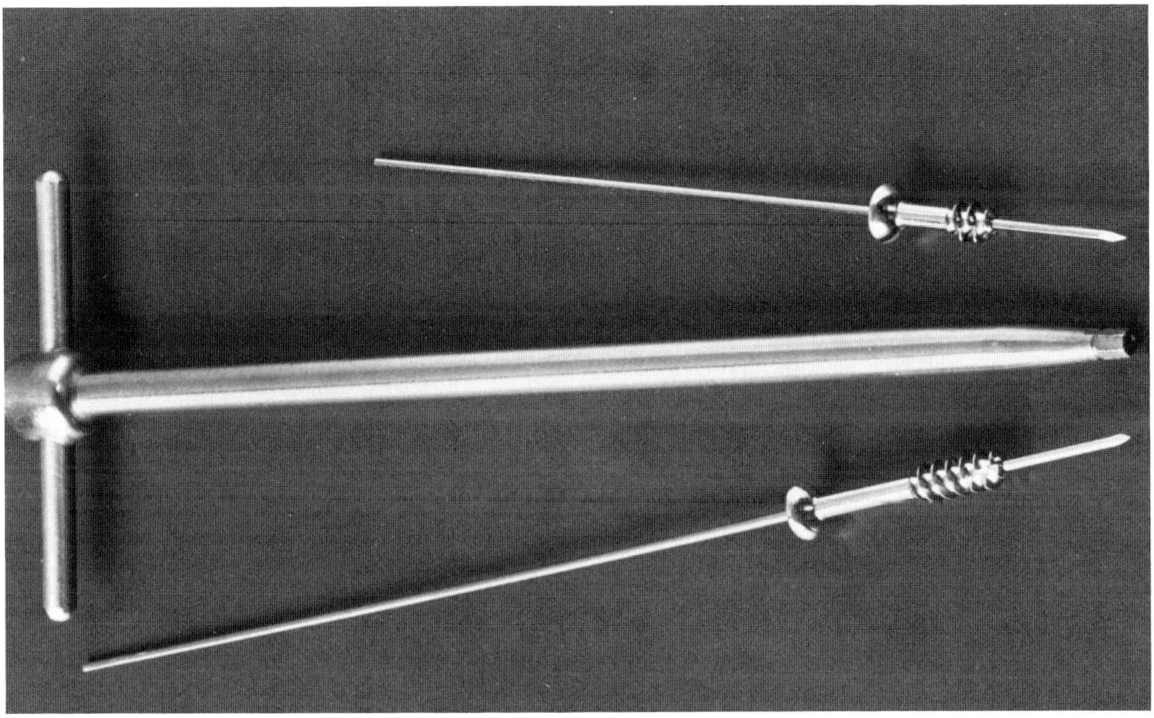

**Figure 6–9** Cannulated cancellous bone screw, wire, and inserter.

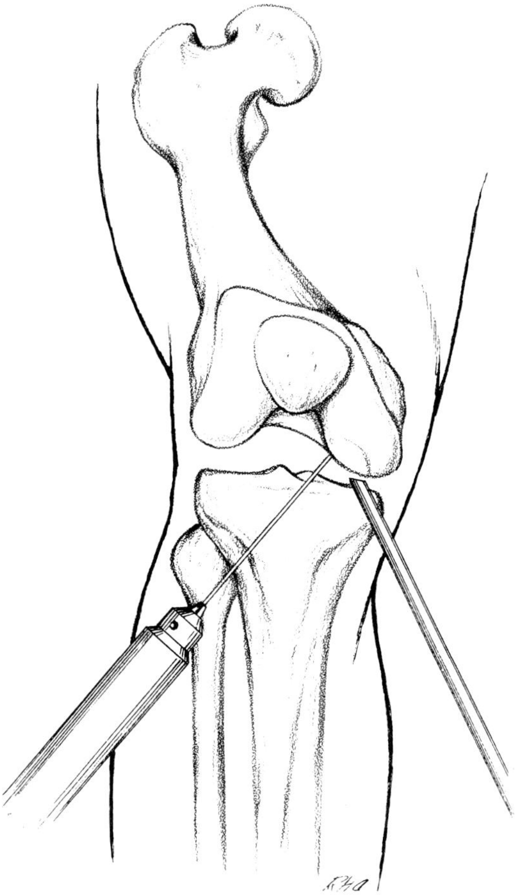

**Figure 6–10** Diagram illustrating arthroscopic pinning technique.

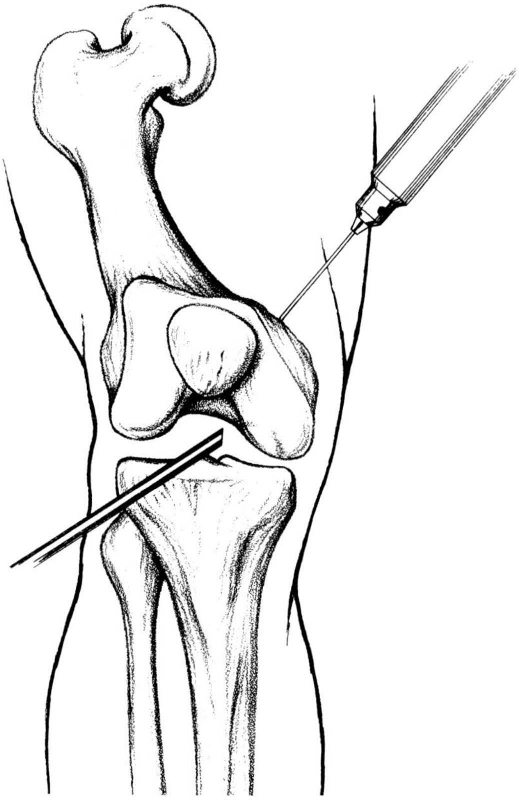

**Figure 6–11** Same diagram showing withdrawal of the pin from a proximal position.

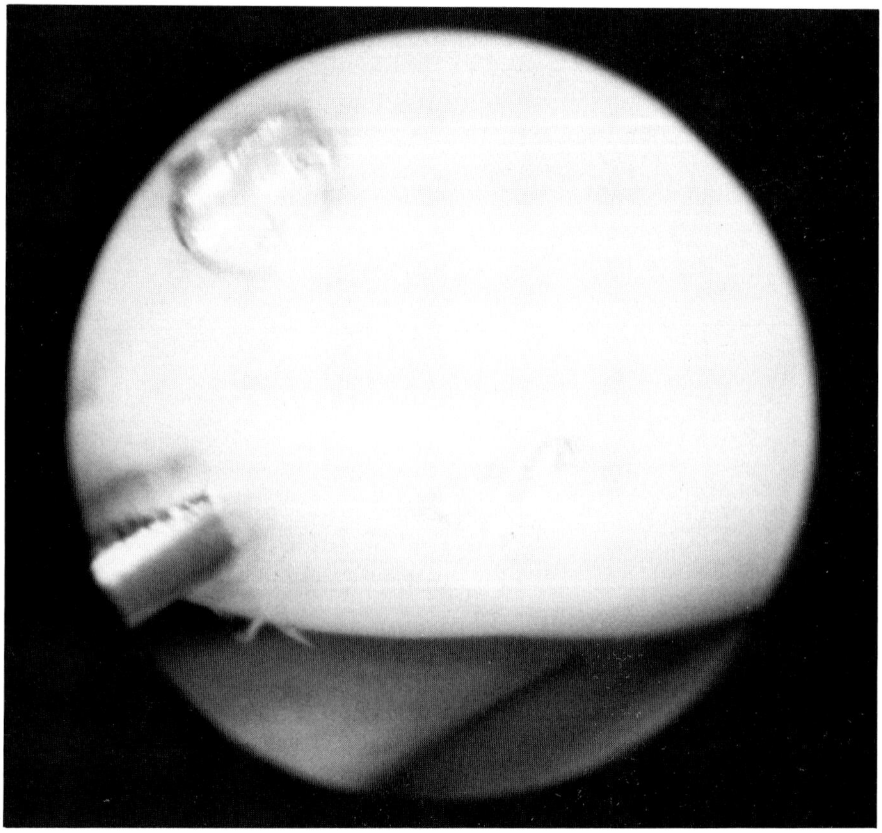

**Figure 6–12** Arthroscopic view of three threaded pins fixing a large lesion in place (left knee). One pin has been countersunk.

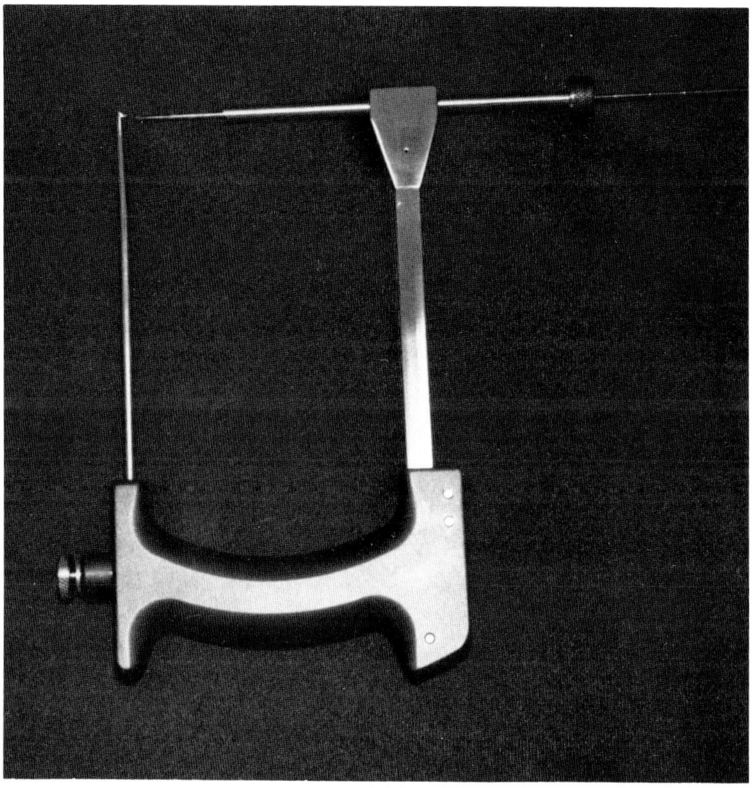

**Figure 6–13** Caspari-designed jig for anterior cruciate reconstruction. (Courtesy of Richard Caspari, M.D., Richmond, Virginia)

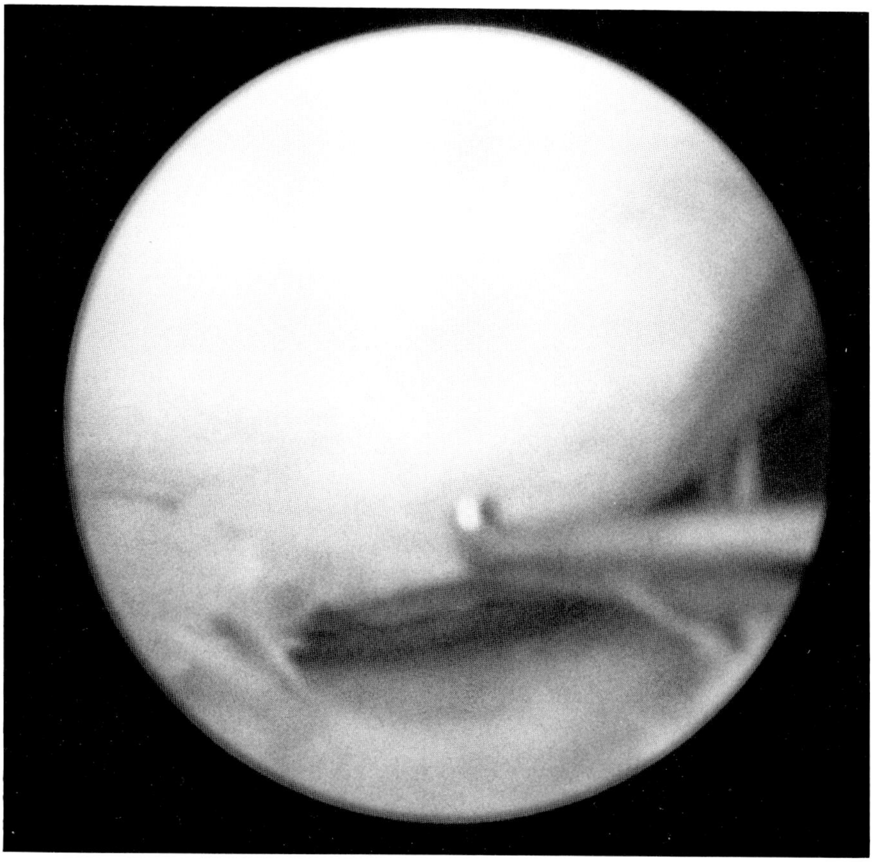

**Figure 6–14** Arthroscopic view of jig point within joint, used for pinning separated lesions of the medial femoral condyle (right knee). Note the fibrous tissue. (Courtesy of Dr. Richard Caspari, Richmond, Virginia)

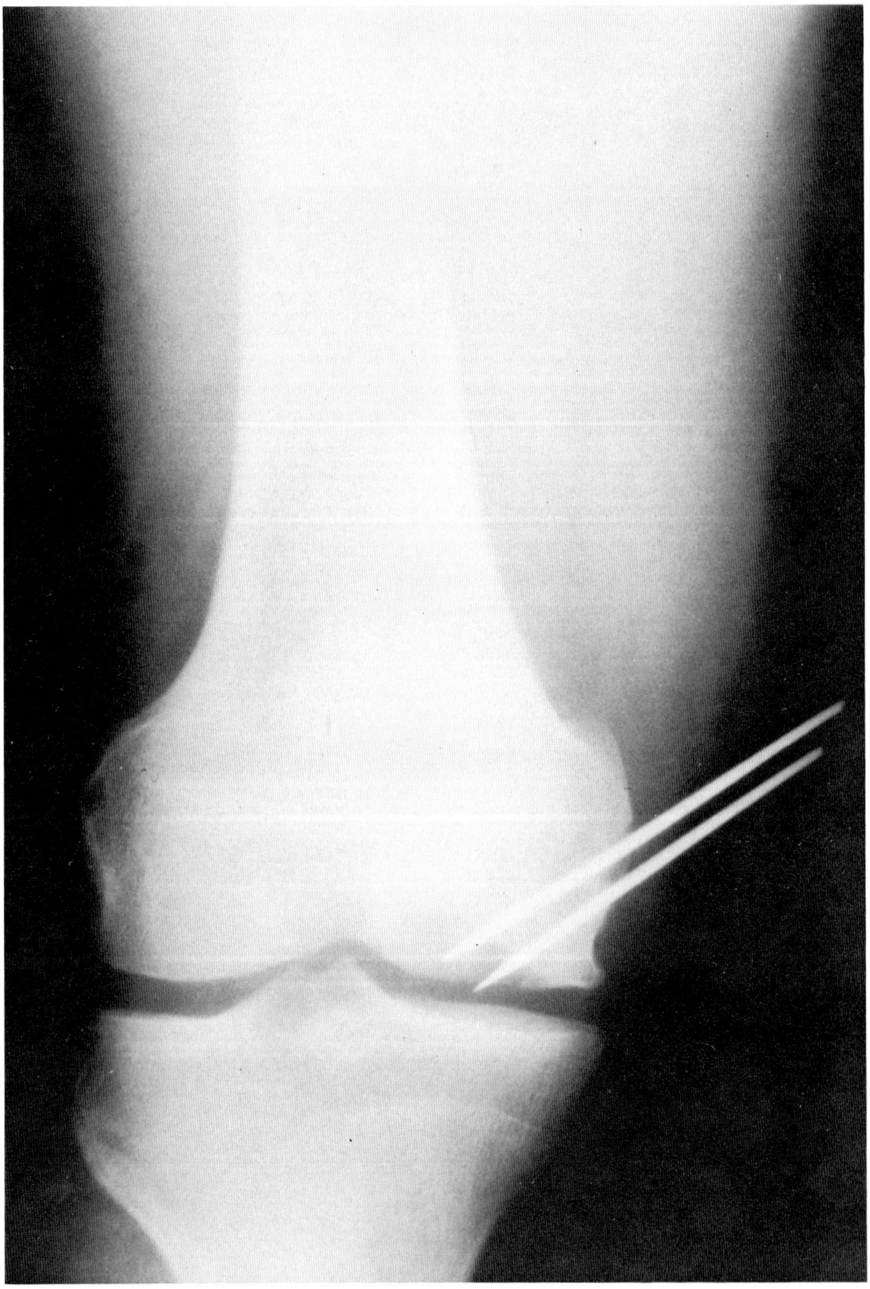

**Figure 6–15** X-ray of the lesion in Figure 6–14 with placement of the wires by employing the anterior cruciate jig (right knee). (Courtesy of Richard Caspari, M.D., Richmond, Virginia)

**Reduction and/or Replacement, Fixation, and Grafting** Lesions that are partially detached must have the undersurface debrided with a rongeur and the crater curetted of fibrous tissue. They are then reduced and pinned or fixed with a screw (Figures 6–16 and 6–17). Cancellous bone can be added from above as an arthroscopically placed graft, as described below, to fill space and obtain a hairline reduction if an incongruity exists.

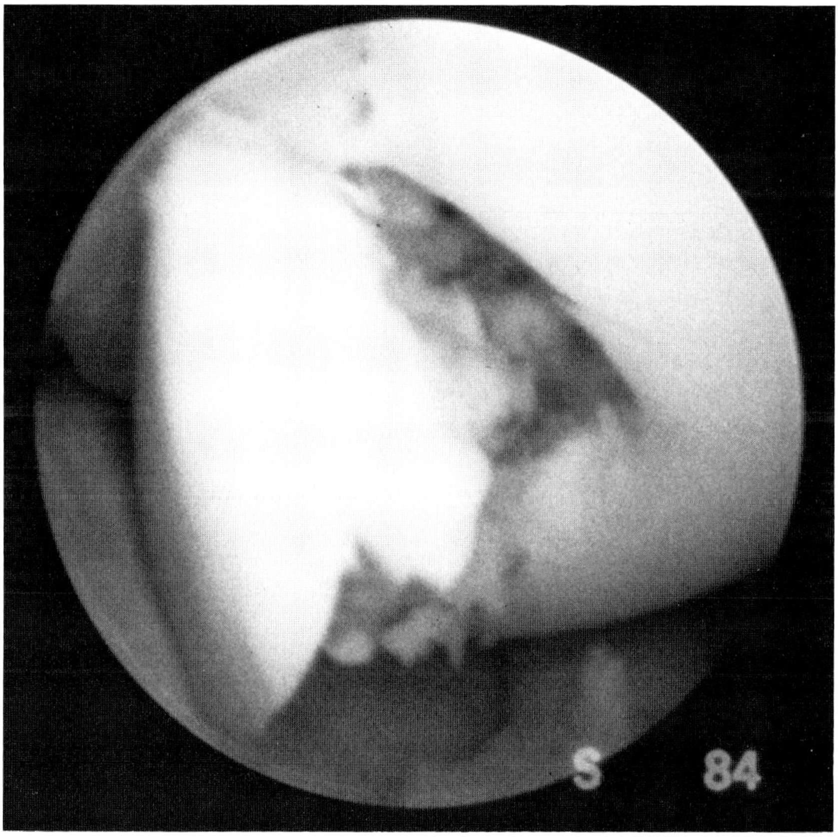


**Figure 6–16** Arthroscopic view of a partially detached lesion of the medial femoral condyle (right knee). (Courtesy of Lanny Johnson, M.D., East Lansing, Michigan)

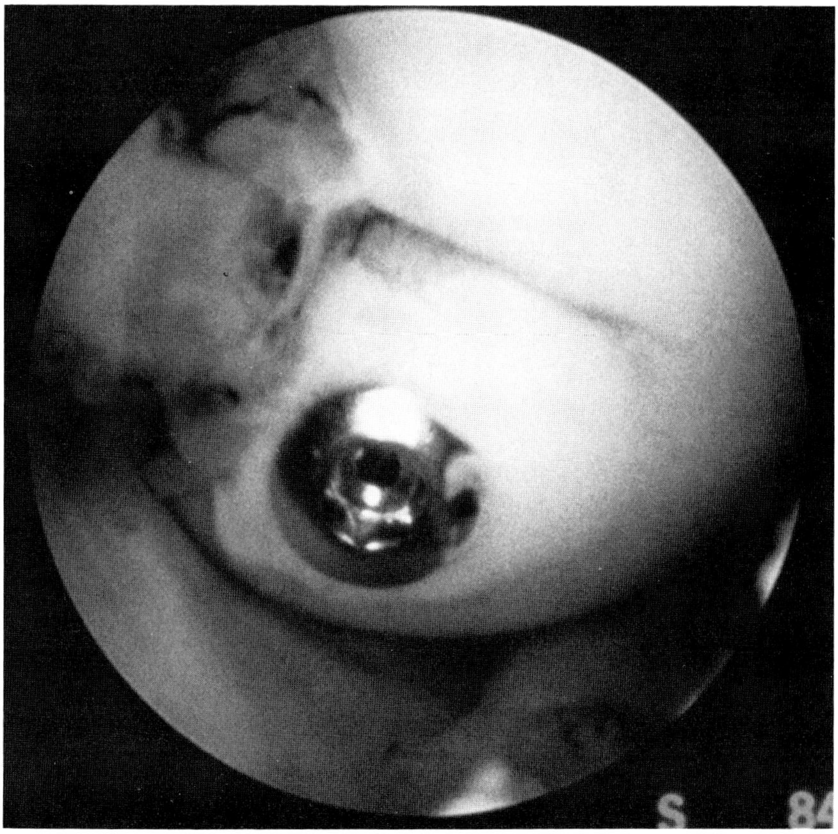

**Figure 6–17** Arthroscopic view of the lesion in Figure 6–16 fixed with a cannulated cancellous bone screw (right knee). (Courtesy of Lanny Johnson, M.D., Lansing, Michigan)

Where there is a large, completely detached fragment 6 weeks or less since separation, a decision must be made to place and fix the lesion either arthroscopically or by open methods. The same principles of debridement apply. Arthroscopic manipulation is tricky but in skilled hands is quite possible. Old, chronic, unsalvageable fragments must be removed, and the crater must be reconstructed since, in these cases, an accurate reduction cannot be obtained.

***Grafting*** Early in the series arthroscopic bone grafting was used where the indications appeared obvious. These were in large, chronic, detached lesions. Later, small bone pegs were used as a means of fixation as well as a stimulus for healing. As time went on, it was noted that drilling alone was not always sufficient in some large intact lesions, usually in the older age group. The need for grafting was anticipated in later cases of this nature by experience.

Arthroscopic grafting can be done proximal (method 1) or distal (method 2) to the lesion. The former is chosen when a large-diameter graft is desired or when filling the channel with cancellous bone to obtain an accurate reduction. Grafting from below is done when the grafts are small cortical pegs used also for fixation. Cortical (and cancellous) bone can be obtained locally from a small incision, or allografts can be used, obtainable from the University of Miami bone bank.

In method 1 a 0.062 mm wire is placed from below, as described for pinning or from above if the anterior jig is used. A small incision is made in the skin where the wire protrudes proximally, and a cannulated reamer ranging from 5 to 10 mm in diameter is passed down over the wire until it reaches a point just proximal to

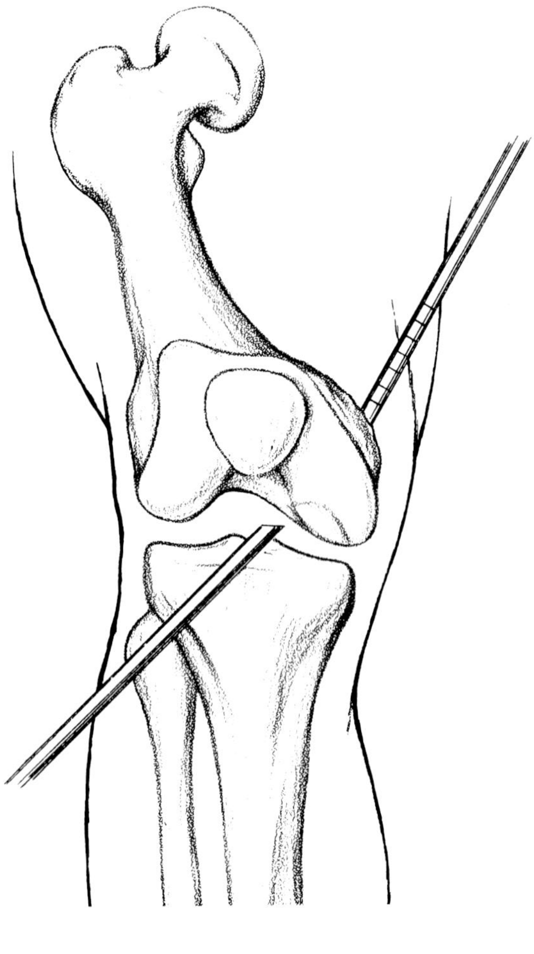

**Figure 6–18** Diagram illustrating grafting from a proximal position.

the articular surface (Figure 6–18). This is done by carefully measuring the wire and the distance to be traversed in bone and also by monitoring under arthroscopic control. Cortical grafts and/or cancellous bone is then packed down from above (Figure 6–19). An additional advantage in the use of the previously mentioned anterior cruciate ligament jigs is that they cannot only attain more accurate placement but also hold the fragment in place during reaming or drilling.

In method 2 the reamer is passed about 5 mm over the wire from below, into the lesion, and beyond and into the condyle to a depth of about 3–4 cm (Figure 6–20). Bone pegs held by a loose-body forceps or passed through a cannula are

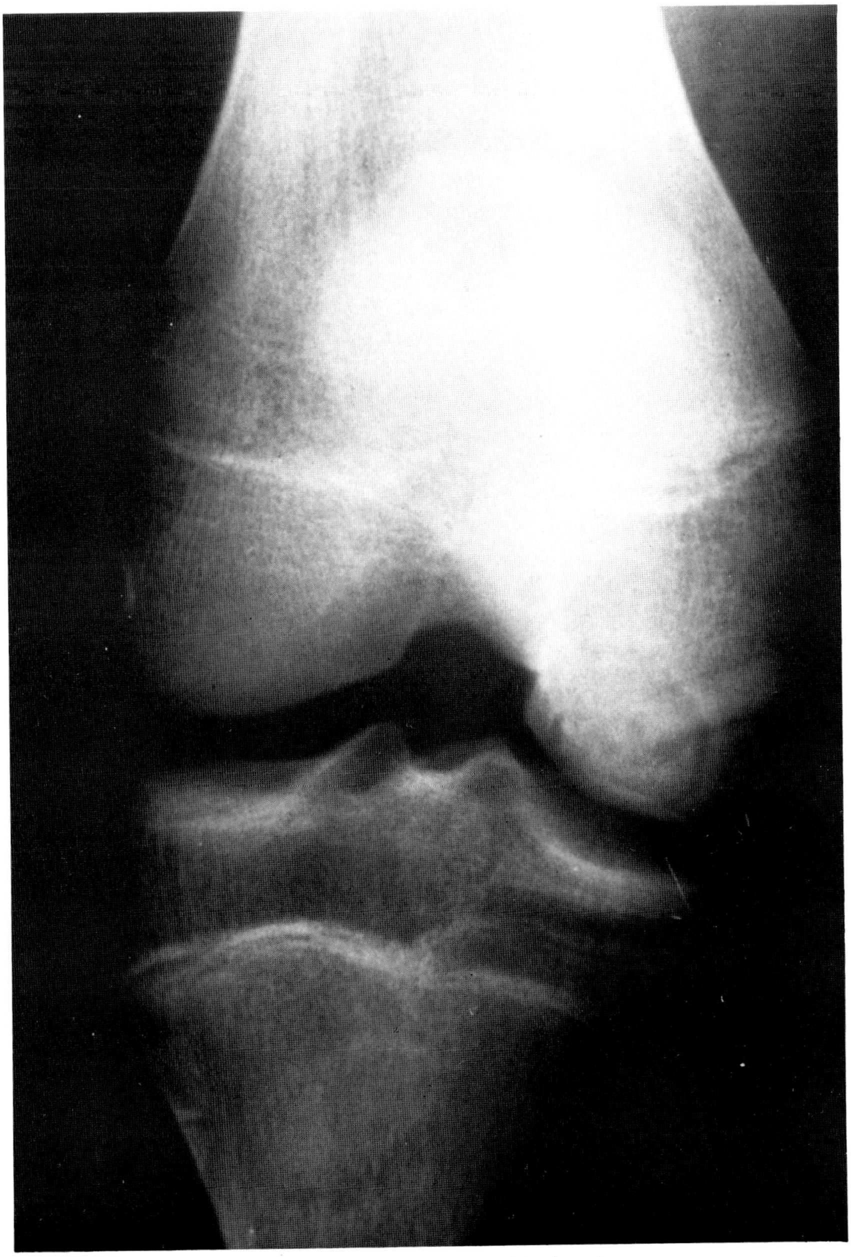

**Figure 6–19** X-ray of graft inserted from above (right knee).

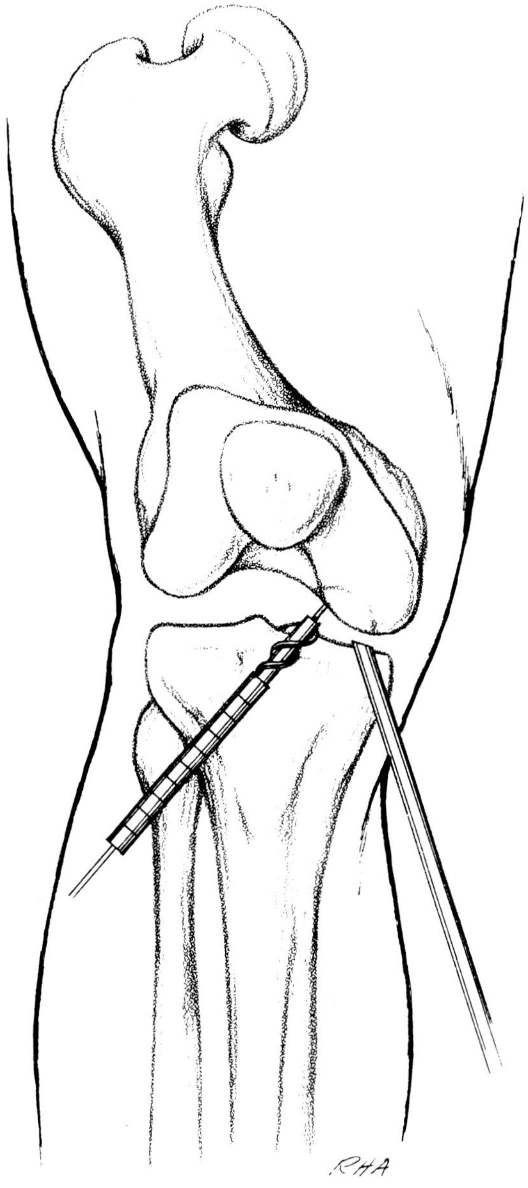

Figure 6–20 Diagram showing a reamer placed over a guidewire for grafting from a distal position.

then carefully placed through an adjacent portal and passed up into the canal. They are tapped into place and slightly countersunk (Figures 6–21 and 6–22). One or possibly two grafts can be done arthroscopically, but when more are used in a large lesion, open techniques are best.

***Reconstruction*** Craters are initially trimmed back to good healthy cartilage arthroscopically by using basket forceps and/or knifes. The edges are cut perpendicular to the articular cartilage. The base is then curetted of fibrous tissue, abraded, and sometimes also drilled. The abrasion and drilling is done down to bleeding bone.

**Arthrotomy** Lesions 4–5 cm in diameter and occupying a large portion of the weight-bearing area are best fixed by peg grafts distally inserted by open methods. Again, the same principles of preparation apply. The technique described by Gillespie (3) has been my choice, as illustrated in Figure 6–23. A medial parapatellar incision is made and the lesion exposed and prepared. A second incision is made

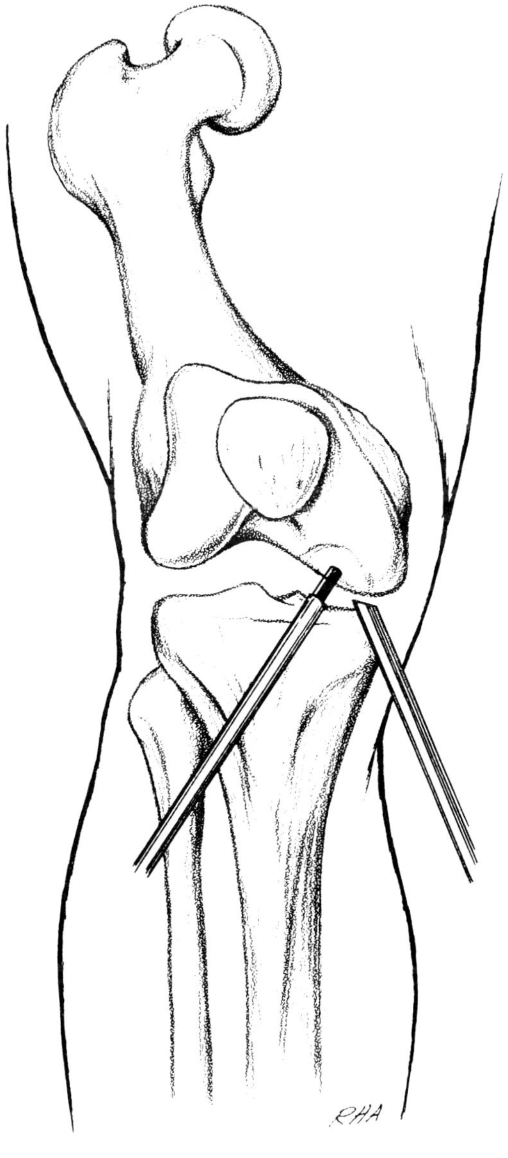

**Figure 6–21** Diagram of the lesion in Figure 6–20 illustrating placement of the graft through a cannula. A loose body forceps can also be used.

below, just adjacent to the tibial tubercle. The periosteum is split to obtain the cortical pegs and cancellous graft. The pegs act as an excellent means of fixation and wires are rarely necessary.

## Postoperative Care and Rehabilitation

Young patients whose intact lesions are drilled are usually immobilized in a cast and walk with crutches for 3–4 weeks. This is followed either by the use of an immobilizer or by restricted activities, judged individually for each case. In large lesions and in older patients, immobilization and non-weight bearing are employed for 2–4 months. Protection must be maintained until the pins are removed, which is usually done at 6 weeks. Non-weight bearing is then maintained until adequate healing is shown on laminagrams. This is best shown by small trabecular lines of bone formation, indicating early incorporation of the graft. Usually about 8 weeks or more are required. Partial weight bearing and protected

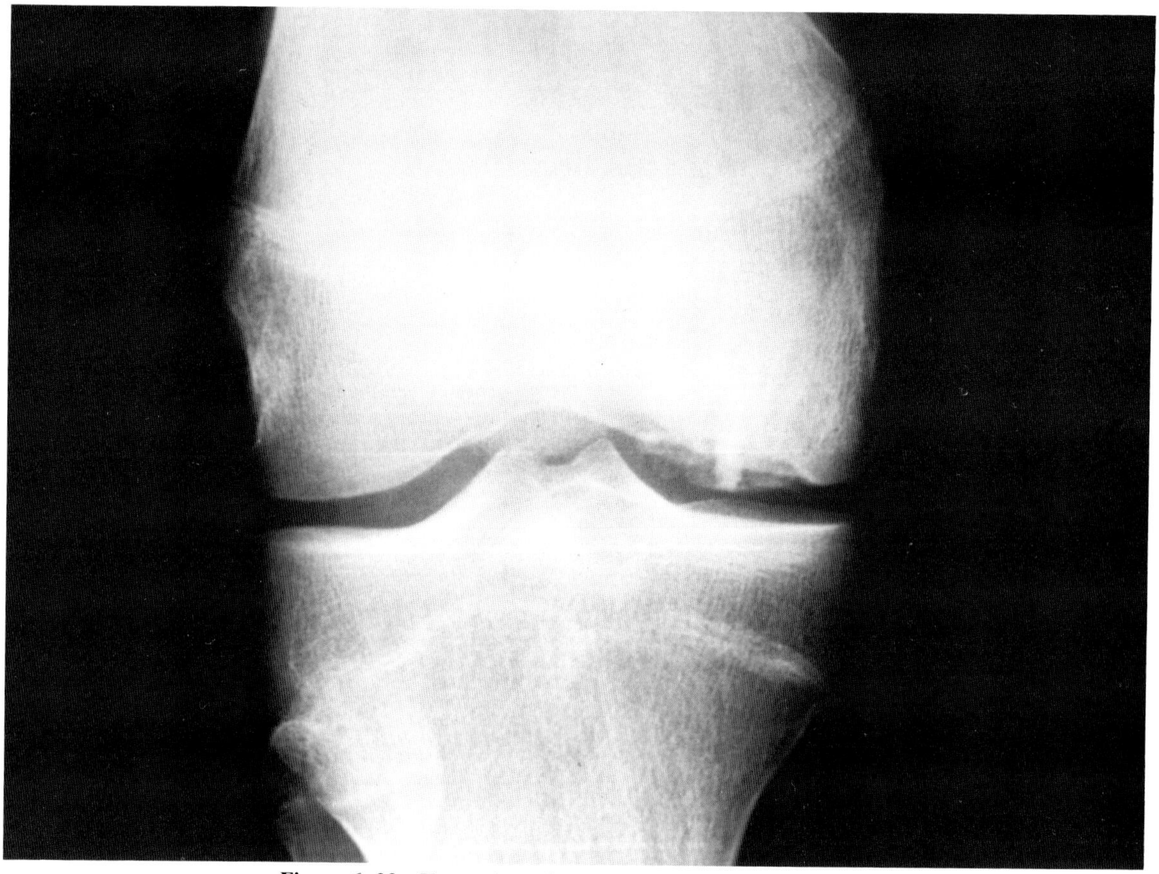

**Figure 6–22** X-ray view of graft inserted from below (right knee).

activities are necessary until more progressive healing is shown on x-ray films, which can be up to 4 or more months. When large craters, over 4–5 cm, have been reconstructed and abraded, non-weight bearing with early motion is employed for 6–8 weeks. Rehabilitation exercises are started on the first postoperative day, as tolerated, especially for older patients.

## Results

The results of 78 knees in 71 patients have been analyzed. Some patients had bilateral treatment arthroscopically. The data from knees treated conservatively or by open techniques was excluded. As of this date, results are available on 58 patients treated arthroscopically. Our survey was done by telephone, letter, personal interview, and examination when at all possible. The latter was employed in about two-thirds of the cases. Most of the telephone or letter interviews were in those out-of-town patients who had already been x-rayed and/or examined some years after treatment.

Of the 58 knees analyzed, 56 healed. The results of the total group were 20 excellent, 26 good, 8 fair, and 2 poor.

Bone scars persisted in most adult cases, even when healing was complete and the result was excellent or good. In children these scars disappeared in most all cases. Articular incongruity when occasionally present persisted, however, and in some cases downgraded the result.

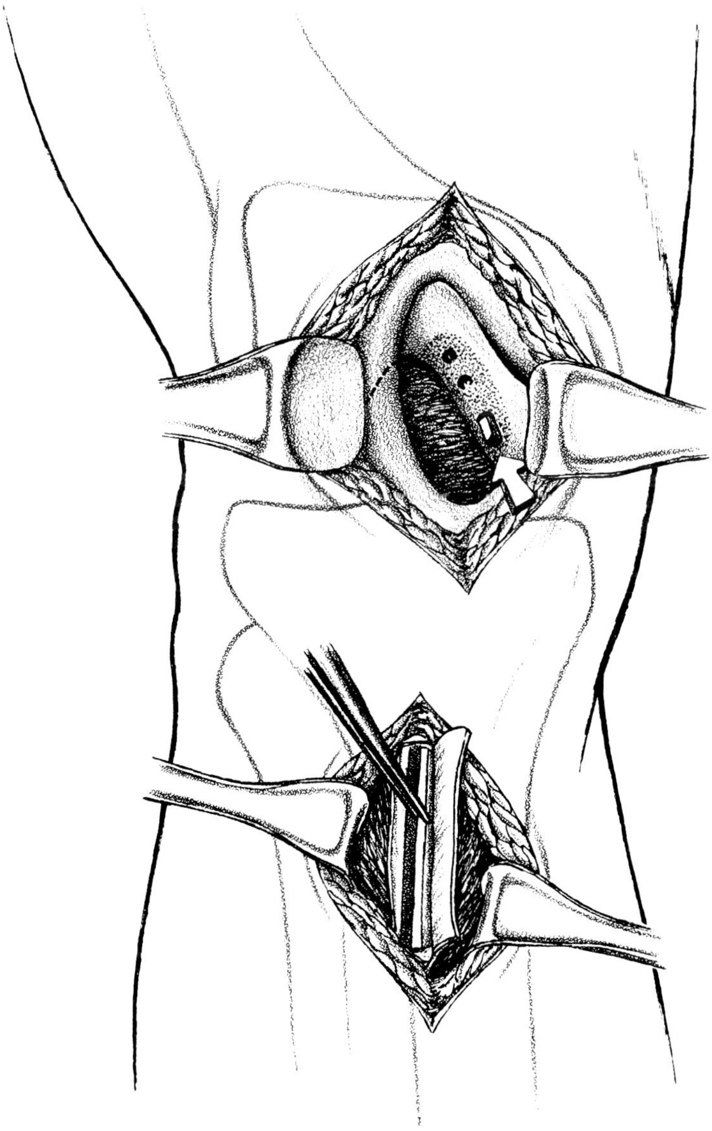

**Figure 6–23** Illustration of open technique for grafting osteochondritis dissecans.

In five cases treatment was repeated. Of these, two were drilled, one was grafted, and two were reconstructed. Six cases were evaluated under local anesthesia to determine the progress of healing.

## Conclusion

The arthroscopic treatment of osteochondritis dissecans has been underway for a decade. In the series discussed, 78 knees were treated in 71 patients, and of these, 58 treated arthroscopically were available for analysis. The remainder were treated either by conservative methods or open methods, and a few were lost to follow-up. Of the 58 knees analyzed, 56 healed. Further valuable information was obtained over the years by personal communication with many surgeons employing this technique. The indications and techniques for conservative treatment, arthroscopic methods, and open techniques have been developed and illustrated. Conservative treatment is employed in patients generally below the age of 12. Intact lesions are drilled only, except in older patients where a bone graft may be added. Partially separated lesions are usually debrided and fixed with a pin or screw except where bone grafts may be added in older patients. In partially detached lesions, the undersurface of the lesion and the crater is thoroughly debrided, the lesion reduced and fixation again done with a pin or screw and/or a bone graft added as necessary. Craters are reconstructed by trimming the margins, debriding the base, abrading and drilling. Loose bodies are occasionally replaced in the early stage, or, in most cases, removed. Open methods are used generally in large lesions over the size of about 4 to 5 cm in diameter. The use of the bone scan and electrical stimulation must be considered and will, in all probability, fit into the future final picture. New devices such as the cannulated bone screw and the numerous jigs now being developed should be helpful in further refining and improving the technique. The intelligent use of these arthroscopic techniques, along with employing the newly developed surgical instrumentation, should result in an increased incidence of healing, thus reducing the amount of total rehabilitation time and upgrading the ultimate results.

## *References*

1. Aichroth P. Osteochondritis dissecans of the knee: A clinical study. J Bone Joint Surg 53:440, 1971
2. Campbell C, Ranawat C. Osteochondritis dissecans: The question of etiology. J Trauma 6:201, 1966
3. Gillespie H, and Day B. Bone peg fixation in the treatment of osteochondritis dissecans of the knee joint. Clin Orthop 143:125, 1979
4. Green J. Osteochondritis dissecans of the knee. J Bone Joint Surg [Br] 48:82, 1966
5. Green W, Banks H. Osteochondritis dissecans in children. J Bone Joint Surg 14:26, 1953
6. Guhl JF. Arthroscopic treatment of osteochondritis dissecans. Preliminary report. Orthop Clin North Am 10:3, 1979
7. Guhl JF. Arthroscopic treatment of osteochondritis dissecans. Clin Orthop 167, 1982
8. Guhl JF. Update in the treatment of osteochondritis dissecans. Orthopedics 7:11, 1984
9. Helfet A. Disorders of the Knee. JB Lippincott, Philadelphia, 1974
10. Lindholm S, Pylkkanen P. Internal fixation of the fragments of osteochondritis dissecans of the knee by means of a bone pin. Acta Chir Scand 140:626, 1974
11. Lipscomb PR Jr, Lipscomb PRS, Byron R. Osteochondritis dissecans of the knee with loose fragments: Treatment by replacement and fixation with readily removed pins. J Bone Joint Surg [Am] 60:235, 1978
12. Scott D, Stevenson C. Osteochondritis dissecans of the knee in adults. Clin Orthop 76:82, 1971
13. Smillie IS. Injuries of the Knee Joint, 4th ed. E & S Livingstone, Edinburgh, 1970

# Blood Supply of the Meniscus

# 7

Steven Paul Arnoczky

The function, injury, and repair of the meniscus have long been topics of interest and discussion among orthopaedic surgeons. Once described as the functionless remains of leg muscle (20), the menisci are now realized to be integral components in the complex biomechanics of the knee (7, 10, 13, 15–18, 21). This fact has stimulated many surgeons to consider primary repair of certain meniscal lesions over traditional meniscectomy (6, 9, 11, 22).

Although Annandale has been credited with the first surgical repair of a torn meniscus in 1883 (1), it was not until 1936, when King (14) published his classic experiment in dogs, that the biological limitations of meniscal healing were set forth. He stated that for meniscal lesions to heal, they must communicate with the meniscal blood supply (14). Whereas the human meniscus has always been considered an essentially avascular structure with only a meager peripheral blood supply, relatively little has been written about its vascular anatomy (8). Such information must predicate a rational approach to the surgical repair of meniscal lesions.

## Vascular Anatomy of the Meniscus

The vascular supply to the medial and lateral meniscus of the human knee originates predominantly from the lateral and medial genicular arteries (both inferior and superior). Branches from these vessels give rise to a perimeniscal capillary plexus within the synovial and capsular tissues of the knee joint. This perimeniscal capillary plexus is an arborizing network of vessels that supplies the peripheral border of the menisci throughout their attachment to the joint capsule (Figure 7–1). These perimeniscal vessels are oriented in a predominantly circumferential pattern with radial branches being directed toward the center of the joint (Figure 7–2).

The middle genicular artery, along with a few terminal branches of the medial and lateral genicular arteries, also supplies vessels to the menisci through the vascular synovial covering of the anterior and posterior horn attachments. This synovial covering appears continuous with the vascular synovial sheath surrounding the cruciate ligaments (Figure 7–3) (2).

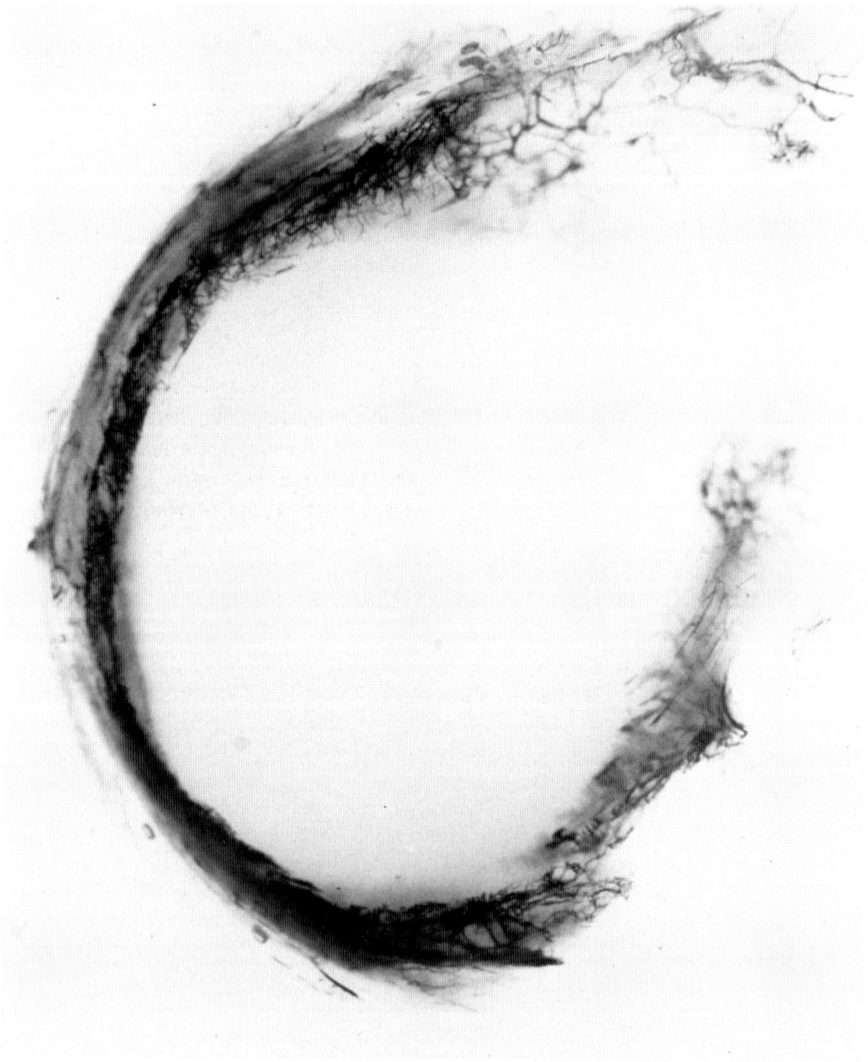

A

**Figure 7–1** Superior aspect of the medial (**A**) and lateral (**B**) meniscus following vascular perfusion with India ink and tissue clearing using a modified Spalteholz technique. Note the vascularity at the periphery of the menisci as well as at the anterior and posterior horn attachments. The absence of peripheral vasculature at the posterolateral corner of the lateral meniscus (arrow) represents the area of passage of the popliteal tendon. [Reproduced with permission from Arnoczky SP, Warren RF. Am J Sports Med 10:90–95, 1982 (3).]

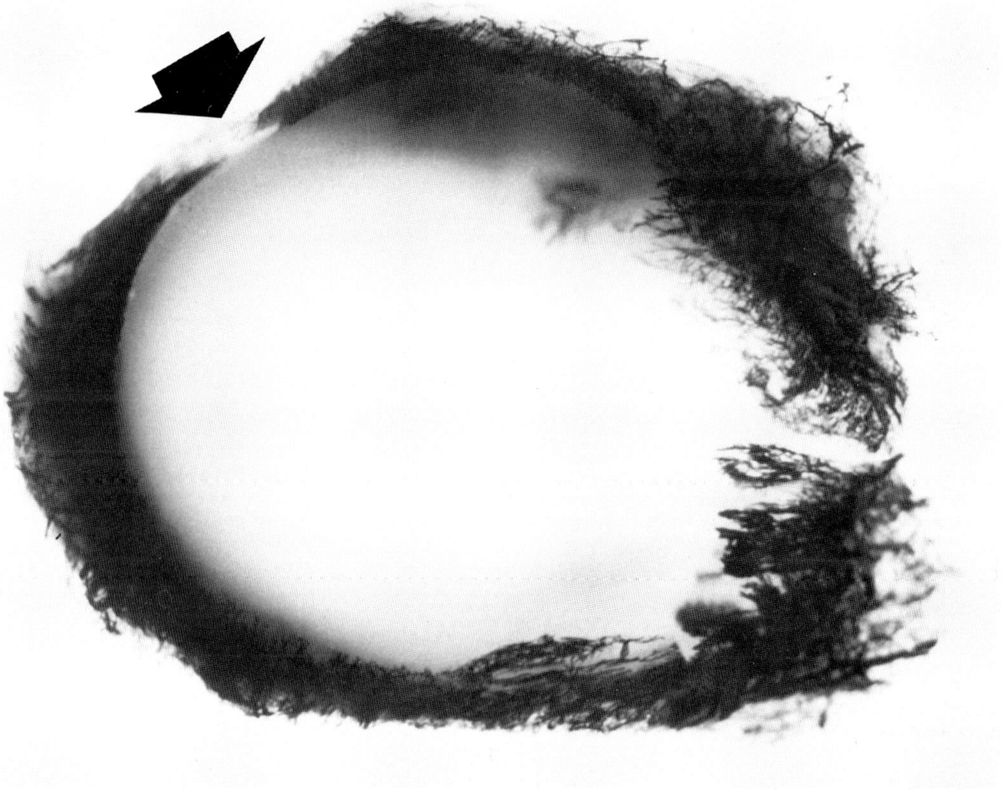

B

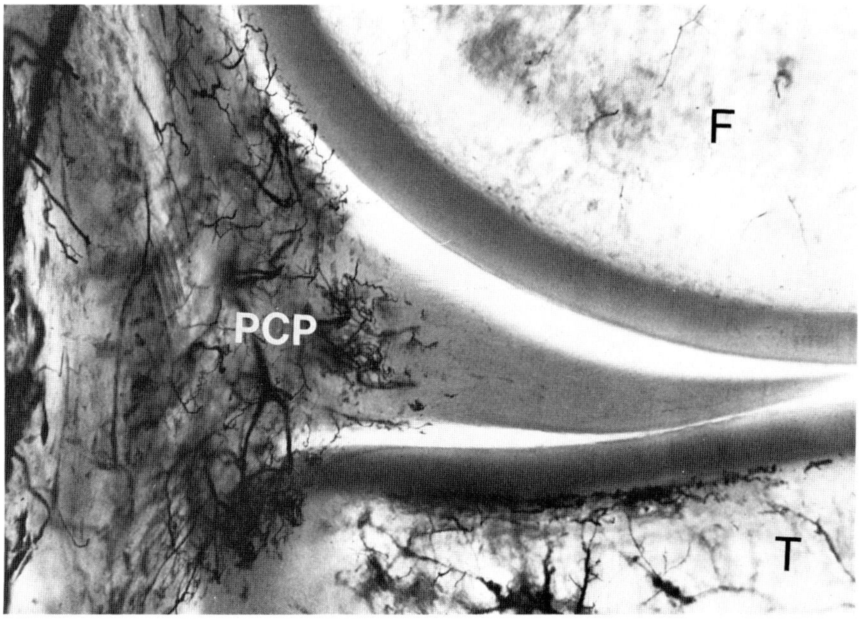


**Figure 7–2** Five-millimeter-thick frontal section (F) of the medial compartment of the knee. Branching radial vessels from the perimeniscal capillary plexus (PCP) can be seen penetrating the peripheral border of the medial meniscus (Spalteholz, ×3). [Reproduced with permission from Arnoczky SP, Warren RF. Am J Sports Med 10:90–95, 1982 (3).]

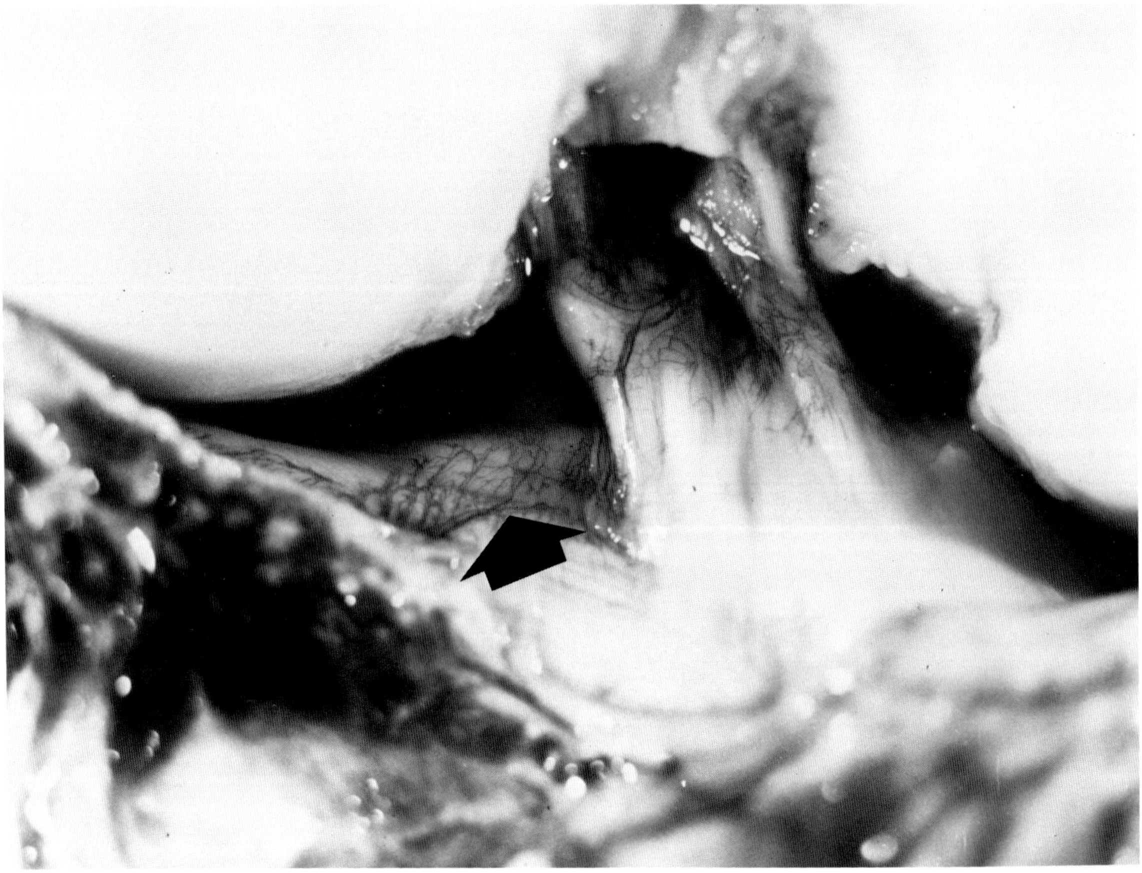

**Figure 7–3** Anterior view of an India ink-perfused knee showing the vascular synovial covering of the anterior cruciate ligament and the anterior horn attachment of the lateral meniscus (arrow). [Reproduced with permission from Arnoczky SP, Warren RF. Am J Sports Med 10:90–95, 1982 (3).]

## Medial Meniscus

The anterior horn attachment of the medial meniscus is covered with a layer of vascular synovial tissue. The vessels in this synovial covering supply branches to the ligamentous attachment of the anterior horn of the meniscus. These endoligamentous vessels, in turn, penetrate the meniscal stroma of the anterior horn for a short distance (2–3 mm) and terminate in small capillary loops (Figure 7–4). The vascular synovial covering of the anterior meniscal attachment extends over the femoral surface of the anterior horn of the meniscus for a short distance but quickly recedes to the peripheral margin of the meniscus.

The body of the medial meniscus receives vessels from its peripheral attachment to the capsular and synovial tissues of the joint. Vessels from the perimeniscal capillary plexus course through this peripheral attachment and give off smaller radial branches that penetrate the meniscal stroma for a short distance and terminate in small capillary loops (Figure 7–5). The degree of vascular penetration into the periphery of the medial meniscus varies between individual specimens as well as within individual specimens, ranging from 10% to 30% of the meniscal width. No correlation could be established for this variation with regard to age, sex, race, or anatomical location (3).

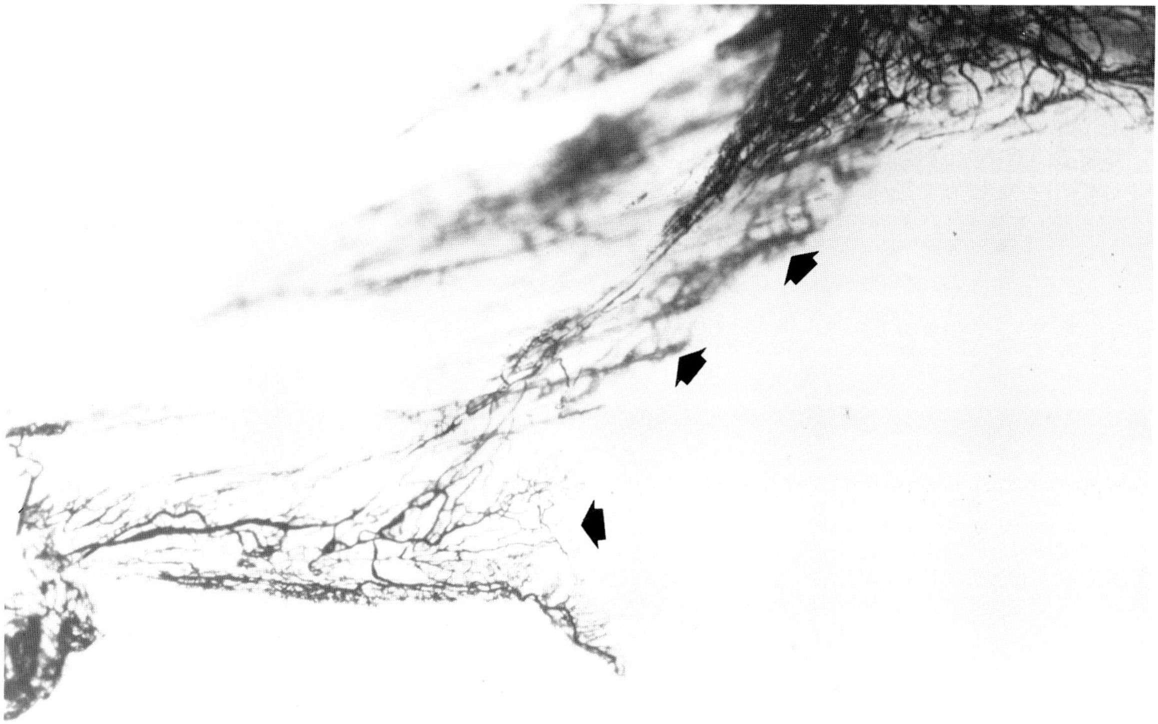

**Figure 7–4** Anterior horn attachment of the medial meniscus demonstrating the capillary vessels that penetrate the anterior horn of the medial meniscus (arrows; Spalteholz, ×5). [Reproduced with permission from Arnoczky SP, Warren RF. Am J Sports Med 10:90–95, 1982 (3).]

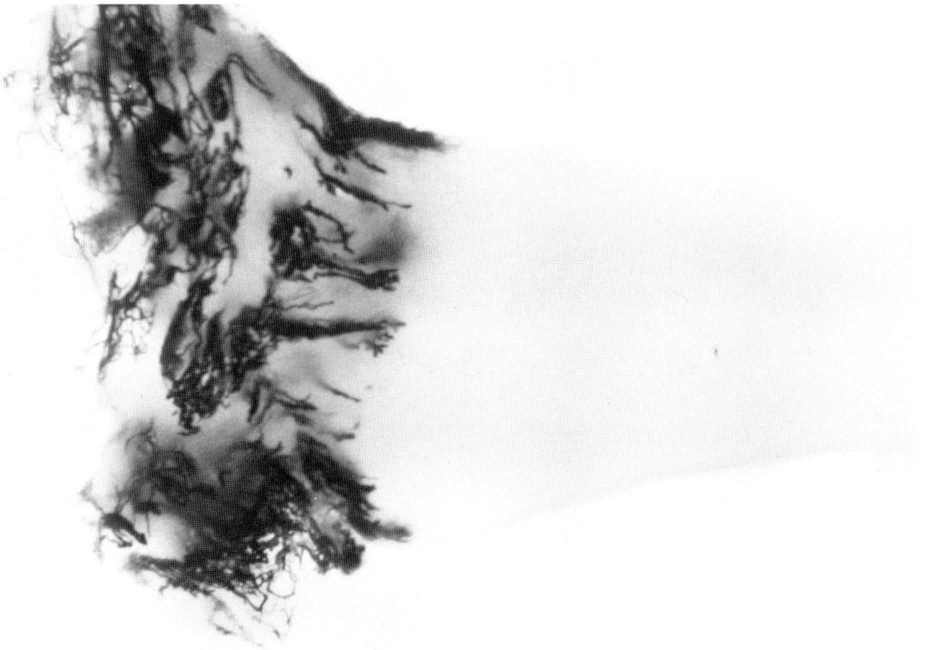

**Figure 7–5** Three-millimeter-thick transverse section of the medial meniscus demonstrating the terminally looped capillary vessels and their penetration into the peripheral border of the meniscus (Spalteholz, ×8). [Reproduced with permission from Arnoczky SP, Warren RF. Am J Sports Med 10:90–95, 1982 (3).]

A small reflection of vascular synovial tissue is present throughout the peripheral border of the medial meniscus on both its femoral and tibial surfaces. This "synovial fringe" extends a short distance (1–3 mm) over the articular surfaces of the meniscus and contains small, terminally looped vessels (Figure 7–6). Histological and cleared tissue injection specimens reveal that although this vascular synovial tissue intimately adheres to the articular surfaces of the menisci, it does not contribute vessels into the meniscal tissues (3). In some specimens, the synovial fringe recedes markedly in the area of the medial collateral ligament and the posteromedial aspect of the meniscus. On the femoral surface of the medial meniscus, this synovial fringe appears continuous with the synovial covering of the anterior horn and anterior horn attachment (Figure 7–7).

The posterior horn attachment of the medial meniscus is also covered with a smooth layer of synovial tissue. As with the anterior horn, these synovial vessels penetrate the posterior attachment and give rise to endoligamentous vessels that enter the posterior horn of the meniscus for a short distance and end in capillary loops.

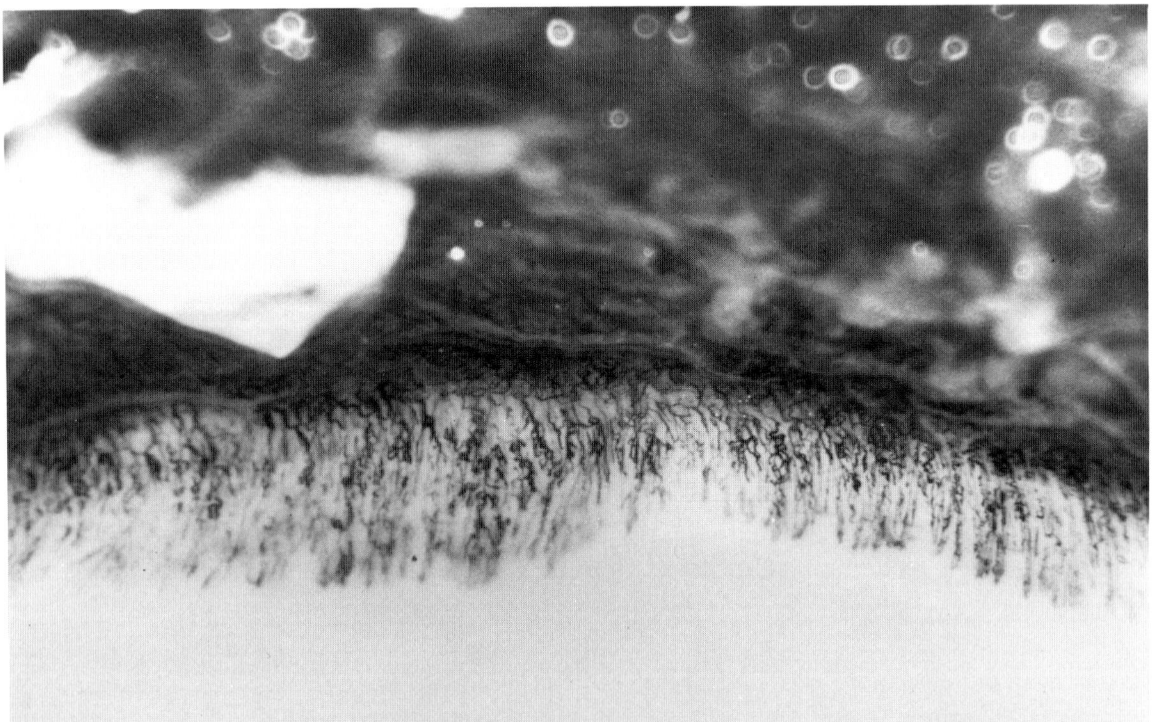

**Figure 7–6** Superior aspect of the medial meniscus demonstrating the terminally looped capillary vessels within the synovial fringe as they extend out from the peripheral border of the meniscus (Spalteholz, ×5). [Reproduced with permission from Arnoczky SP, Warren RF. Am J Sports Med 10:90–95, 1982 (3).]

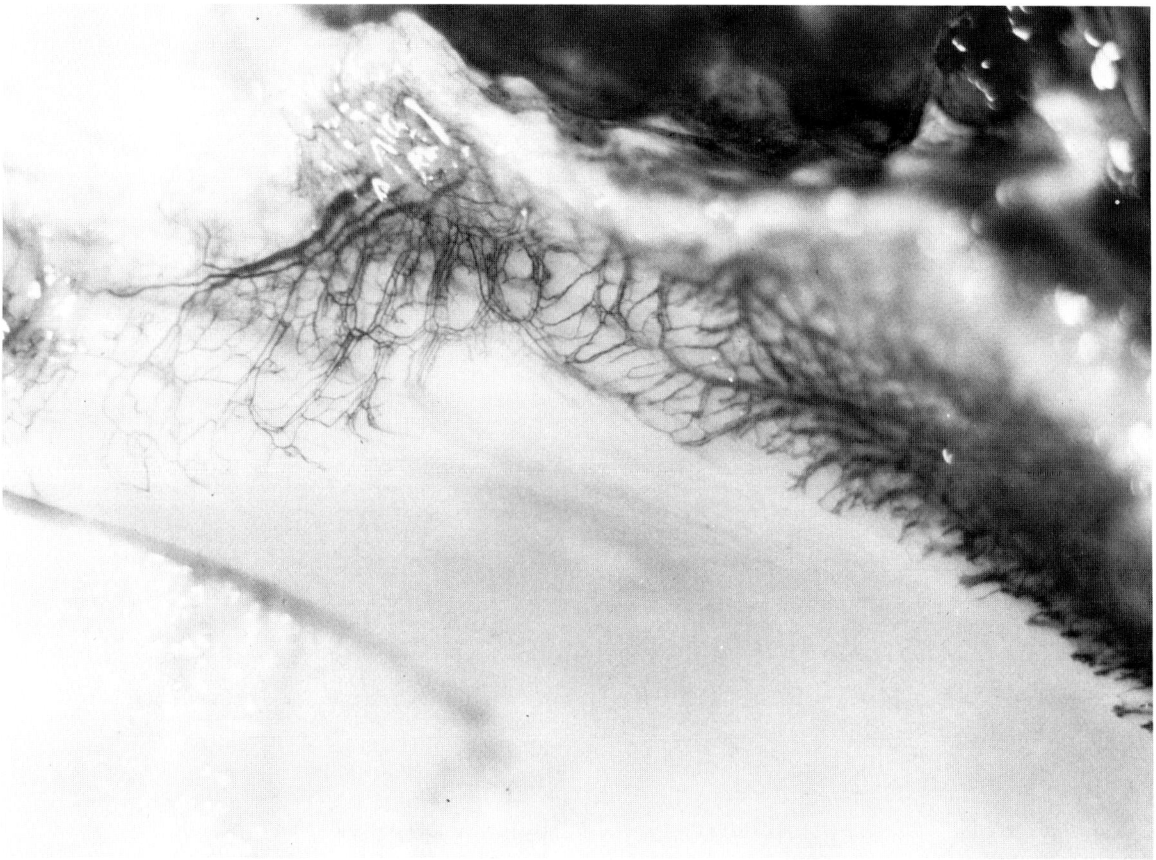

**Figure 7–7** Anterior horn of an India ink-perfused medial meniscus showing the extension of the vascular synovial fringe into the synovial covering of the anterior horn attachment. [Reproduced with permission from Arnoczky SP, Warren RF. Am J Sports Med 10:90–95, 1982 (3).]

## Lateral Meniscus

The vascular anatomy of the lateral meniscus is very similar to that observed in the medial meniscus. Both anterior and posterior horn attachments are covered with a layer of vascular synovial tissue that appears to be continuous with that of the vascular synovial sheath surrounding the cruciate ligaments (2). Vessels within these horn attachments penetrate the meniscal tissue for a short distance and end in terminal capillary loops (Figure 7–8).

The body of the lateral meniscus is supplied by circumferential and radial branches of the lateral inferior genicular artery, which courses adjacent to the peripheral border of the lateral meniscus and deep to the lateral collateral ligament (Figure 7–9). (The lateral inferior genicular artery is a fairly large-caliber vessel at this location, and because of its proximity to the peripheral border of the lateral meniscus, extreme care should be taken when performing a total lateral meniscectomy.) As in the medial meniscus, these radial vessels penetrate the peripheral meniscal stroma for a short distance, ending in terminal capillary loops. The degree of vascular penetration in the lateral meniscus ranges from 10% to 25% of the meniscal width. This peripheral vascular supply is altered at the posterolateral aspect of the lateral meniscus. In this area the popliteal tendon lies adjacent to the peripheral border of the meniscus and in between the meniscus and the lateral

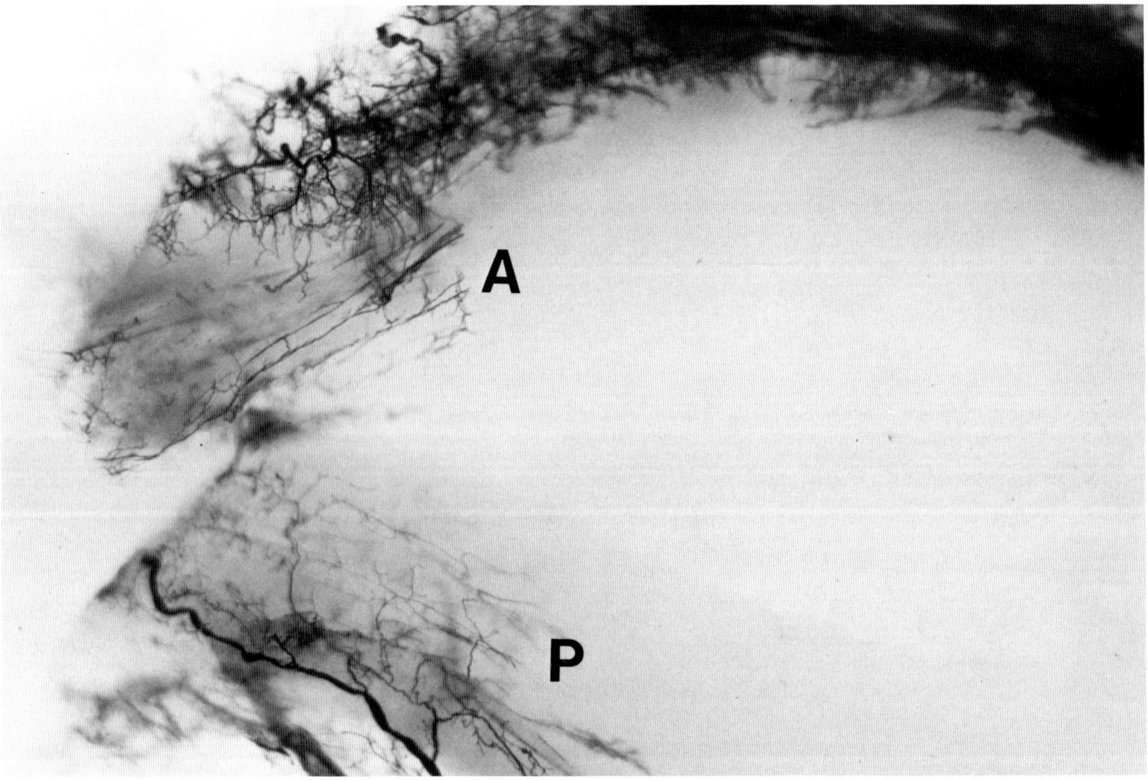


**Figure 7–8** Anterior (A) and posterior (P) horn attachments of the lateral meniscus showing the vascularity of the attachments and their penetration into the horns of the meniscus (Spalteholz, ×2). [Reproduced with permission from Arnoczky SP, Warren RF. Am J Sports Med 10:90–95, 1982 (3).]

**Figure 7–9** Transverse section of a lateral meniscus just anterior to the level of the popliteal tendon showing the location of the lateral inferior genicular artery (arrow) adjacent to the peripheral border of the lateral meniscus. Note the penetration of small capillary vessels into the meniscus (Spalteholz, ×2). [Reproduced with permission from Arnoczky SP, Warren RF. Am J Sports Med 10:90–95, 1982 (3).]

capsular tissues. This posterolateral corner of the lateral meniscus is supplied by a ventral fascicle of capsular tissue that provides small vascular branches to the lateral wall of the meniscus (Figure 7–10). Circumferential vessels from the capsular tissues anterior and posterior to this segment also extend along the lateral wall of the meniscus in a horizontal fashion but do not appear to penetrate the meniscal stroma. In all lateral menisci examined, there existed an avascular area on the peripheral wall of the meniscus immediately adjacent to the popliteal tendon (Figure 7–11) (3). It has been suggested that this avascular area is a result of intermittent reciprocal pressures between the tendon and the meniscus during joint motion (8).

A synovial fringe is also present on the femoral and tibial surfaces of the lateral meniscus. This fringe extends a short distance over the articular surfaces of the meniscus and appears continuous with the vascular synovial covering of the anterior and posterior horn attachments. As in the medial meniscus, this vascular fringe is intimately attached to the meniscal surface but does not contribute vessels into the meniscal tissue. This synovial fringe is absent in the area of the popliteal tendon (Figure 7–12).

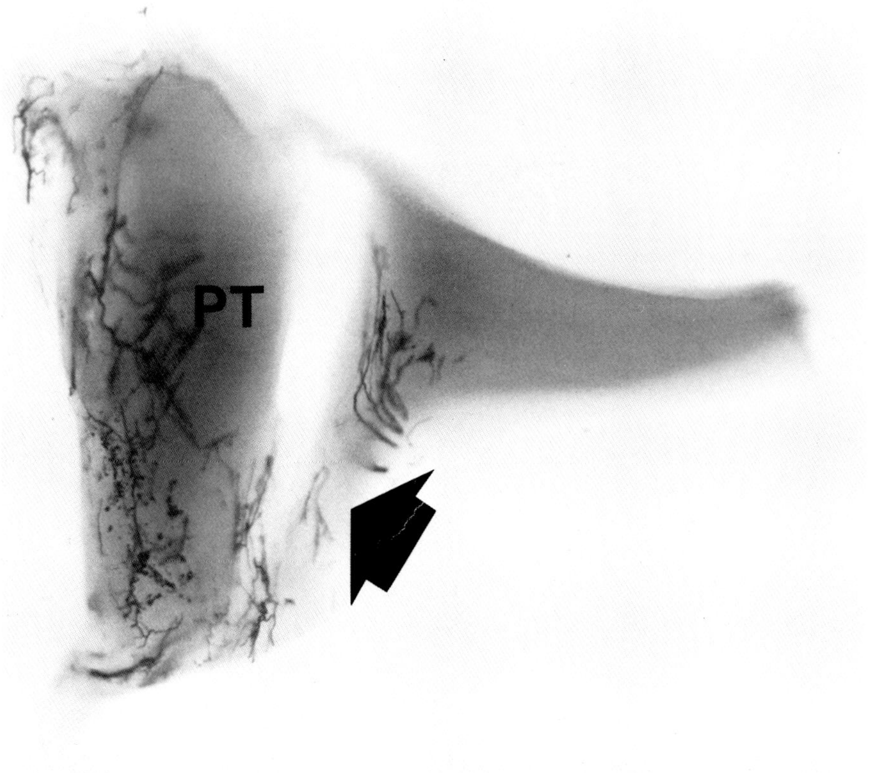


**Figure 7–10** Transverse section of the lateral meniscus adjacent to the popliteal tendon (PT) showing the ventral capsular attachment in this area and the vascular pedicle (arrow) that supplies surface vessels to the periphery of the meniscus in this area (Spalteholz, ×2). [Reproduced with permission from Arnoczky SP, Warren RF. Am J Sports Med 10:90–95, 1982 (3).]

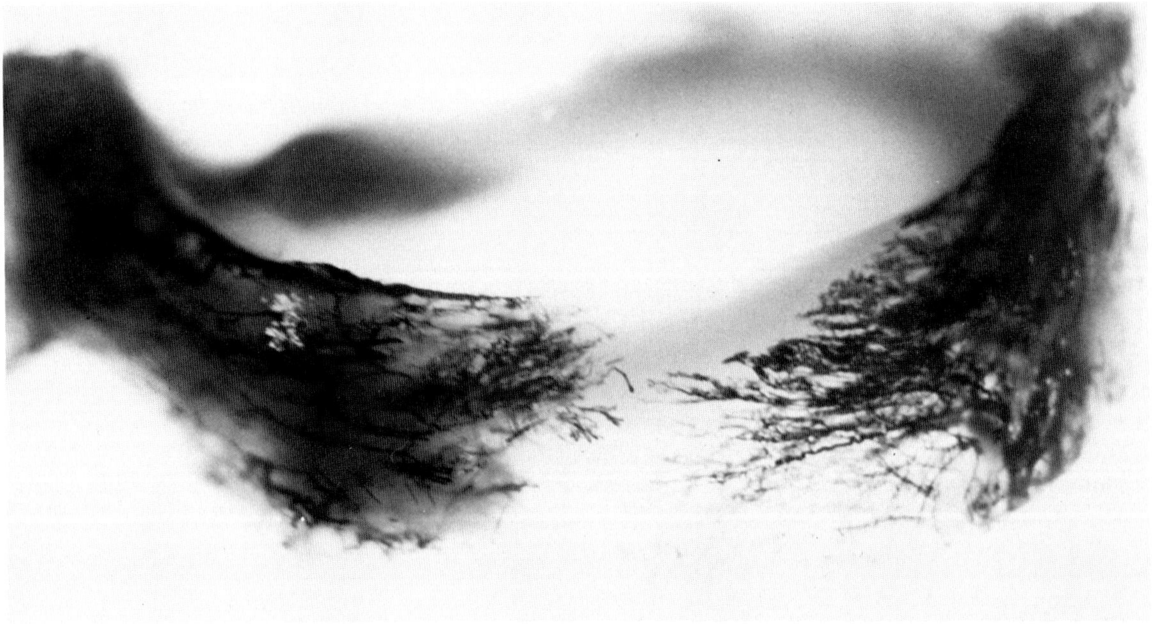

**Figure 7–11** Peripheral surface of the lateral meniscus immediately adjacent to the popliteal tendon. Note the avascular area on the peripheral surface of the meniscus where the tendon passes across the meniscus (Spalteholz, ×2). [Reproduced with permission from Arnoczky SP, Warren RF. Am J Sports Med 10:90–95, 1982 (3).]

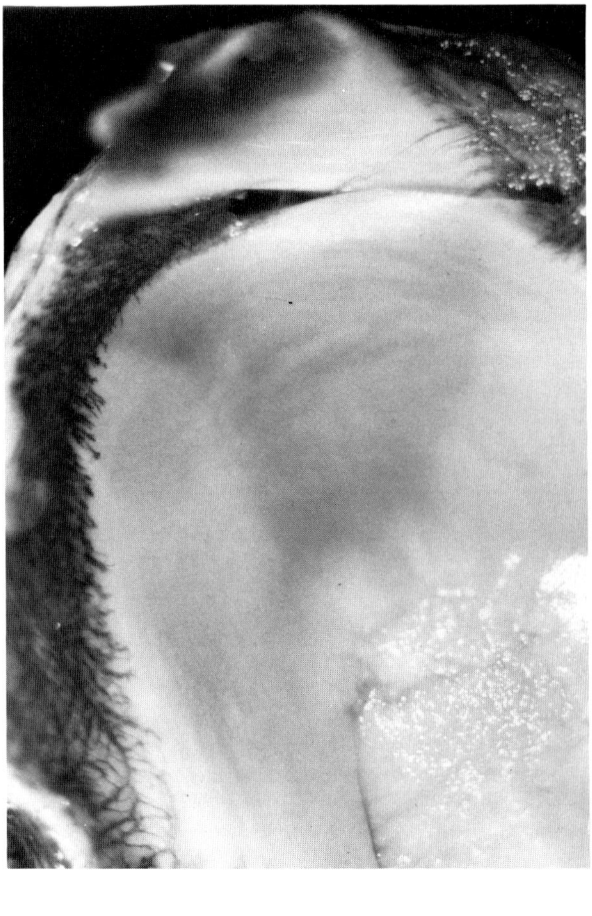

**Figure 7–12** Photograph of an India ink-injected specimen showing the absence of the synovial fringe in the area of the popliteal tendon. [Reproduced with permission from Arnoczky SP, Warren RF. Am J Sports Med 10:90–95, 1982 (3).]

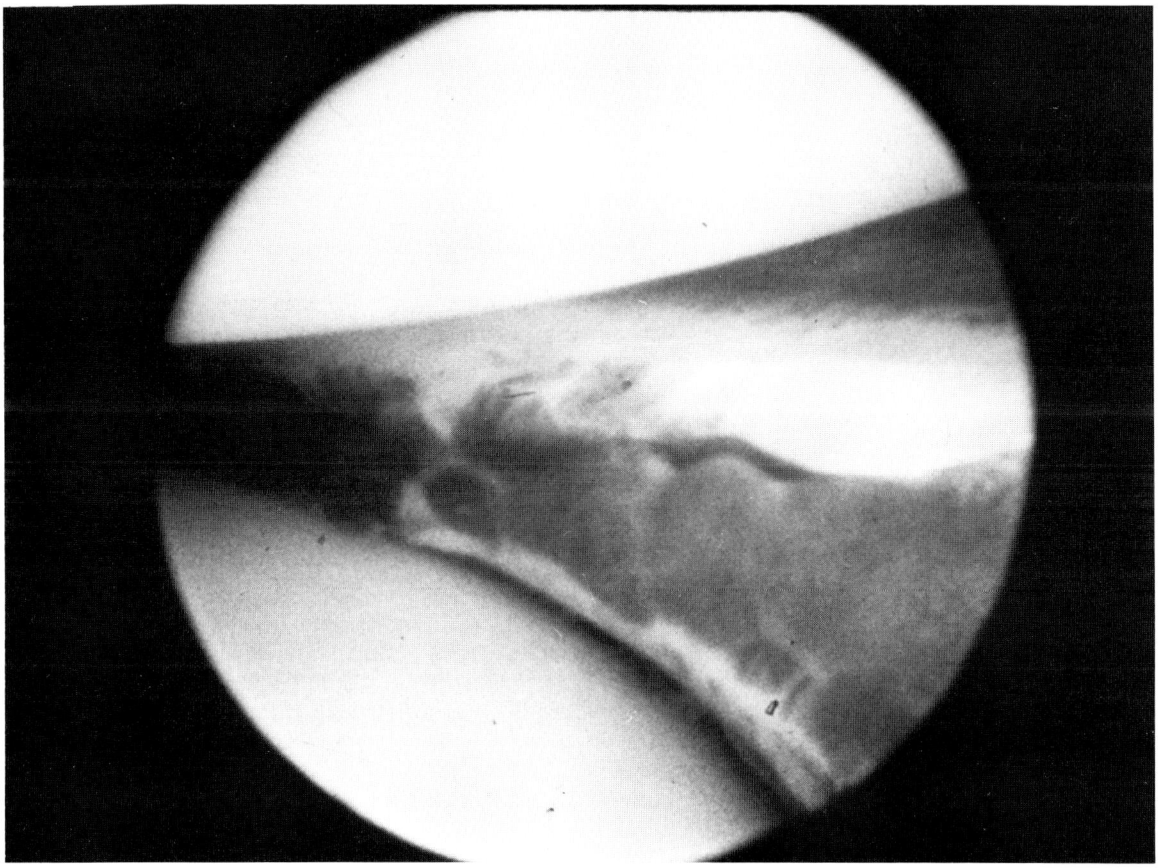

**Figure 7–13** Arthroscopic view of a peripheral tear of a human meniscus. Note the granulation tissue present at the margin of the lesion as well as the synovial fringe over the femoral surface of the meniscus. (Courtesy of Robert Jackson, M.D., Toronto, Ontario, Canada)

# Conclusion

The importance of the peripheral meniscal vasculature with regard to meniscal healing and repair in animals has been stressed by King (14) and others (4, 5, 12). Several cases of naturally healed meniscal lesions that have communicated with the peripheral meniscal vasculature have also been reported in man (19, 22). These observations have led to increasing efforts by orthopaedic surgeons to repair certain meniscal lesions (6, 9, 11, 22). From the above description it would appear that lesions of the peripheral attachment of the menisci, as well as those involving the anterior or posterior horn attachments, have access to a vascular supply that may be adequate enough to support a healing response (Figure 7–13). An exception would be lesions in the posterolateral aspect of the lateral meniscus, where the blood supply is tenuous.

## *References*


1. Annandale T. An operation for displaced semilunar cartilage. Br Med J 1:779, 1885
2. Arnoczky SP. The anatomy of the anterior cruciate ligament. Clin Orthop 172:19–25, 1983

3. Arnoczky SP, Warren RF. Microvasculature of the human meniscus. Am J Sports Med 10:90–95, 1982
4. Arnoczky SP, Warren RF. The microvasculature of the meniscus and its response to injury—An experimental study in the dog. Am J Sports Med 11:131–141, 1983
5. Cabaud HE, Rodkey WG, Fitzwater JE. Medial meniscus repairs: An experimental and morphological study. Am J Sports Med 9:129–134, 1981
6. Cassidy RE, Shaffer AJ. Repair of peripheral meniscal tears. Am J Sports Med 9:209–214, 1981
7. Cox JS, Nye CE, Schaffer WW, Woodstein IJ. The degenerative effects of partial and total resection of the medial meniscus in dogs' knees. Clin Orthop 109:178–183, 1975
8. Davies DV, Edwards DAW. The blood supply of the synovial membrane and intra-articular structures. Ann R Coll Surg Engl 2:142–156, 1948
9. DeHaven KE. Peripheral meniscal repair—An alternative to meniscectomy. Orthop Trans 5:399–400, 1981
10. Fairbanks TJ. Knee joint changes after meniscectomy. J Bone Joint Surg [Br] 30:664–670, 1948
11. Hamberg P, Gillquist J, Lysholm J. Suture of new and old peripheral meniscal tears. J Bone Joint Surg [Am] 65:193–197, 1983
12. Heatley FW. The meniscus—Can it be repaired? An experimental investigation in rabbits. J Bone Joint Surg [Br] 62:397–402, 1980
13. King D. The function of semilunar cartilages. J Bone Joint Surg 18:1069–1076, 1936
14. King D. The healing of semilunar cartilages. J Bone Joint Surg 18:333–342, 1936
15. Krause WR, Pope MH, Johnson RJ, Wilder DG. Mechanical changes in the knee after meniscectomy. J Bone Joint Surg [Am] 58:599–604, 1976
16. Levy IM, Torzilli PA, Warren RF. The effect of medial meniscectomy on anteroposterior motion of the knee. J Bone Joint Surg [Am] 64:883–890, 1982
17. Seedhom BB. Loadbearing function of the meniscus. Physiotherapy 62:223–226, 1976
18. Seedhom BB, Dowson D, Wright V. Functions of the meniscus. A preliminary study. J Bone Joint Surg [Br] 56:381–382, 1974
19. Smillie IS. Injuries of the Knee Joint, 1st ed. ES Livingstone, Edinburgh, 1946
20. Sutton JB. Ligaments, Their Nature and Morphology. MK Lewis and Co, London, 1897
21. Tapper EM, Hoover NW. Late results after meniscectomy. J Bone Joint Surg [Am] 51:517–526, 1969
22. Wirth CR. Meniscal repair. Clin Orthop 157:153–160, 1981

# Arthroscopic Meniscus Repair

# 8

Charles E. Henning
Mary A. Lynch
Ben L. Jolly
Gary A. Scott

A combined arthroscopic and limited open approach allows the surgeon to repair nearly all meniscus tears in a young, athletic population. We have progressed from repairing 50% of the meniscus tears encountered in 1980 to over 95% of these tears by 1983. More than 70% of the tears have occurred in an anterior cruciate-deficient knee.

Although our initial results from partial meniscectomy in the anterior cruciate-deficient knee were promising at 1 year, Lynch reported that by 3 years Fairbank's changes developed in these knees nearly as often as in the open meniscectomy group (4). In patients with two or more Fairbank's changes, there was a 68% incidence of pain.

More difficult meniscus tear problems such as tears in the body of the meniscus, double longitudinal tears of the medial and lateral meniscus, and the posterior radial split of the lateral meniscus are quite amenable to repair by the transarticular arthroscopic approach. A posteromedial or posterolateral dissection and a popliteal retractor are always used to protect the popliteal neurovascular structures and to aid in recovering and tying the sutures.

## Vascularity and Healing

Clark reported that the vascularity of the meniscus in patients 14 years and under is good and may be sufficient for healing (3). In patients over 14 years of age, significant vascularity is limited to the very peripheral part of the meniscus (1, 2). The parameniscal synovium can be abraded by using the arthroscopic rasps. The result is an increase in vascular panus growing out over the surface of the meniscus, frequently to within 1 mm of the free margin. The rasp is the preferred method of roughening the parameniscal synovium and is statisticly superior to use of a basket forcep.

## Instrumentation

Instrumentation includes a 30-degree fore-oblique arthroscope, popliteal retractor, arthroscopic rasps, distractor (medial meniscus), and arthroscopic needle holder (Figure 8–1). The arthroscope is placed in the anterolateral portal. The popliteal retractor is placed to expose the posterior capsule and protect the popliteal neurovascular structures. Rasps are placed through posterior (medial or lateral) arthrotomies and the anteromedial portal. The arthroscopic needle holder with the prebent needle is placed through a cannula in the anteromedial portal (Figure 8–2).

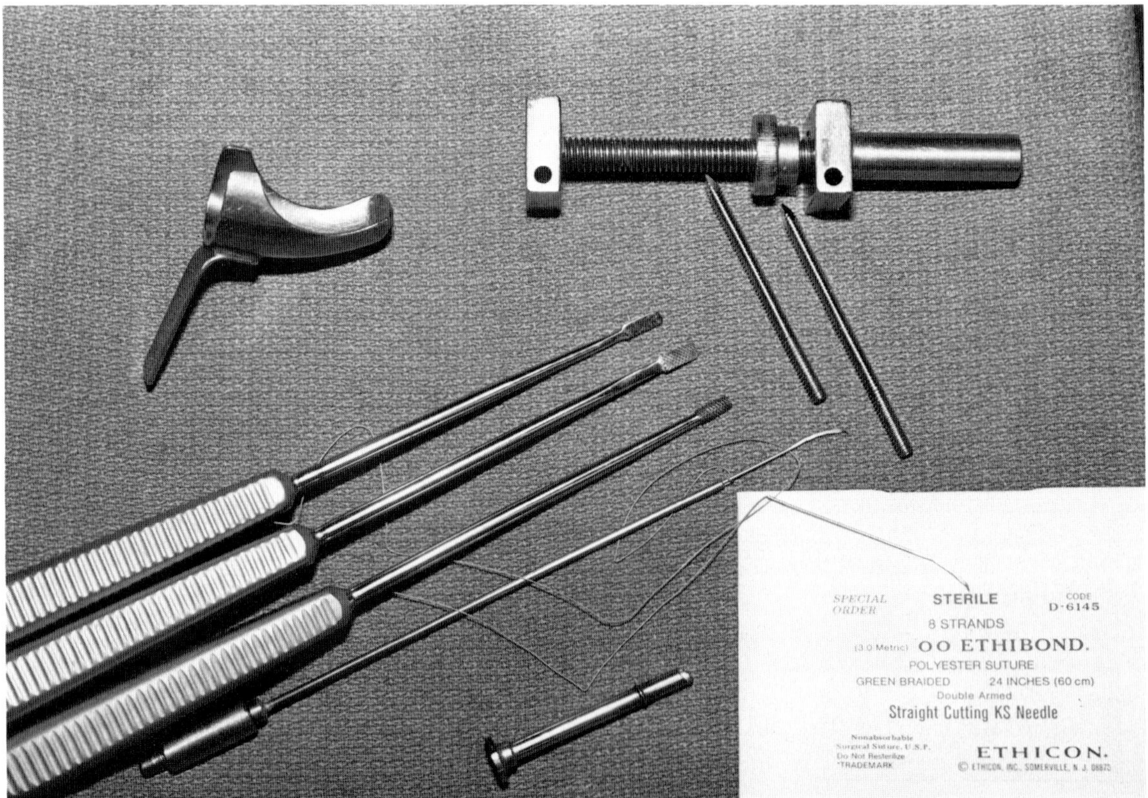


**Figure 8–1** *Upper left:* Popliteal retractor for protection of the popliteal neurovascular structures. *Lower left:* Arthroscopy rasps used for abrading the parameniscal synovium and peripheral white rim. *Upper right:* The joint distractor used for medial meniscus repair. *Lower central:* The arthroscopic needle holder used to hold the needle of the double armed 2-0 Ethibond suture, which is passed through the 5-mm port shown below the needle holder.

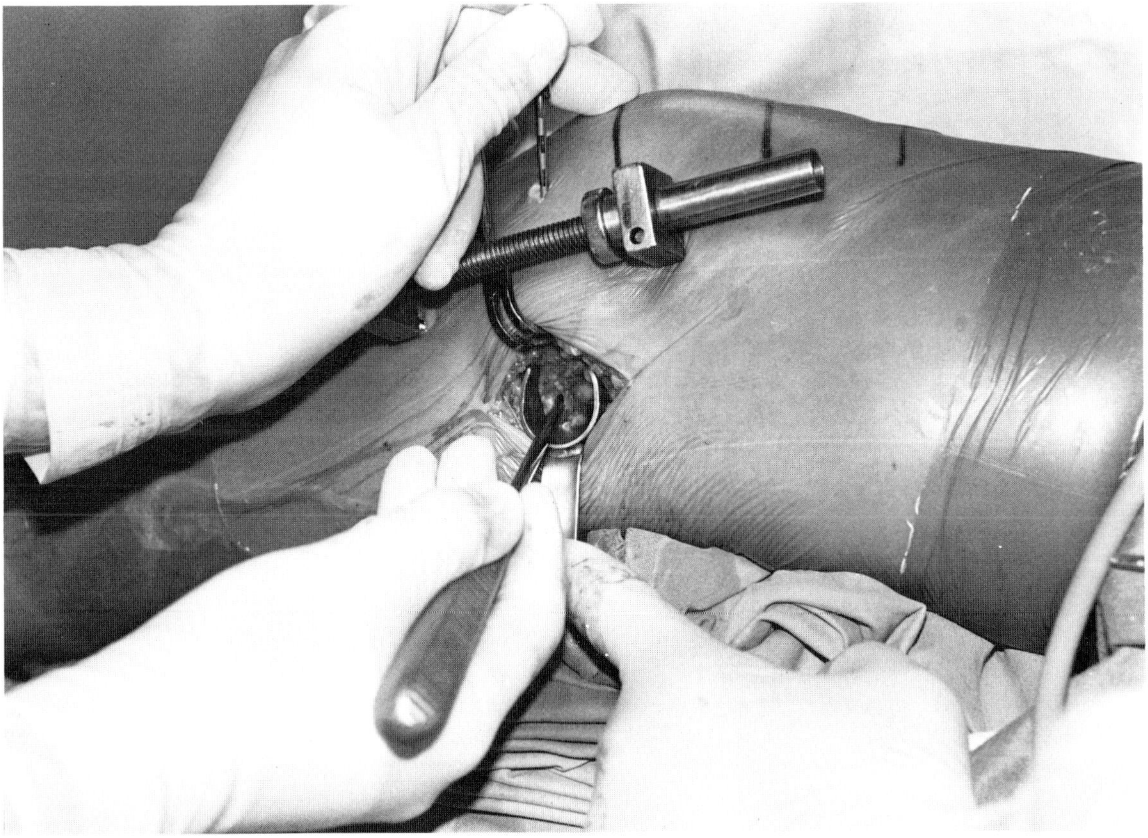

**Figure 8–2** Medial aspect of a right knee. The posterior dissection between the posterior capsule and the semimembranous and medial aspect of the medial head of the gastrocnemius has been done. The popliteal retractor is then placed to protect the neurovascular structures. The medial joint distractor is then placed to facilitate visualization of the medial joint space with the knee flexed 30 degrees. A probe is used to find the superior aspect of the meniscus at the posteromedial corner. A small arthrotomy is made, and the arthroscopy rasp is used to roughen the perimensical synovium and peripheral white rim of the posterior one-third of the meniscus.

## Evaluation of Meniscus

The meniscus tear is probed to determine the start, end, and rim width (Figure 8–3). A longitudinal tear of 10-mm or greater in length and a white rim of 5-mm or less is suitable for repair.

## Parameniscal Synovial Abrasion

Parameniscal synovial abrasion is performed through a posterior (medial or lateral) incision. A 1-cm. arthrotomy is made and the parameniscal synovium is abraded using the arthroscopic rasp on both the superior and inferior surface of the synovium and meniscus rim. When more than a 1-mm rim is present, it is necessary to make

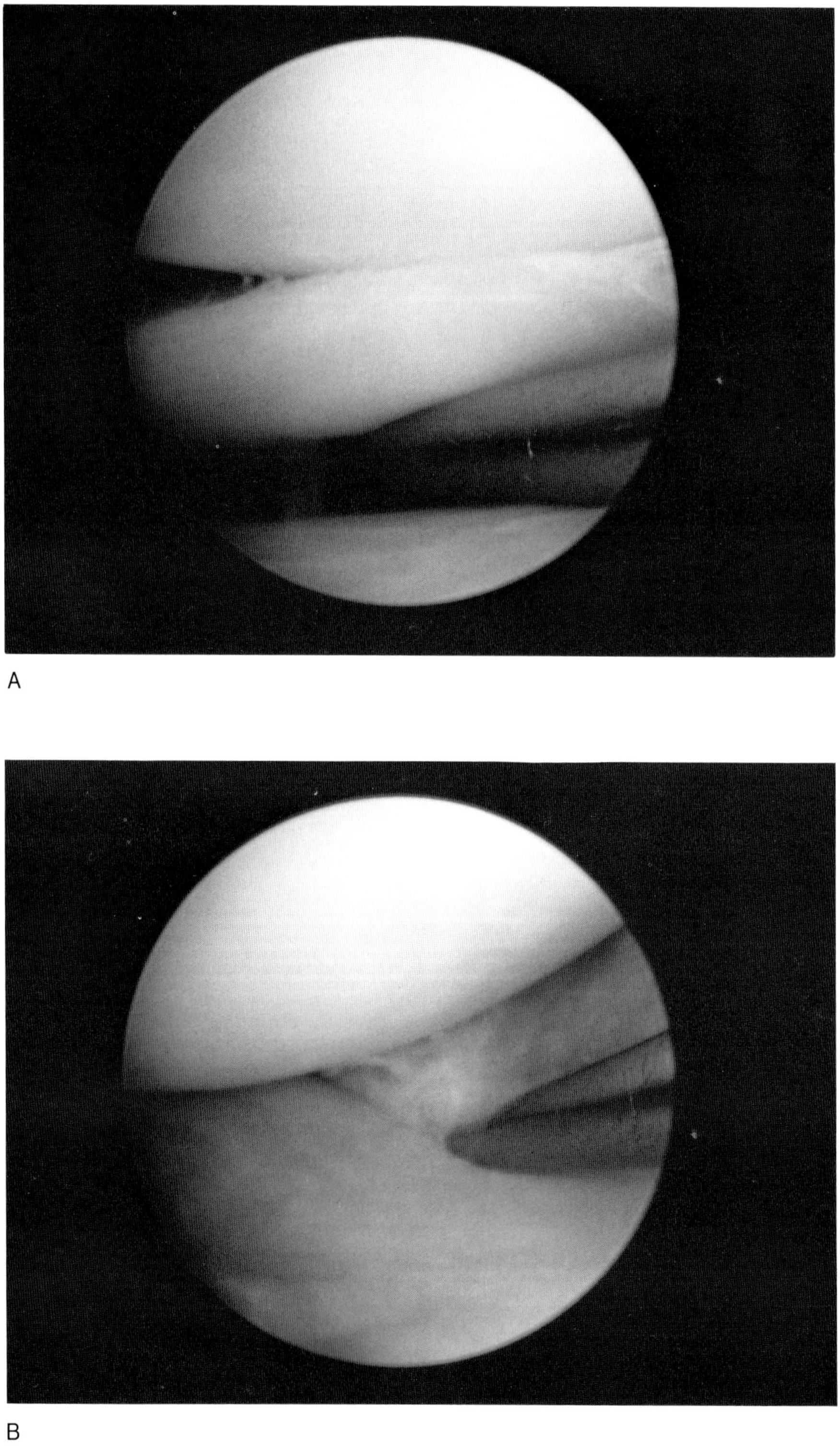

**Figure 8–3** **A** An arthroscopic view of the medial meniscus from the anterolateral portal, demonstrating the instability of a meniscus tear beginning at 10-mm from the posterior horn. **B** The view of the anterior aspect of the longitudinal tear of the medial meniscus ending at 35-mm from the posterior horn. The peripheral white rim measures 2-mm.

a separate, smaller arthrotomy inferior to the meniscus to abrade the inferior surface. Although the peripheral white rim is abraded on both the top and bottom surface, none of the white rim material is resected.

When the meniscus tear extends anteriorly into the middle third, the parameniscal synovium is abraded under arthroscopic control on both the superior and inferior surface, with the rasp introduced through the anteromedial portal (Figure 8–4).

## Stable Suture Fixation

Stable suture fixation is obtained by using multiple sutures of nonabsorbable material (2-0 Ethibond) and placing the sutures to oppose both the superior and inferior margin of the meniscus tear. Suturing begins at the extreme posterior aspect of the tear, typically 5–10 mm from the posterior horn attachment.

The needles of the double-armed suture can be bent 10 to 25 degrees near the tip to allow precise placement of the sutures with the arthroscopic needle holder. The first needle is placed on the inferior surface of the meniscus 3–4 mm from the tear margin and directed superiorly to cross the tear near the superior surface (Figure 8–5, A). The needle is recovered in the popliteal retractor. The second needle of the double-armed suture is introduced on the inferior surface of the mobile fragment and is directed across the tear surface near the tibial surface of the meniscus tear, and this needle is also recovered in the space of the popliteal retractor (Figure 8–5, B). This procedure is repeated placing the sutures at 2-mm intervals throughout the length of the tear (Figure 8–6). For a typical 15-mm tear of the posterior third of the medial meniscus, five sutures would be used.

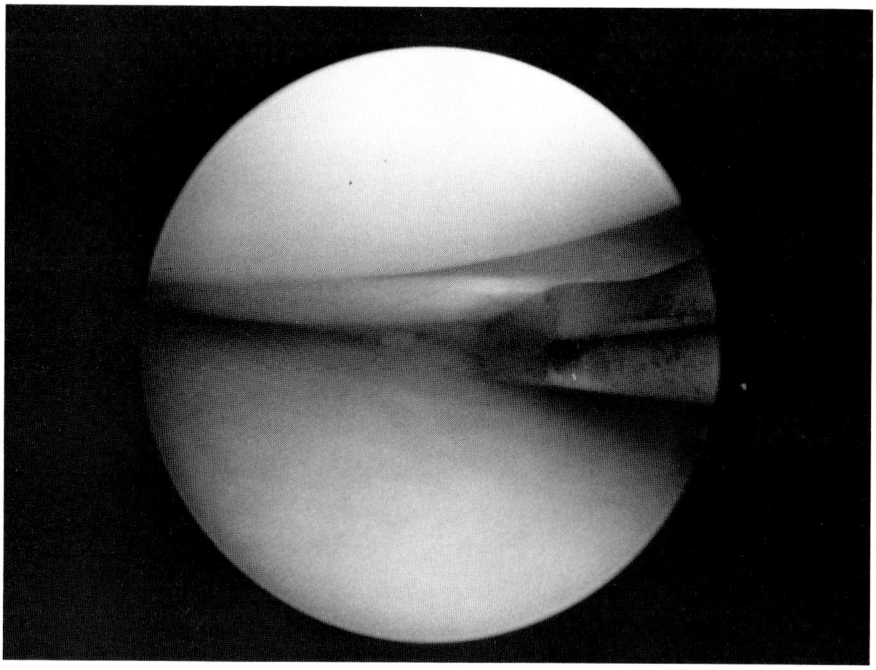

**Figure 8–4** With the rasp in the anteromedial portal, the inferior parameniscal synovium and inferior surface of the peripheral white rim are abraded with the edge cutting arthroscopy rasp. The superior parameniscal synovium and peripheral white rim are also abraded.

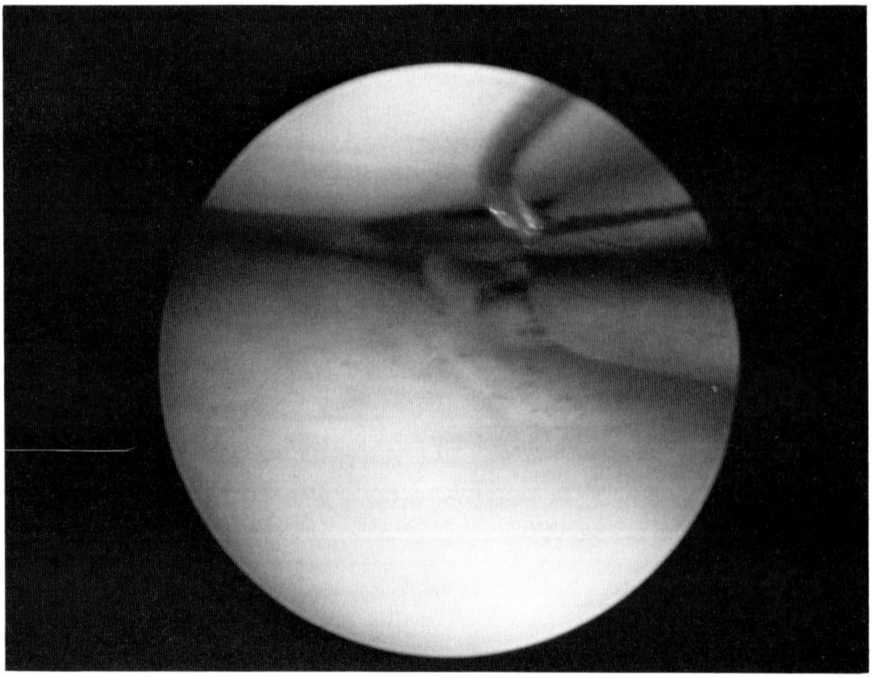

A

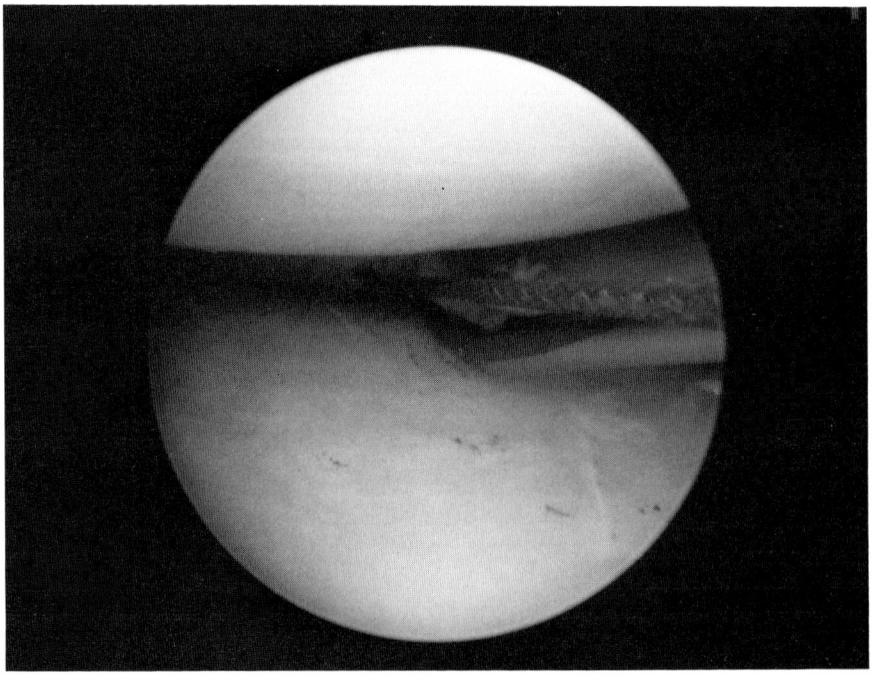

B

**Figure 8–5** **A** Suturing the meniscus. The needle is given a gradual bend over the distal 0.5-cm as shown in Figure 8–1. The first needle of the double-armed suture is placed at the inferior surface of the mobile fragment, with the needle directed proximally and medially so that the tip will enter the space of the popliteal retractor. **B** The second needle of the double-armed suture is introduced into the inferior surface of the meniscus and directed horizontally and medially so that the tip of the needle will enter the space of the popliteal retractor. Each suture is tagged for tying later.

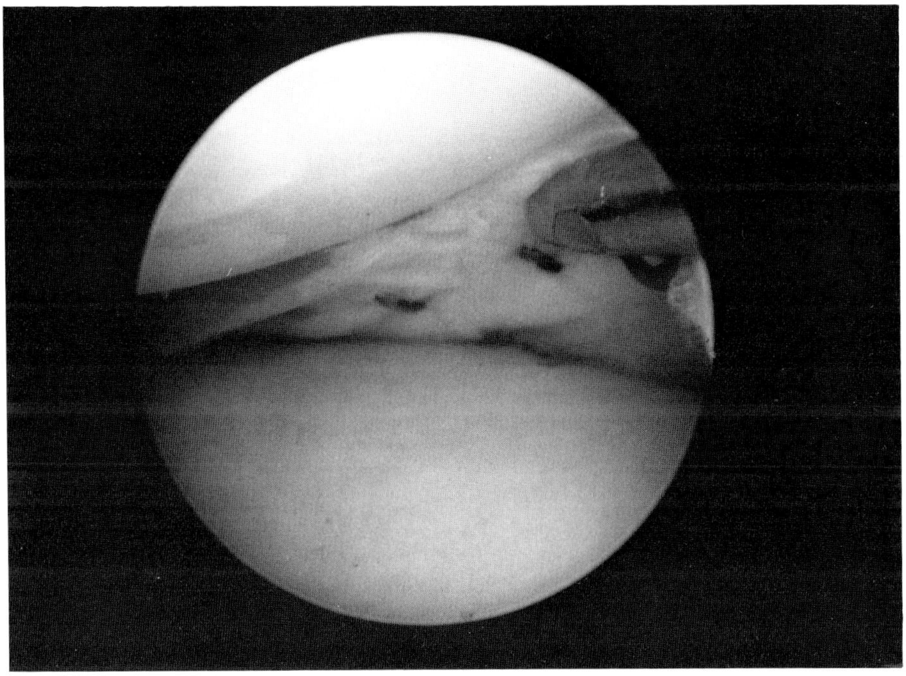

**Figure 8–6** Completion of suturing. Each suture is individually checked to verify that no suture has been abraded by a subsequent needle and that the meniscus is held stable as all sutures are held taut.

To stabilize a radial split, one needle is placed on the posterior horn side and the second needle in the opposite side of the radial split. The needles are recovered in the space of the popliteal retractor. When the suture is pulled taut, the radial split is held together.

# Surgical Procedures

## Medial Meniscus Technique

The arthroscope is placed in the anterolateral portal. The anteromedial portal is used initially for probing and later for passing the sutures for repair of the meniscus tear in the posterior third.

The open posterior dissection for the medial meniscus repair progresses through the posterior aspect of the sartorius, the interval between the posterior capsule and the semimembranosus, and is continued to the midportion of the medial gastrocnemius tendon (Figure 8–2). The surgeon should avoid dissection closer to the midline of the knee because of potential injury to the popliteal vessels. Care should be taken in dissection of the sartorius to avoid injury of the saphenous nerve and its branches.

The popliteal retractor is used to protect the popliteal neurovascular structures. If the tear extends into the middle third of the meniscus, the sartorius is elevated from the medial collateral ligament, taking care to protect the sartorial branch of the saphenous nerve.

A medial distractor is used to improve visibility for the medial meniscus repair. A posteromedial arthrotomy is done and the parameniscal synovium is roughened using the arthroscopic rasp. When the meniscus tear extends into the middle third, the parameniscal synovium is roughened on the superior and inferior surface with the rasp in the anteromedial portal.

Sutures are placed in the posterior third of the medial meniscus through the anteromedial portal (Figure 8–5). An anterolateral portal is used for suturing the middle third of the medial meniscus. Sutures are placed under arthroscopic control, as described in the section on suture fixation (Figure 8–7).

Sutures in the anterior half of the menisci are placed from the superior surface to the inferior surface (Figure 8–8, A). The second needle is placed at the same entry point, and the prebent needle is directed superiorly. As the suture is pulled taut, it disappears just under the surface to avoid abrasion by the moving femoral condyle (Figure 8–8, B and C).

## Lateral Meniscus Technique

The arthroscope is placed in the anterolateral portal and the 3.8-mm sheath is placed in the anteromedial portal. The open posterolateral dissection is begun just behind the fibular collateral ligament. Dissection is continued between the posterior aspect of the iliotibial band and the anterior aspect of the biceps and continued on the posterior capsule-arcuate complex to the midpoint of the lateral gastrocnemius tendon. Dissection is not done more medially to avoid injury of the neurovascular structures. The peroneal nerve is protected only by a thin layer of

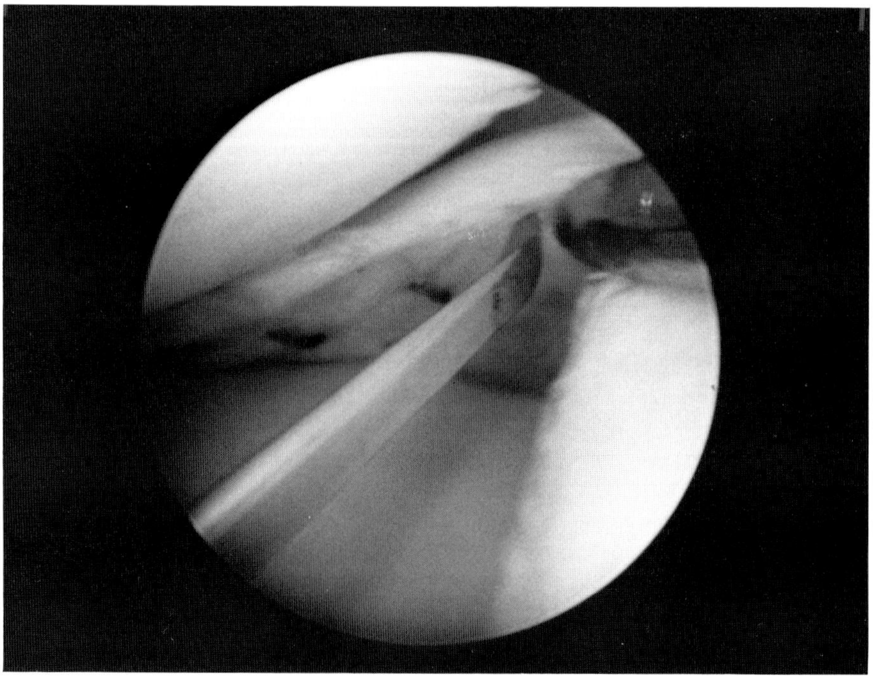

**Figure 8–7** Suturing the meniscus in the middle one-third. A 3.8-mm sheath parallel with the arthroscope in the anterolateral portal is used. The arthroscopic needle holder is used to introduce the first suture superiorly and posteriorly on the inferior surface. The second needle will be directed inferiorly and posteriorly. Three sutures previously placed are visible on the inferior surface of the posterior third of the meniscus.

fascia in the interval between the lateral margin of the gastrocnemius and the medial margin of the biceps. The popliteal retractor is used to protect the neurovascular structures.

Parameniscal synovial abrasion is done through a small arthrotomy just posterior to the fibular collateral ligament and anterior to the popliteus tendon. When the meniscus tear communicates with the popliteus hiatus, the surface of the popliteus tendon is abraded and the meniscus will be attached back directly to the popliteus tendon, as well as to the superior fascicle of the hiatus. When the tear is in the substance, the parameniscal synovium on both the superior and inferior aspect of the white rim is abraded, as well as the superior and inferior surface of the white rim. None of the white rim material is excised. When the tear extends anteriorly to the popliteus hiatus, the arthroscopy rasp can be placed through the anteromedial portal, and the parameniscal synovium on the superior and inferior aspect of the meniscus is abraded under arthroscopic control.

Suture fixation is done using the arthroscopic needle holder through the 3.8-mm portal placed anteromedially. The sutures are placed as described under the section on suture fixation. Sutures should be placed at 2- to 3-mm intervals throughout the entire length of the tear. A radial split is repaired by placing one needle on either side of the radial split. A flap tear would be treated as a combination of a radial split and a longitudinal tear.

The needles are recovered in the space of the popliteal retractor. It is improper to advance a needle more than 15-mm through the meniscus without having control of the tip of the needle within the space of this retractor.

### Common Errors

Parameniscal synovial abrasion of the peripheral white rim must be complete to obtain a high incidence of healing. This portion of the operation requires as much time as placing the sutures.

Suture placement is important for stable meniscus fixation. Common errors include placing the sutures too close to the tear margin with the suture cutting out of the mobile fragment, placing the sutures too close to the free margin with puckering of the free margin, and placing the suture on the superior surface of the meniscus, which is subject to breakage from abrasion by the moving femoral condyle.

## Postoperative Management

The leg is immobilized in the operative splint at about 30 degrees of flexion. The patient must be non-weight bearing through the first 2 months, and weight bearing is gradually increased over the next month. It is our opinion that sheer strain in a meniscus repair is very high with weight bearing, and restriction of weight bearing is critically important to healing, particularly of the substance tears.

Cycle riding is begun at 3 months. Running is begun at 5–6 months, and sports participation is allowed between 9 and 12 months.

## Results

During the period of 1980 through 1982, 168 meniscus repairs were done using the basket forcep for parameniscal synovial abrasion. Over 90% of the repairs were clinically stable but only three-fourths were satisfactorily healed by the time follow-

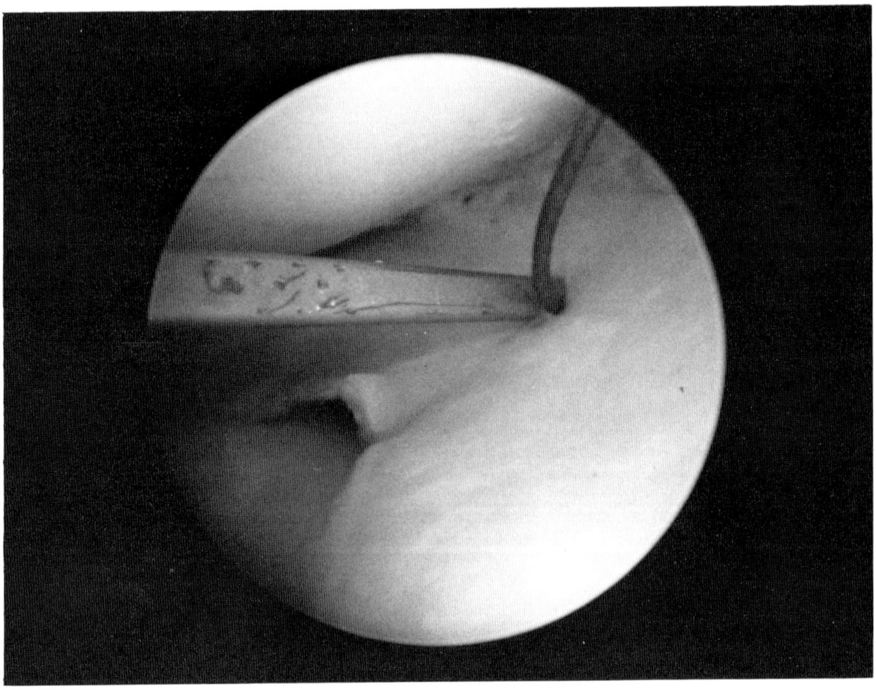

A

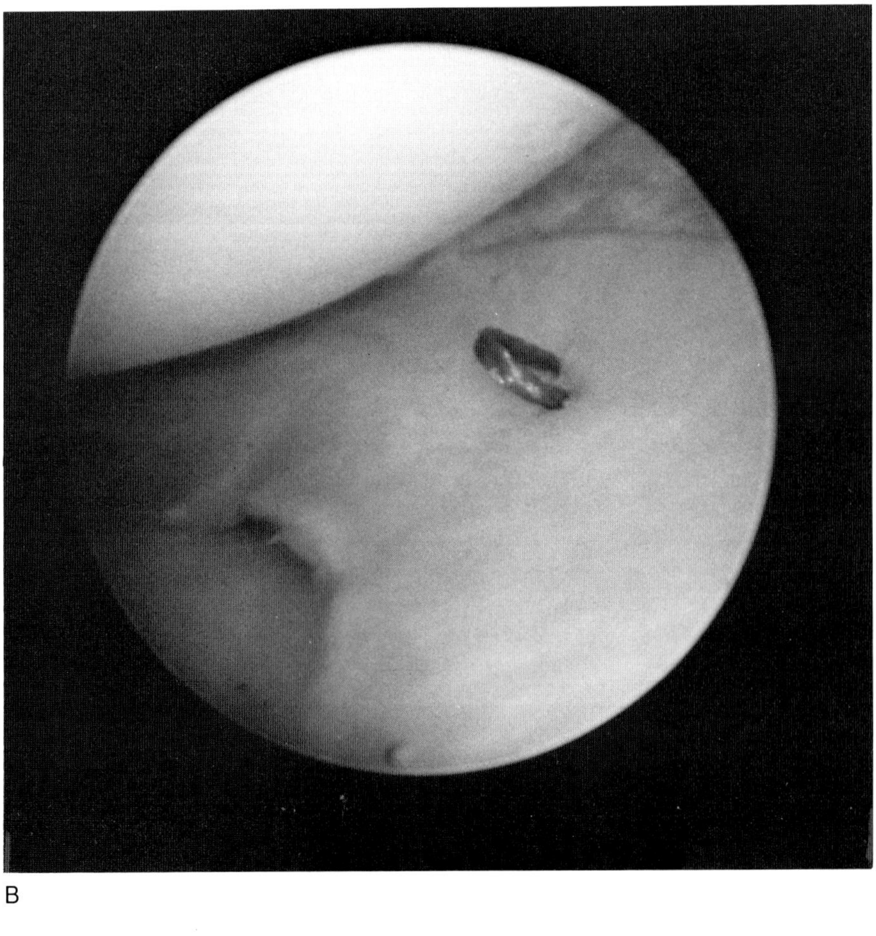

B

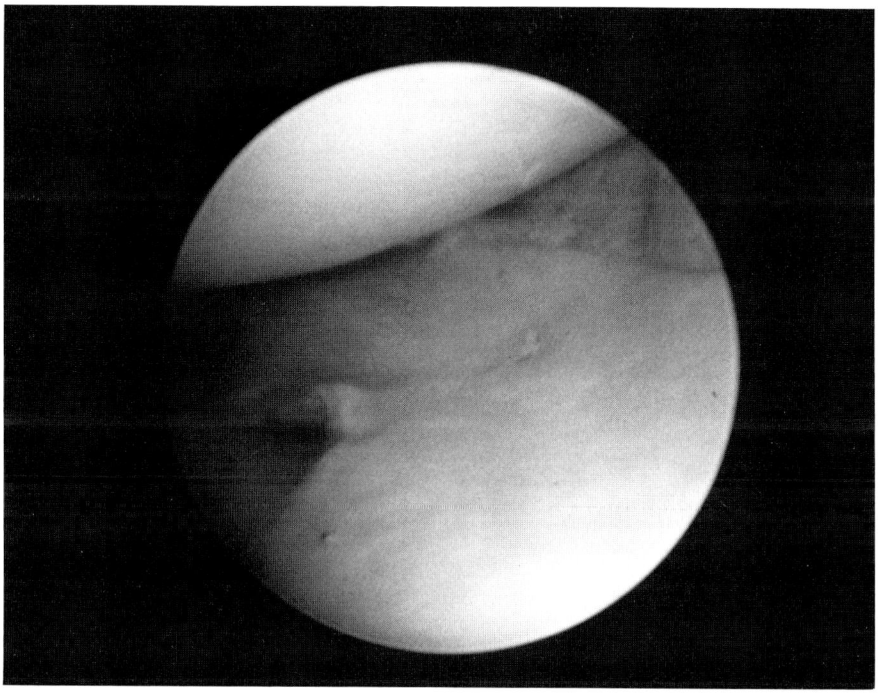

C

**Figure 8–8** **A** Suturing the anterior aspect of the meniscus. The sutures are introduced through the sheath parallel with the arthroscope in the anterolateral portal. The first needle is directed inferiorly and then posteriorly through the capsule. The second needle (shown in the photo) enters the meniscus at the same hole and is immediately directed superiorly and posteriorly to create a vertical suture in the substance of the meniscus. **B** and **C** As the anteriorly placed suture is pulled taut, it disappears just under the surface of the meniscus so that it will not be subject to abrasion by the moving femoral condyle.

up arthrography or arthroscopy was done. Although not statistically significant, there was slightly better healing of the lateral meniscus and of all meniscus tears with white rims of 0–2 mm. Tear length was not significant.

There was a statistically significant increased rate of meniscus healing when the rasp was used for parameniscal synovial abrasion and when the meniscus repair was associated with a normal anterior cruciate ligament. Patients with a combined anterior cruciate ligament reconstruction have a lower incidence of meniscus healing, but there is a low incidence of clinical instability of the ''not healed'' meniscus. Although the reconstructed anterior cruciate ligament and presence of the meniscus protects the knee from rapidly progressive degenerative changes, patients with ''not healed'' meniscus repairs probably should be permanently restricted from involvement in deceleration sports.

Since November 1983 the rasp has been used for parameniscal synovial abrasion. Satisfactory meniscus healing has improved to 90 percent. I would like to thank Dr. Dilworth Cannon for his contribution of the rasp technique.

## Complications

Subsequent to this series of patients, we have had a popliteal artery laceration requiring a reverse saphenous vein graft. It was not clear when the injury occurred during the operation. Although we originally recommended using the Doane knee retractor, we feel this is no longer satisfactory. We have developed a popliteal retractor that makes it easier to protect the neurovascular structures and to retrieve the sutures.

### Discussion

In this series of patients, 70% of the meniscus repairs were done in conjunction with an anterior cruciate ligament reconstruction. These reconstructed knees as well as anterior cruciate-deficient knees are extremely sensitive to loss of any of the meniscus substance. Our best results both subjectively and objectively are obtained in knees with intact or reconstructed anterior cruciate ligaments.

Even arthroscopic partial meniscectomy results in a four times greater incidence of Fairbank's changes and a two times greater incidence of pain at 3-year follow-up compared to knees with normal or repaired menisci.

The arthroscopic approach to meniscus repair enables the surgeon to repair any meniscus tear that can be probed. Over a period of 4 years, we have gradually developed the technique to allow repair of more than 95% of all meniscus tears encountered. Minimal additional instrumentation is necessary for proper meniscus repair technique and safety of the popliteal neurovascular structures.

## Summary

From the period of 1980 through 1982, 168 meniscus repairs were done. More than 90% of these tears were clinically stable, and three-fourths of the repairs were satisfactorily healed by the time arthrography or arthroscopy was done. The combined arthroscopic and limited open approach allows repairing of more than 95% of meniscus tears encountered. Safety of the popliteal neurovascular structures is improved with the small, posterior, open dissection and the popliteal retractor.

### *References*

1. Arnoczky SP, Warren RF. Microvasculature of the human meniscus. Am J Sports Med 10:90–95, 1982
2. Arnoczky SP, Warren RF. The microvasculature of the meniscus and its response to injury: An experimental study in the dog. Am J Sports Med 11:131–141, 1983
3. Clark CR, Ogden JA. Development of the menisci of the human knee joint. Morphological changes and their potential role in childhood meniscal injury. J Bone Joint Surg [Am] 65:538–547, 1983
4. Lynch MA, Henning CE, Glick KR. Knee joint surface changes. Long-term follow-up meniscus tear treatment in stable anterior cruciate ligament reconstructions. Clin Orthop 172:148–152, 1983

# Functions of the Meniscus 9

John B. McGinty

Because of the recent attitudes and advances in meniscus surgery, particularly the change from total meniscectomy to repair in the management of meniscus tears, it is of value to review the literature and look at the functions of the semilunar cartilages of the knee. The approach to problems with the semilunar cartilages has changed dramatically with the development of arthroscopic surgical techniques.

Not more than fifteen years ago, it was established by one of the pioneers and great teachers of knee surgery that total meniscectomy was the answer to all meniscal tears because "these observations offered evidence in favor of total rather than partial meniscectomy, no matter what lesion is encountered, for if it be accepted that the meniscus performs any function, that function can best be performed by the most perfect replica of the original. The most perfect replica possible follows total meniscectomy" (24). This observation has not stood the test of time. In this author's experience with viewing arthroscopically several hundred knees that have had a meniscectomy, the regenerated meniscus was either thin, frail fibrous tissue less than 5 mm in width or there was no indication of regeneration. It has subsequently been shown that clinical results are significantly better following partial meniscectomy (5, 21).

In a classic paper it was shown that long-term results of meniscectomy showed an increased incidence radiologically of joint space narrowing, chondral flattening, and osteophyte formation (11). Several long-range studies showed a significant incidence of deterioration of good clinical results following total meniscectomy (7, 12, 15–17, 19, 25). In dogs it has also been shown that total resection of the meniscus results in degenerative changes in the knee (8). Therefore it has become increasingly apparent that the meniscus is an important structure in the knee and that preservation of the meniscus is a goal worth striving for.

In the knee there are basically three motions that work in a synchronous fashion: flexion-extension, anterior and posterior gliding, and external and internal rotation. As the knee flexes the tibia internally rotates in the femur. If stress is applied during these rotary motions, it is transmitted to the meniscus and its peripheral attachments. This stress can be considerably increased if the restraining influence of the anterior cruciate ligament is absent (22). In fact, the incidence of torn meniscus in the anterior cruciate-deficient knee is greater than 50%. This author has found the combination of a bucket-handle tear of the medial meniscus with a posterior longitudinal tear of the lateral meniscus to be very common in the anterior cruciate-deficient knee.

The meniscus is a semilunar piece of fibrocartilage that is concave on the superior surface and flat on the inferior surface to mate with the femoral condyle and tibial articular surface, respectively, thereby providing a mechanism for a convex surface to articulate with another surface of considerably less concavity. The lateral meniscus is larger, C-shaped, and more mobile than the medial meniscus. To fill the space between the femoral and tibial surfaces, the meniscus must be wedge shaped, wider in the periphery, and taper to a slim, free edge. The peripheral fibers of the menisci have a circumference orientation to resist "hoop-stresses." Both menisci are tethered to the tibial surface by the meniscotibial ligaments. This circumferential ligament combined with the meniscofemoral ligament forms the deep medial collateral ligament. The anterior horns are connected to each other by the transverse ligament. The posterior horn of the lateral meniscus is attached to the posterior cruciate ligament anteriorly and posteriorly by the ligaments of Humphrey and Wrisberg. There is also a variable ligament, the ligament of Barkow, that sometimes connects the posterior horn of the lateral meniscus to the anterior horn of the medial meniscus.

It has been recently established that the blood supply of the meniscus is more extensive than had been previously thought. In microvascular studies blood vessels have been shown to extensively supply the peripheral 40–50% of the meniscus (2, 3, 9). This information has considerable bearing on meniscal healing and therefore influences recent work on meniscal repair. Repair of peripheral detachments and even repair of structural tears of the meniscus appears to be feasible (4, 6, 10, 13, 14, 18, 27).

Significant evidence has been established to demonstrate the role of the meniscus in sharing load with the articular cartilage in the weight-bearing function of the knee. It has been established that the menisci transmit over 50% of the joint compression force, the lateral more than the medial. Contact stress is increased after partial meniscectomy (1). It has also been shown with cadaver-testing machines that joint space narrowing in response to compression forces is greater after meniscectomy and that the contact area is 2.5 times greater in the presence of the menisci or 40% less after meniscectomy (23). Therefore meniscectomy results in greater force per unit area of articular cartilage or a greater predeliction for wear.

Finally, there is evidence to suggest that the menisci have a function in stabilizing the knee. Rapid deterioration has been shown in the anterior cruciate-deficient knee with loss of both menisci (22). In cadaver studies in the anterior cruciate-deficient knee, anterior tibial displacement is greater when the menisci have been removed (20, 26). Therefore the menisci are a secondary restraint for anterior tibial displacement. If the anterior cruciate ligament is absent, forward motion of the tibia may create a "wedge effect" in the posterior horn of the meniscus, producing a longitudinal tear.

It is therefore concluded that the semilunar cartilages of the knee fundamentally have three functions:

1. maintenance of mechanical congruity of the knee by mating the greater convexity of the femoral surface to the tibial surface, particularly in gliding and rotary motion;
2. sharing load bearing with the femoral and tibial joint surfaces by spreading the forces of weight bearing over a greater area and decreasing the force per unit area;
3. contributing to rotary stability of the knee by acting as a secondary restraint in conjunction with the primary restraint of the cruciate ligaments.

In the management of meniscal lesions, stable meniscal tissue should be preserved whenever possible. This may be accomplished by partial meniscectomy or meniscal repair, whichever seems more appropriate, depending on a variety of clinical factors.

## *References*


1. Ahmed AH, Burke DJ. In review of measurements of static pressure distribution in synovial joints. J Biomech Eng 105:201, 1983
2. Arnoczky SP, Warren RF. Microvasculature of the human meniscus. Am J Sports Med 10:90, 1982
3. Arnoczky SP, Warren RF. The microvasculature of the meniscus and its response to injury—an experimental study in the dog. Am J Sports Med 11:131, 1983
4. Cabaud HE, Rodkey WG, Fitzwater, JE. Medial meniscus repairs: An experimental and morphological study. Am J Sports Med 9:129, 1981
5. Cargill, AO'R, Jackson JP. Bucket-handle tears of the medial meniscus. A case for conservative surgery. J Bone Joint Surg [Am] 58:248, 1976
6. Cassidy RE, Shaffer, AJ. Repairs of peripheral meniscal tears. Am J Sports Med 9:209, 1981
7. Charnley RK. Late joint changes, a result of internal derangement of the knee. Am J Surg 76:496, 1948
8. Cox JS, Nye CE, Shaffer WW, Woodstein IJ. The degenerative effects of partial and total resection of the medial meniscus in dogs' knees. Clin Orthop 109:178, 1975
9. Davies DV, Edwards DAW. The blood supply of the synovial membrane and intra-articular structures. Ann R Coll Surg Engl 2:142, 1948
10. DeHaven KE. Peripheral meniscal repairs—An alternative to meniscectomy. Orthop Trans 5:399, 1981
11. Fairbanks TJ. Knee joint changes after meniscectomy. J Bone Joint Surg [Br] 30:664, 1948
12. Gear MWL. The late results of meniscectomy. Br J Surg 54:270, 1967
13. Hamberg P, Gillquist J, Lyshocm J. Suture of new and old peripheral meniscal tears. J Bone Joint Surg [Am] 65:193, 1983
14. Heatley FW. The meniscus—Can it be repaired? An Experimental investigation in rabbits. J Bone Joint Surg [Br] 62:397, 1980
15. Huckell JR. Is meniscectomy a benign procedure? A long-term followup study. Can J Surg 8:254, 1965
16. Jackson JP. Degenerative changes in the knee after meniscectomy. Br Med J 2:525, 1968
17. Johnson RJ, Kettlekamp DB, Clark W, Leaverron P. Factors affecting late results after memiscectomy. J Bone Joint Surg [Am] 56:719, 1974
18. King D. The healing of semilunar cartilages. J Bone Joint Surg 18:333, 1936
19. Krause WR, Pope MH, Johnson RJ, Wilder DG. Mechanical changes in the knee after meniscectomy. J Bone Joint Surg [Am] 58:599, 1976
20. Levy IM, Torzilli PA, Warren RF. The effect of medial meniscectomy in anterior-posterior motion of the knee. J Bone Joint Surg [Am] 64:883, 1982

21. McGinty JB, Geuss LF, Marvin RA. Partial or total meniscectomy. J Bone Joint Surg [Am] 59:763, 1977
22. Noyes FR. The symptomatic anterior cruciate deficient knee. J Bone Joint Surg [Am] 65:2, 1983
23. Shrive NG, O'Connor JJ, Goodfellow JW. Load bearing in the knee joint. Clin Orthop 131:279, 1978
24. Smillie IS. Injuries of the Knee Joint. ES Livingston, Edinburgh, 1970
25. Tapper EM, Hoover NW. Late results after meniscectomy J Bone Joint Surg [Am] 51:517, 1969
26. Warren RF, Levy IM. Meniscal lesions associated with anterior cruciate injury. Clin Orthop 172:32, 1983
27. Wirth CR. Meniscal repairs. Clin Orthop 157:153, 1981

# The Techniques for Arthroscopic Management of Tibial Plateau Fractures

# 10

Richard B. Caspari

There has been a history of controversy over the appropriate techniques of management for tibial plateau fractures. Options range from complete conservative treatment with closed reduction and casting to open exposure of the entire knee with anatomical reduction of intra-articular fragments and sophisticated internal fixation (1–3, 5, 10, 16, 20, 21, 22, 23). The morbidity of tibial plateau fractures is not inconsequential. Decreased range of motion, pain, instability, and eventual degenerative arthritis are all well-known sequelae.

Several classification systems for tibial plateau fractures have been suggested (8–11, 20). Common patterns of fractures do occur and basically involve varied combinations of splitting and depression of the tibial plateau. Accurate classification and identification of the fracture allows the surgeon to make critical decisions regarding fracture management and to preplan an operative approach. Routine anteroposterior and lateral X-rays, anteroposterior views of the knee angled 15 degrees caudad to parallel the slope of the tibial plateau, and tomograms are all part of the surgeon's armamentarium for more precisely defining these fractures (6, 7, 14,17). Even so, it is a common experience for a surgeon to open the knee and find the fracture to be more severe than he had anticipated based on these diagnostic tests.

Soft tissue injuries have also been reported in association with tibial plateau fractures (2, 13, 15, 18, 19, 23, 24). These include injury to the menisci, collateral and cruciate ligaments, and articular surfaces that are not directly involved with the fracture. The conventional methods of diagnosing these soft tissue injuries are severely limited in the presence of a tibial plateau fracture. Physical examination and double contrast arthrography are both of limited use because of the patient's pain associated with the fracture.

Arthroscopy is a modality that addresses the problems of precise fracture identification and soft tissue injury in the presence of a tibial plateau fracture (4, 12, 18). In addition, arthroscopy is a low-risk procedure and does not alter future considerations with regard to fracture management. This technique also allows the surgeon to drain the joint of hemarthrosis and debride bony debris. Appropriate fractures may be reduced under arthroscopic control, bone grafted, and/or fixed percutaneously. Following any of these techniques, the patient's postoperative regimen may be tailored based upon the stability of the fracture.

## Diagnostic Arthroscopy

The procedure is performed with a general or spinal anesthetic and utilizes a standard operating room table. Initially we performed some of these procedures on a fracture table to make use of fluoroscopy; however, this step is unnecessary and the use of a fracture table is quite cumbersome for arthroscopy. An examination of the knee under anesthesia should be performed prior to prepping and draping the patient, and may provide valuable information with regard to ligamentous injury. Stress x-rays should be obtained as appropriate. One of the standard substantial and circumferential thigh holders should be utilized to affix the femur to the operating table and allow adequate stress to be applied to the knee. A tourniquet is routinely utilized for these procedures because excessive bleeding from the fracture fragments is a significant problem and cannot be controlled by the hydrostatic pressure of saline in the joint. Also, if elevation, bone grafting, and fixation are to be accomplished, limited incisions must be made and bleeding will need to be controlled.

Following these preliminary steps the extremity is sterilely prepared and draped so that the leg may be freely moved. If there is even the smallest possibility that a bone graft will be necessary, the area of the contralateral iliac crest should also be sterilely prepared and draped. A sandbag under the buttocks will also facilitate obtaining a bone graft. Following sterile preparation the donor site should be covered until the graft is taken.

The method of direct visualization through the arthroscope by the surgeon is crucial. Every effort should be made to maintain sterility since the technique of arthroscopy converts a closed to an open fracture. A sterilely draped or gluteraldehyde-soaked camera should be used at all times, and if the scope is to be changed, sterile technique should be maintained.

A large-bore inflow cannula is placed in the suprapatellar pouch to allow initial drainage of the hemarthrosis. A continuous inflow system of either Ringer's lactate or saline is established with 3-liter bags of solution suspended approximately 1 meter above the level of the knee. The use of distilled water in this circumstance is to be condemned, as the fracture may communicate with the closed fascial compartments of the lower leg, producing the potential for a compartment syndrome. In this regard, it is advisable to wrap the lower leg with an elasticized bandage.

The arthroscopic cannula is generally placed in the anteromedial or anterolateral portal opposite the side of the fracture. The transpatellar tendon portal may also be utilized. Following placement of the cannula, suction should be applied prior to insertion of the arthroscope, thereby clearing any hemarthrosis. Once the effluent is clear, the arthroscope is inserted and diagnostic arthroscopy commences. Suction should continue to be applied to the side arm of the arthroscope, or visualization will gradually become diminished due to further bleeding in the joint.

Large fragments of coagulated blood can usually be removed by suctioning through the arthroscopic cannula with removal and reinsertion of the arthroscope. Small fragments of articular cartilage and bone should also be removed.

The arthroscopic examination begins in the suprapatellar pouch with removal of all debris and examination of the patella. One case of patellar dislocation in association with the tibial plateau fracture has been reported, and it is not unusual to observe articular injury to the surface of the patella (J. Andrews, L. L. Johnson, T. Rosenberg, S. Springer, J. Toft, and T. L. Whipple, personal communications). As a routine the compartment opposite to the side of the fracture is next examined. Once again debris is removed and careful attention is given to the articular surfaces and the meniscus of this compartment. Extension of the fracture into this compartment should be ruled out. Meniscal injuries are handled in the routine fashion with balanced resection of meniscal body tears and repair of appropriate meniscal injuries. The collateral ligament and capsule may also be observed for interstitial bleeding. The intercondylar notch is next examined, and resection of the ligamentum synovium and some fat pad may be necessary in order to obtain visualization. A probe is used to palpate the cruciate ligament and as a retractor so that the posterior cruciate may also be observed. At this point it is important to visualize the posterior compartments, as this is a likely site for gravitation of small fragments of cartilage and bone.

Finally, one turns attention to the fractured compartments. Usually access to this compartment is quite easy, especially if there is depression of the tibial plateau, which results in rather marked widening of the compartment. The surgeon should bear in mind, however, that he is presented with a two-dimensional visualization of this fracture, and therefore it is essential to have a calibrated hook probe to judge the displacement and size of fracture fragments. In addition, the fracture fragments may be palpated and moved with the hook probe so that better visualization and understanding of the fracture is achieved. Observation of the femoral condyle for articular damage, the meniscus, and capsular structures is carried out at this juncture. On occasion a bucket-handle tear of the meniscus is found to be driven into the fracture itself and will have to be delivered into the field, utilizing the hook probe. The torn fragment of meniscus can then be removed in the con-

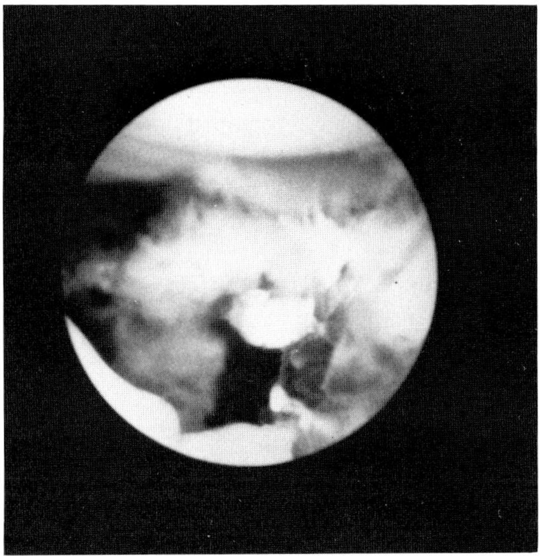

**Figure 10–1** View into the depths of a lateral plateau split fracture with depression.

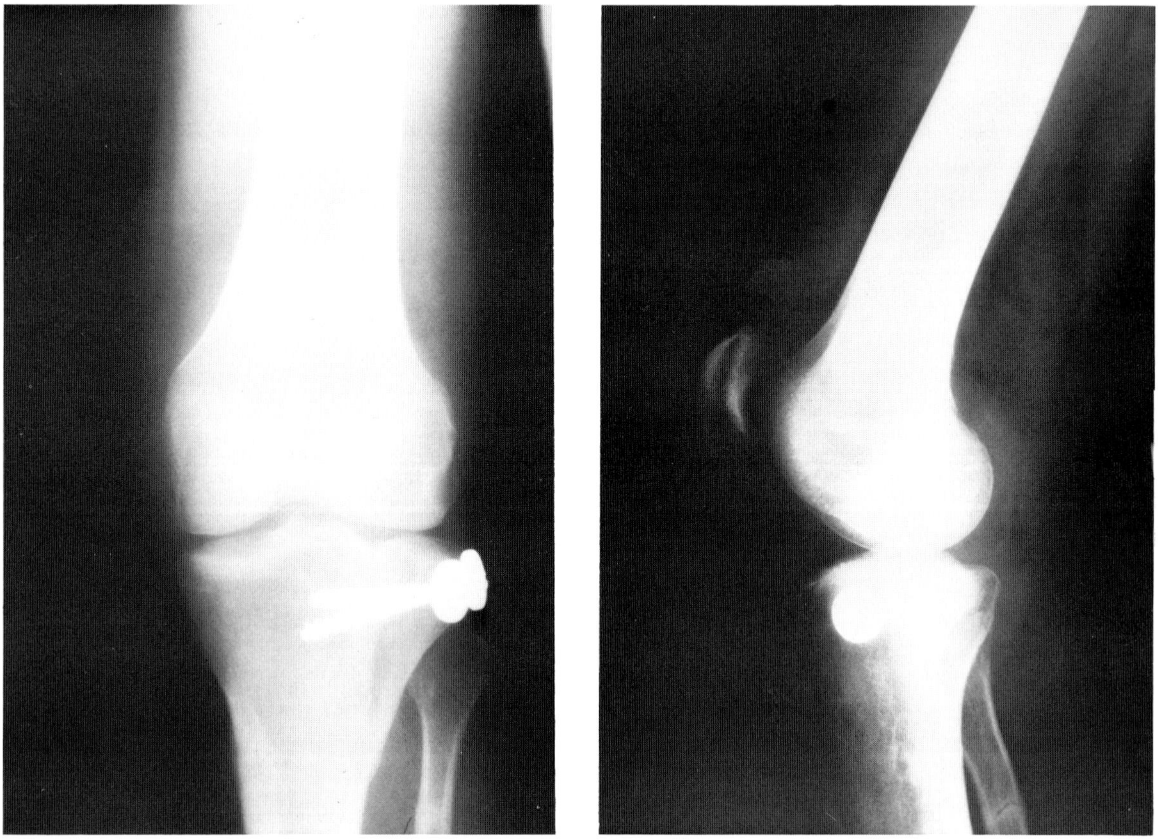

A B

**Figure 10–2** X-rays after arthroscopic elevation, reduction, and percutaneous fixation of a lateral plateau fracture.

ventional manner. Menisci that can be repaired should be because the presence of the meniscus will afford some protection to the surface of the joint. An intact meniscus is elevated with the hook probe so that the extent of the fracture underneath the meniscus can be determined. Palpation of the medial or lateral and posterior walls of the proximal tibia externally with a finger will provide valuable clues as to the stability of the cortex. At this point it is valuable to compare the findings on arthroscopic examination with the preoperative x-rays.

After thorough investigation of all intra-articular injuries, decisions regarding management must be made. No treatment modalities should be excluded. Closed reduction and institution of traction may still be the most efficacious method of treatment, and this modality has not been ruled out after a diagnostic arthroscopy. Both open and arthroscopic techniques may be utilized, and indeed, in some instances a combination of the two techniques may be necessary. Frequently, soft tissue injuries may be handled arthroscopically, allowing the open reduction and fixation to be performed via a more directed and limited arthrotomy. All treatment modalities should be considered and the most appropriate means of management should be selected.

## Operative Arthroscopy

As a general rule, soft tissue injuries are handled before approaching the fracture itself. Tears of the body of the menisci are resected arthroscopically and peripheral detachments are repaired. Articular surfaces that have been injured but not directly involved with the fracture are debrided with powered instrumentation. Removal of debris is usually accomplished during the diagnostic phase of the arthroscopy.

If major ligamentous injuries have occurred, repair may be instituted immediately or delayed at the surgeon's discretion. Arthroscopic techniques for ligament reconstruction and substitution are now being introduced and undoubtedly will have an impact on the management of the tibial plateau fractures in which these injuries occur (J. Andrews, L. L. Johnson, T. Rosenberg, S. Springer, J. Toft, and T. L. Whipple, personal communications). The present state of art, however, would dictate open repair or reconstruction of severe ligamentous injuries, and in these cases open reduction and fixation of the tibial plateau fracture is accomplished at the same time.

Selected tibial plateau fractures may be reduced, grafted, and fixed percutaneously utilizing arthroscopic techniques. Fluoroscopy during the procedure may be of some value as one begins to develop expertise; however, in time this step becomes unnecessary. Certain fractures may be managed by closed reduction alone with direct observation of the reduction via the arthroscope. In many fractures elevation of the plateau will be necessary, and in some of these, bone grafting to maintain the reduction will also be necessary. Percutaneous fixation has generally been accomplished with either a Web bolt or cancellous lag screw.

Fracture types that have been amenable to arthroscopic reduction and fixation include the longitudinal split, which may be displaced or nondisplaced and be in any plane. Depressed fractures are also amenable to elevation, bone grafting, and percutaneous fixation. Perhaps one of the most common fracture types is the combined longitudinal split with central depression. These fracture types, even though somewhat complex, may also be elevated, grafted, and fixed arthroscopically. The severely comminuted fracture, however, is very difficult to handle arthroscopically. Good fracture management would dictate the application of one or more buttress plates which, of course, requires an open procedure. Also in these severely comminuted fractures, landmarks for reference may be absent, making accurate reduction extremely difficult.

The simple split fracture is the easiest of the tibial plateau fractures to treat arthroscopically. If the split is simply widened and the fragment is not depressed, a closed reduction may be obtained by manual compression and then assessed arthroscopically. One or more Web bolts or lag screws are then placed transversely across the fracture, and as compression is applied, the fracture line will be seen to close. Usually an anatomical reduction can be obtained with these fractures. If the split fragment is depressed, it may be secured with a smooth Steinman pin and elevated; then the pin is driven across the fracture site. Once again Web bolts or lag screws are placed percutaneously to apply compression and secure internal fixation. The Steinman pin is then removed.

Depressed fractures are somewhat more difficult to manage arthroscopically and require a limited incision anteriorly. After thorough study of the fracture, a ½- to 1-inch transverse incision is made anteriorly just below the flare of the tibia and under the same compartment as the fracture. The anterior cortex of the tibia is exposed subperiosteally, and two to three small drill holes are placed through the anterior cortex and connected with a ½-inch osteotome. The osteotome is then driven under the fracture and the fragments are elevated. Initially one may wish to utilize fluoroscopy to place this osteotome under the fracture fragment; however, with experience this step will become unnecessary. Each fragment can be elevated individually while being viewed with the arthroscope. This technique has been termed "indirect triangulation."

The meniscus, if present, will act as a landmark to determine the proper amount of elevation. In most cases a satisfactory reduction may be obtained by overelevating the fracture, releasing the stress on the knee, and placing the joint through a range of motion. The femoral condyle will then "mold" the fragments, resulting in a fairly close approximation of the normal shape of the tibial plateau. The fracture fragments may then be manipulated from above with a hook probe as necessary, and each fragment is then tested with the probe to determine its stability. If the depression has been more than 5 mm, a bone graft will generally be required. A cancellous and cortical graft is taken from the previously prepared iliac crest and placed through the small window in the anterior cortex under the fracture until stability has been obtained.

The most common type of tibial plateau fracture encountered in our series was a Hohl type III, involving both depression and fracture of the medial or lateral wall of the tibia. These fractures are managed by utilizing both of the techniques just described. Elevation and bone grafting of the fracture should be accomplished first, and then a lag screw or Web bolt fixation should be performed as the last step.

In all cases biplaner x-rays should be obtained to determine and document reduction of the fracture and placement of internal fixation devices. Hemovac tubes are utilized routinely to drain the knee postoperatively.

Postoperative management should be tailored to the individual patient and based on the final stability of the fracture. Early motion is beneficial but not at the expense losing the reduction of the fracture. Accordingly, the fracture may be managed with a continuous passive motion machine, traction with or without motion, or a cast brace. In some instances early motion with non-weight bearing on crutches will be appropriate. In other cases, a period of immobilization in a cast will be necessary.

## Summary

The arthroscope has proven to be a particulary useful tool in the management of tibial plateau fractures. The ability to accurately define the fracture and diagnose concomitant soft tissue injuries is most valuable in planning management. Selected fractures may be reduced, internally fixed, and/or grafted arthroscopically; however, these techniques are demanding and require considerable arthroscopic experience. In all cases the surgeon should adhere to principles of good fracture management and should not hesitate to open these fractures or treat them in a more conventional manner. Finally, arthroscopy allows the postoperative management of fractures to be tailored to the individual patient and fracture.

### *References*

1. Apley AG. Fractures of the lateral tibial condyle treated by skeletal traction and early mobilization: A review of sixty cases with special reference to long term results. J Bone Joint Surg [Br], 38:699–708, 1956
2. Bowes DN, Hohl M. Tibial condylar fractures: Evaluation of treatment and outcome. Clin Orthop 171:104–108, 1982

3. Brown GA, Sprague BL. Cast brace treatment of plateau and bicondylar fractures of the proximal tibia. Clin Orthop 119:184–193, 1976
4. Caspari RB, Hutton PMJ, Whipple TL, Meyers JF. The role of arthroscopy in the management of tibial plateau fractures. Paper presented at the Semiannual Meeting of the American Orthopaedic Society for Sports Medicine, Anaheim, CA, 1984
5. Drennan B, Locher FG, Maylahn DJ. Fractures of the tibial plateau: Treatment by closed reduction and spica cast. J Bone Joint Surg [Am] 61:989–995, 1979
6. Elstrom J, Pankovich AM, Sasoon H, Rodriguez J. The use of tomography in the assessment of fractures of the tibial plateau. J Bone Joint Surg [Am] 58:551–555, 1976
7. Fagerberg S. Tomographic analysis of depressed fractures within the knee joint and of injuries to the cruciate ligaments. Acta Orthop Scand 27:219–227, 1958
8. Hohl M. Tibial condylar fractures. J Bone Joint Surg [Am] 49:1455–1467, 1967
9. Hohl M. Tibial condylar fractures—Long term follow up. Tex Med 70:46–54, 1974
10. Hohl M. Treatment methods in tibial condylar fractures. South Med J 68:985–991, 1975
11. Holh M, Luck J. Fractures of the tibial condyle: A clinical and experimental study. J Bone Joint Surg [Am] 38:1001–1018, 1956
12. Jennings JE. Arthroscopic management of tibial plateau fractures. Paper presented at the Annual Meeting of the Arthroscopy Association of North America, New Orleans, 1984
13. Martin AF. The pathomechanics of the knee joint, the medial collateral ligament and lateral tibial plateau fractures. J Bone Joint Surg [Am] 42:13–22, 1960
14. Moore TM, Harvey JP Jr. Roentgenographic measurement of tibial plateau depression due to fracture. J Bone Joint Surg [Am] 56:155–160, 1974
15. Moore TM, Meyers MH, Harvey JP Jr. Collateral ligament laxity of the knee: Long term comparison between plateau fractures and normal. J Bone Joint Surg [Am] 58:594–598, 1976
16. Neviaser JS, Eisenberg SH. Diagnostic and therapeutic obstacles encountered in tibial plateau fractures. Bull Hosp Joint Dis 17:48–57, 1956
17. Newburg AH, Greenstein R. Radiographic evaluation of tibial plateau fractures. Radiology 126:319–323, 1978
18. Reiner MJ. The arthroscope in tibial plateau fractures: Its use in evaluation of soft tissue and bony injury. J Am Osteopath Assoc 81:704–705, 1982
19. Rasmussen PS. Tibial condylar fractures: Impairment of knee joint stability as an indication for surgical treatment. J Bone Joint Surg [Am] 55:1331–1350, 1973
20. Rockwood CA, Green DP. Fractures in Adults, 2nd ed. JP Lippincott, Philadelphia, 1984
21. Rombold C. Depressed fractures of the tibial plateau: Treatment with rigid internal fixation and early mobilization—A preliminary report. J Bone Joint Surg [Am] 42:783–797, 1960
22. Sarmiento A, Kinman PG, Latta L. Fractures of the proximal tibia and tibial condyles: A clinical and laboratory comparative study. Clin Orthop 145:136–145, 1979
23. Waddell JP, Johnson DWC, Neidre A. Fractures of the tibial plateau: A review of ninety-five patients and comparison of treatment methods. J Trauma 21:376–381, 1981
24. Wilppula E, Bakalim G. Ligamentous tear concomitant with tibial condyle fracture. Acta Orthop Scand 43:292–300, 1972

# Arthroscopic Management of Anterior Cruciate Ligament Tears

# 11

Joe W. Tippett

Dealing with the anterior cruciate ligament tear has been a controversial subject over the past twenty years and still remains unresolved as no one treatment or procedure provides the end results of a "normal knee." Identifying structural anatomy and its importance to joint function has resulted in more aggressive reparative procedures in order to achieve a higher percentage of stable functional knees.

## Anatomy and Biomechanics

The anterior cruciate ligament, averaging 38 mm by 11 mm, originates from the anterior surface of the tibial plateau lateral to the tibial spine and passes beneath the transverse meniscal ligament, to blend with the attachment of the lateral meniscus. This ligament transverses the lateral portion of the intercondylar notch to insert with a broad attachment over the posterior medial surface of the lateral femoral condyle. The tibial attachment is somewhat wider and stronger than the femoral insertion, probably resulting in the tendency for more tears in the proximal portion. The anterior cruciate ligament is not a single synovia-encased cord but consists of twisted bundles of individual fibers (Figure 11–1) divided into an anterior medial band and a larger posterior lateral bundle. The spiral orientation of the fibers provides tension on some portion of the ligament throughout the entire range of flexion and extension (8, 12). With the knee in extension, the posterior lateral bundle is tight with varying degrees of anterior medial band relaxation. In flexion the opposite occurs as the femoral attachment moves from a vertical to a

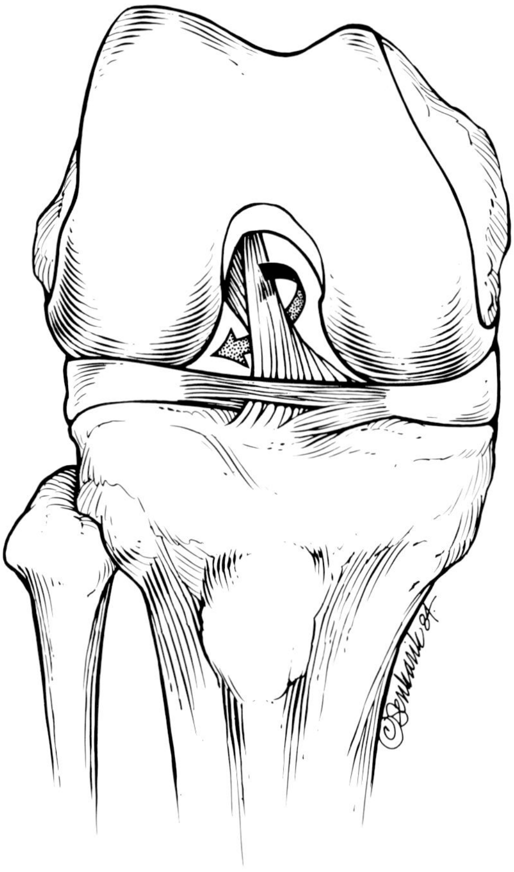

**Figure 11–1** Schematic demonstrating a multifascicular structure. [Adapted from Arnoczky (2).]

horizontal orientation (Figure 11–2). It is clinically important in management and rehabilitation to recognize that some portion of the anterior cruciate ligament remains under tension throughout the range of motion, with no known correlation, however, between the degree of flexion and tension distribution.

The major vascular supply of the anterior cruciate ligament is from the synovial fold that is generously provided by the middle genicular artery (16). This rich network of capillaries penetrates the ligament, making it totally independent of the blood supply from the ligamentous attachment to the femoral and tibial epiphyses. This suggests the preservation and utilization of synovium in the repair of the anterior cruciate ligament and accounts for the rapid synovial overgrowth encountered soon after injury in the acutely traumatized knee.

The anterior cruciate ligament is a very complex ligament with multiple functions that vary depending on the position of the knee. It is important as a constraint to joint motion, being the first line of defense against hyperextension (2) and anterior displacement of the tibia on the femur (9). A rupture of the anterior medial band functionally allows a positive anterior drawer in flexion, whereas a positive anterior drawer in extension suggests a torn posterior lateral bundle. Besides the forward motion, the tibia rotates on the femur during the entire range of motion. The anterior cruciate ligament predominately limits its external rotation in flexion, with slightly less control of internal rotation in extension and during valgus stress.

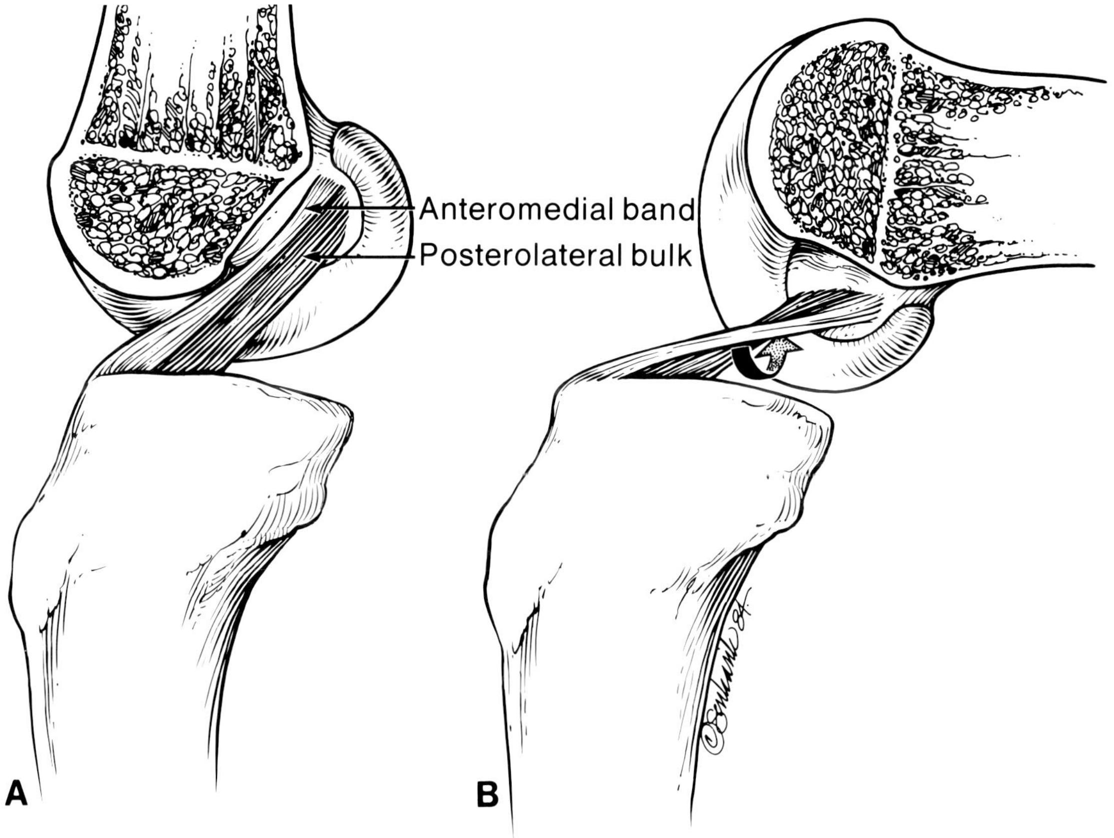


**Figure 11–2** Schematic drawing of the anterior cruciate representating the tension on the anteromedial band and posterolateral bulk in flexion and extension. [Adapted from Girgis et al. (8).]

Due to the spatial orientation of the bundles in the anterior cruciate ligament and the arrangement of the secondary restraints, there are two predominant basic mechanisms that will produce tears. First, hyperextension of the knee with the leg internally rotated usually causes the "isolated" anterior cruciate ligament tear. This type of rupture may or may not be associated with a contact force to the knee since it can occur while jumping, as in basketball or volleyball. Second, external rotation of the tibia with the knee flexed and a valgus stress applied will tear the anterior cruciate ligament, but usually with some medial collateral ligament injury and meniscal damage. This stress does not have to be an external force but may be due to body rotation on the fixed foot. More than 90% of these anterior cruciate ligament tears occur in the main substance, usually the proximal one-half of the ligament; about 7% of the ligaments are pulled from the femur as a periosteal avulsion; and the remaining 3% are avulsed from the tibia, frequently with a fragment of bone attached.

The occurrence of isolated lesions of the anterior cruciate ligament is doubtful. A significant number of cases will have associated interstitial damage in the ligament and the capsule itself. In his acute anterior cruciate series, DeHaven (4) has reported 65% with associated medial or lateral meniscal tears and 6% with osteochondral fractures.

## Clinical Evaluation

A traumatic episode to the knee during athletics, occupation, or vehicle injury that results in severe pain, a popping sensation, inability to further participate, a giving way, and swelling within a few hours should alert us to be highly suspicious of an "isolated" anterior cruciate ligament tear. A systematic examination usually reveals an intense effusion due to hemarthrosis. The bloody fluid that is aspirated should be examined for fat, which indicates àvulsion of the anterior cruciate ligament bony attachment. Instillation of Marcaine or Xylocaine into the acute knee will provide a less painful knee and thus a more accurate examination. Deep palpation of the joint lines and ligament attachments for tenderness and swelling delineates associated ligament pathology. The anterior drawer test is reliable in only 10% of the acute cases because it requires flexion which is usually too painful in the acute knee. In contrast, a Lachman test may be performed with 80% accuracy in awake patients and 100% accuracy in patients under general anesthesia (4). In the acute knee a pivot shaft, indicating anterolateral rotatory instability, is diagnostic but will be difficult to determine in 90% of the cases because the knee cannot extend fully secondary to hemarthrosis with attendant spasm of the hamstring and injured secondary restraints. Examination under general anesthesia, therefore, is recommended in all doubtful cases.

X-rays should be taken to rule out fractures and resultant articular cartilage involvement, but very little information can be gained from the plain film with reference to the anterior cruciate ligament injury. The double contrast arthrogram is not more than 90% accurate in cruciate ligament tears (10, 13, 14), whereas clinical examination under anesthesia can be 100% accurate. The former technique is limited because only the synovial surface of the ligament is outlined and not the ligament substance itself (20). A significant number of substance tears are missed because they do occur with the synovial sheaths still intact.

The treatment of the anterior cruciate ligament is still controversial. Patients with acute partial tears and minimal instability who are in a low-risk category, consisting of the older age group with sedentary occupations and no athletic inclinations, may be treated by immobilization with a hinged brace. This allows secondary restraints, such as the collateral, the oblique, and the capsular ligaments, to heal rather than to be continuously stretched. After an intense rehabilitation program, the patient may return to normal activity. If any athletic endeavors are contemplated, a derotational brace should be worn.

Those patients who are very unstable and in a high-risk category with strenuous demands on the knee, such as athletics and certain physically active occupations, should have an arthroscopic examination. The value of arthroscopy in diagnosing the acute anterior cruciate ligament was described by O'Connor (19). Today, the arthroscope is considered an efficient instrument for removing blood from the joint to decrease synovitis and scarring, contrary to earlier opinions that arthroscopy of the acute knee was contraindicated (3). It eliminates missed or undiagnosed tears (5), helps evaluate partial or complete tears, establishes the location of the tear, and confirms associated meniscal lesions. These findings of meniscal and associated pathology can be treated expediently and precisely through the arthroscope by partial excision, meniscoresis, or nonintervention, thus allowing healing by immobilization.

The active individual who has a partial tear and a moderate degree of instability may be treated by one of the extra-articular procedures, such as described by Andrews or Ellison, to create a lateral dominant knee and stability for the injured secondary restraints (1, 6). The grossly unstable knee with a midsubstance cruciate tear in the young high-risk patient requires the maximum amount of stabilization, either by a primary repair (7, 17, 23) being reinforced by an intra-articular stint, or by a tendon substitution such as the semitendinosus muscle (18), a vascularized patellar tendon graft (21), or an iliotibial band (15). In conjunction, an extra-articular procedure may also be required. Investigators are studying an endoscopic technique of graft insertion in these cases, using fresh tendons, freeze-dried tendons, fascia lata, or synthetic materials.

The anterior cruciate ligament partially avulsed with a bony fragment from the tibia usually is reduced with extension after the bloody effusion is aspirated. If the x-ray examination shows no significant separation on extension, the injury is treated with a hinged knee brace for approximately 1 month. If reduction is imperfect, then it should be repaired surgically, either through an arthrotomy incision or through an arthroscope with sutures brought out through drill holes over the anterior medial aspect of the tibia.

The ligament avulsed from the femoral insertion cannot be treated in a closed manner due to its inability to reduce spontaneously in the anatomical position with aspiration and leg positioning. This type of injury has been diagnosed more frequently since routine arthroscopy was initiated. These lesions require a primary repair, again either by means of an arthrotomy or arthroscope.

## Clinical Experience

Over the past 5 years, 19 isolated anterior cruciate ligament tears from the tibial or femoral insertion were repaired arthroscopically. We believe that midsubstance tears or those associated with collateral ligament damage still require the standard arthrotomy approach. Arthroscopic repair of these is technically difficult, although it is still under intense investigation. In this series 58% were males with an average age of 25 years (range, 7–43 years). They were all repaired within 15 days of injury, which classifies them as acute knees. The causes of injury ranged from simple twisting and falling off a horse to strenuous competitive athletics.

Ninety-four percent of the patients presented with effusion and inability to participate further in various activities, with 88% suffering severe pain. The sensation of giving way and popping was only occasionally present in this series (Table 11–1). On examination under local anesthesia, the abduction and adduction tests were 100% negative, denoting no medial or lateral instability. The pivot shift test could be carried out in only one patient while the Lachman was impossible in one-third of the group due to pain and discomfort. However, in those patients who could tolerate it, it was positive in 92%. Difficulty in relaxing the hamstring muscles hindered the reliability of the anterior drawer test (Table 11–2). Under general anesthesia 100% of the pivot shift and Lachman tests became positive while 79% of the anterior drawer tests were positive (Table 11–3).

## Examination Procedures

Under general anesthesia the knee is prepped and draped with impermeable sheeting, and a tourniquet is applied to minimize bleeding, thus producing optimal conditions for viewing and suturing. A 5-mm arthroscope is inserted through the inferior lateral portal with a 4-mm perforated cannula as outflow in the superior lateral portal. The acute hemarthrosis, or bloody effusion, can be evacuated rapidly with a constant inflow of saline from 3-liter bags through the arthroscope itself, providing a clear visual field.

**Table 11–1** Multiple Symptomatic Complaints in Percentages for the Acutely Torn Anterior Cruciate

| PATIENTS INITIALS | TIME AFTER INJURY TO SURGERY DAYS | COMPLAINTS | | | | |
|---|---|---|---|---|---|---|
| | | Giving Way | "Pop" | Effusion | Severe Pain | Inability to Participate |
| LA | 1 | NO | NO | NO | YES | YES |
| BB | 0 | NO | NO | YES | YES | YES |
| MB | 1 | NO | YES | YES | YES | YES |
| CB | 8 | NO | NO | YES | YES | YES |
| MB | 7 | NO | NO | YES | NO | YES |
| DB | 1 | NO | NO | YES | NO | YES |
| TB | 2 | NO | NO | YES | YES | YES |
| JC | 2 | NO | NO | YES | YES | YES |
| KH | 2 | NO | YES | YES | YES | YES |
| PH | 1 | NO | NO | YES | YES | YES |
| RJ | 2 | YES | NO | YES | YES | YES |
| DJ | 15 | YES | NO | YES | YES | YES |
| DK | 0 | NO | NO | YES | YES | YES |
| DM | 5 | NO | YES | YES | YES | YES |
| JR | 4 | NO | NO | YES | YES | YES |
| LR | 4 | NO | NO | YES | NO | NO |
| DR | 1 | NO | NO | YES | YES | YES |
| JW | 2 | NO | NO | YES | YES | YES |
| BZ | 7 | NO | NO | YES | YES | YES |
| | | 10% | 15% | 94% | 84% | 94% |

Once the knee is cleared of blood, the leg is brought off the side of the table and flexed 70 degrees at the knee with the foot resting on the operator's lap. The arthroscope is inserted into the transpatellar portal, leaving the inferior medial and

**Table 11–2** Pre-anesthetic Examination Reveals that Adduction and Abduction Tests Were Negative, but Only Able to Perform One Pivot Shift*

| PATIENTS INITIALS | TIME AFTER INJURY TO SURGERY DAYS | PRE-ANESTHETIC PHYSICAL EXAMINATION | | | | |
|---|---|---|---|---|---|---|
| | | Abduction | Adduction | Pivot (ALRI) | Lachman | Anterior Draw |
| LA | 1 | NEG | NEG | CT* | CT | CT |
| BB | 0 | NEG | NEG | CT | + | CT |
| MB | 1 | NEG | NEG | CT | + | CT |
| CB | 8 | NEG | NEG | CT | CT | CT |
| MB | 7 | NEG | NEG | CT | + | CT |
| DB | 1 | NEG | NEG | CT | CT | CT |
| TB | 2 | NEG | NEG | CT | + | CT |
| JC | 2 | NEG | NEG | CT | CT | CT |
| KH | 2 | NEG | NEG | CT | + | CT |
| PH | 1 | NEG | NEG | CT | + | CT |
| RJ | 2 | NEG | NEG | CT | CT | CT |
| DJ | 15 | NEG | NEG | CT | + | + |
| DK | 0 | NEG | NEG | CT | CT | CT |
| DM | 5 | NEG | NEG | CT | + | + |
| JR | 4 | NEG | NEG | CT | NEG | NEG |
| LR | 4 | NEG | NEG | CT | + | CT |
| DR | 1 | NEG | NEG | CT | CT | CT |
| JW | 2 | NEG | NEG | + | + | CT |
| BZ | 7 | NEG | NEG | CT | + | NEG |
| *CANNOT TEST | | ALL NEG | ALL NEG | 18 CT | 7 CT | 15 CT |

*The Lachman test performed 12 times, with the anterior draw test performed in only four cases.

**Table 11–3** Under General Anesthesia the Pivot Shift and Lachman Test Was Positive 100%, with the Anterior Draw Positive 79%

| PATIENTS INITIALS | PHYSICAL EXAMINATION UNDER ANESTHETIC | | |
|---|---|---|---|
| | Pivot | Lachman | Anterior Draw |
| LA | 1+ | 2+ | 1+ |
| BB | 1+ | 1+ | 1+ |
| MB | 2+ | 2+ | 2+ |
| CB | 3+ | 3+ | 3+ |
| MB | 1+ | 1+ | 1+ |
| DB | 1+ | 1+ | – |
| TB | 2+ | 2+ | 2+ |
| JC | 1+ | 1+ | – |
| KH | 2+ | 2+ | 2+ |
| PH | 1+ | 1+ | 1+ |
| RJ | 2+ | 2+ | 2+ |
| DJ | 3+ | 3+ | 2+ |
| DK | 1+ | 1+ | – |
| DM | 2+ | 2+ | 1+ |
| JR | 3+ | 3+ | 2+ |
| LR | 2+ | 2+ | 1+ |
| DR | 1+ | 1+ | – |
| TW | 1+ | 1+ | 1+ |
| BZ | 2+ | 2+ | 1+ |
| | 100% | 100% | 79% |

inferior lateral portals open for instrumentation. The synovium over the anterior border of both menisci and the infrapatellar plica (ligamentous mucosa) must be resected by a synovial resector to allow the fat pad to retract with saline distension and afford an unobstructed anterior view of all three compartments. Associated meniscal lesions are then evaluated. Peripheral tears in the zone of vascularity usually will heal spontaneously. Double buck-handle, major flap, and radial tears are excised with basket forceps. In all cases a posterior medial portal is made to examine the posterior one-third of the meniscus for flap tears that appear behind the femoral condyle and can so easily be missed on routine examination. Direct visualization of the posterior cruciate ligament is also possible through this portal, and it found to be involved in about 3% of the acute knee injuries.

In our series arthroscopy demonstrated the cruciate ligament to be torn from the tibia in 26% of cases and from the femur in 74% of cases. There were 10 associated meniscal tears or a 53% occurrence. The one vertical tear in the inner one-third of the posterior horn of the medial meniscus and the six vertical tears of the lateral menisci were excised with a basket forcep, while the three tears of the meniscoligamentous junction of the posterior portion of the lateral meniscus were treated with no surgical intervention. There were no osteochondral fractures or associated ligamentous injuries.

## Repair Techniques

In describing our technique of arthroscopic repair of the anterior cruciate ligament, the right leg will be considered. The reverse of this method would be applicable if the injury were on the left knee. Once the intercondylar compartment is cleared, an Ethicon no. 0 Prolene suture on a M07 needle is passed through the inferior medial portal with the tip and base of the needle covered by a Pilling vascular needle holder (Figure 11–3). The needle, free inside the joint, is grasped to start a reverse Bunnell stitch on the medial edge of the ligament from the torn surface

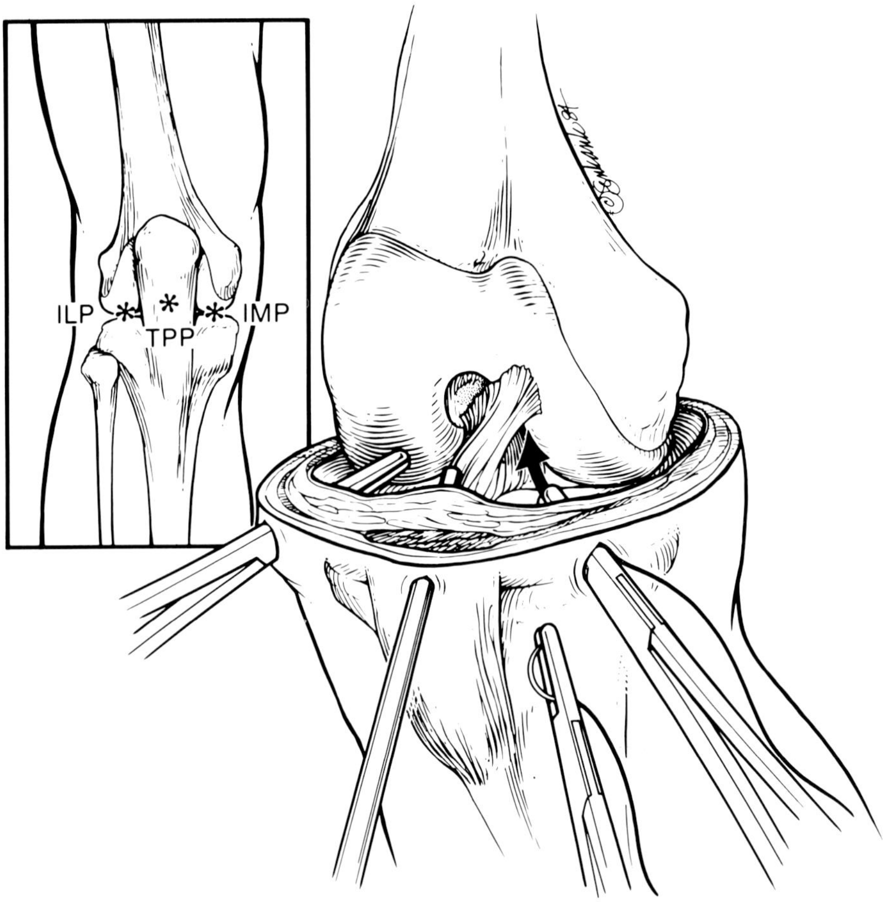


**Figure 11–3** Drawing demonstrating technique of multiple portals with placement of the needle into the joint ILP, inferior lateral portal; IMP, inferior medial portal; TPP,.

to the synovial surface (Figure 11–4, A and B). The tip is then grasped by a second needle holder inserted through the inferior lateral portal for needle rotation. Similar stitches continue down one limb of the anterior cruciate ligament and back up the other side until there are two suture ends exiting from the torn surface (Figure 11–4, C). The tip and base of the needle is then covered and pulled out the inferior lateral portal, leaving a piece of suture out of each inferior portal (Figure 11–5). The avulsed bed of the tibia or femur is then prepared by a curette for reinsertion of the cruciate ligament (Figure 11–6). Two suture passers, which are converted

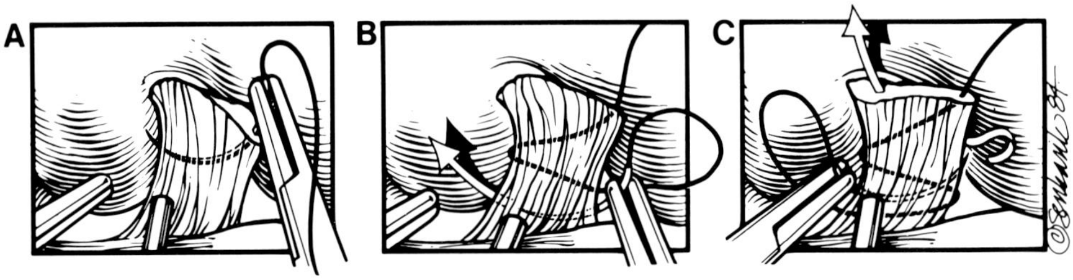


**Figure 11–4** **A** and **B** Drawing of reverse Bunnel suturing of anterior cruciate ligament. **C** Completed suturing with two sutures out the torn end.

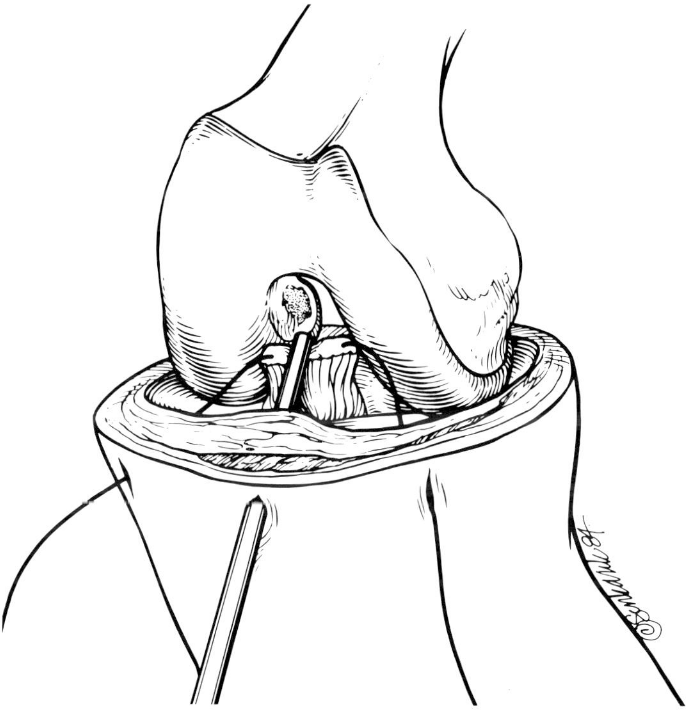

**Figure 11–5** Suture exiting out each inferior portal.

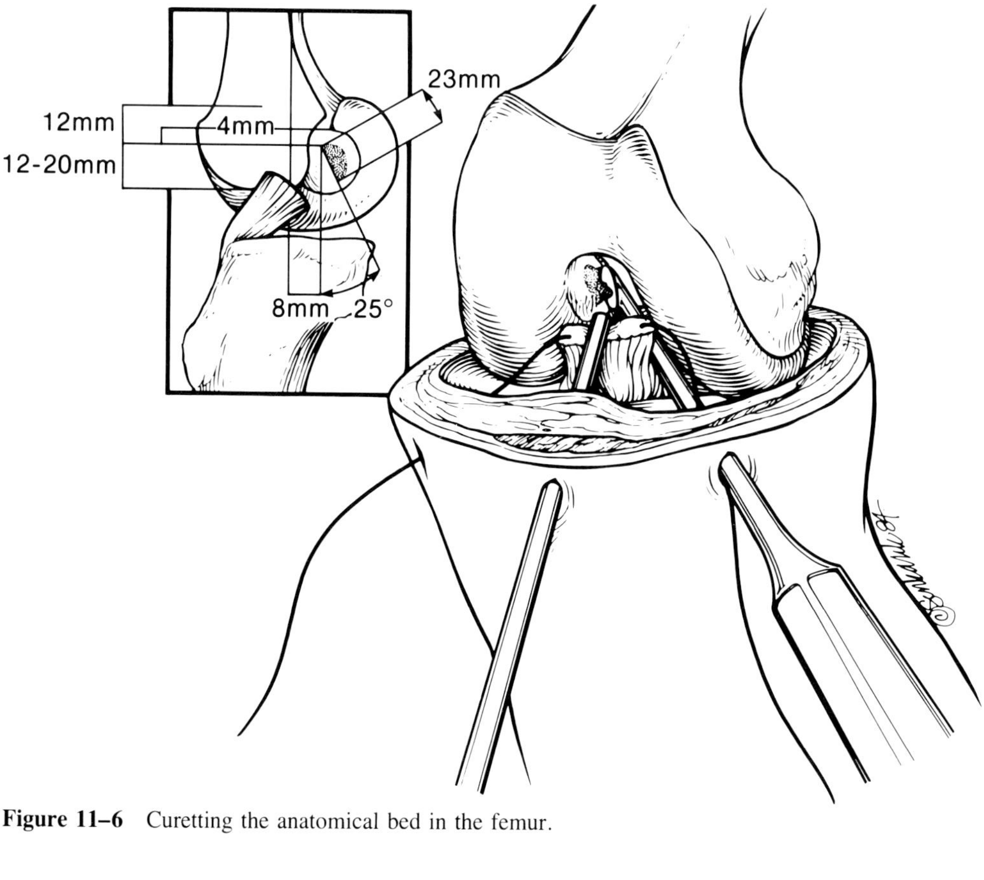


**Figure 11–6** Curetting the anatomical bed in the femur.

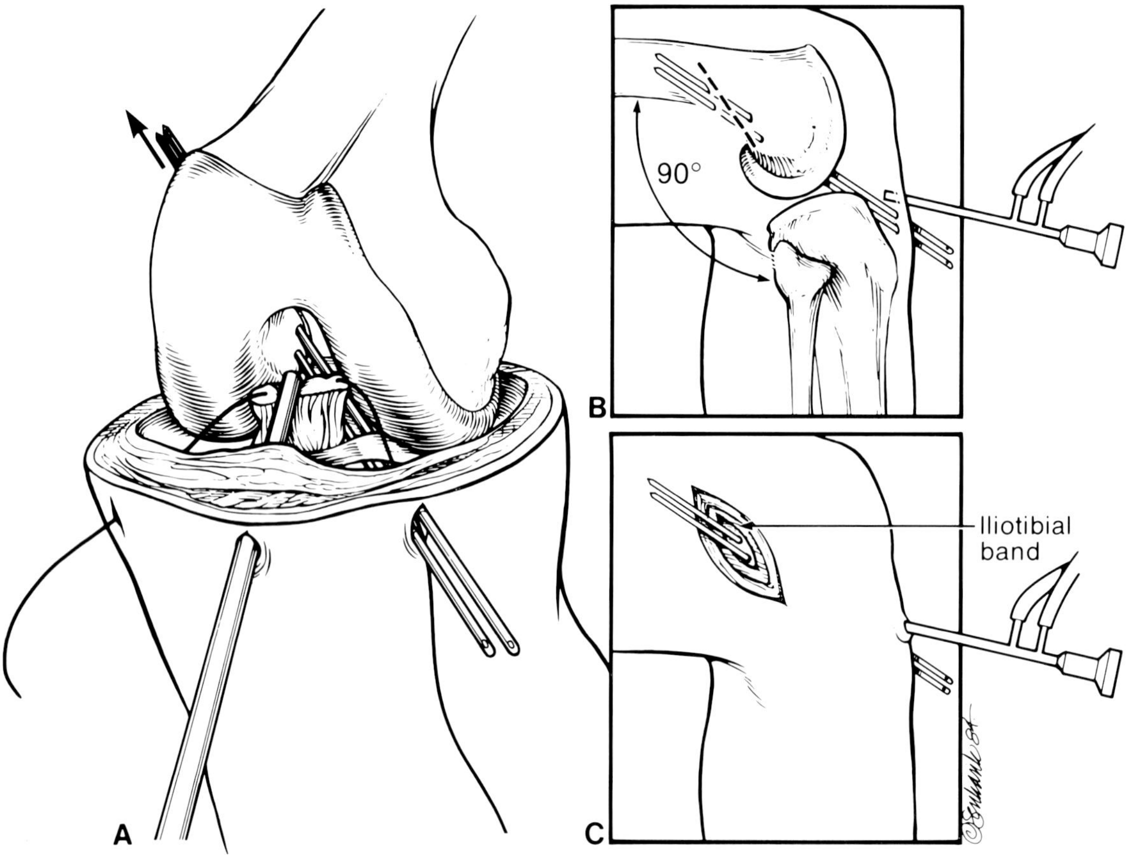


**Figure 11–7** **A** Suture passers underneath the anterior horn of the medial meniscus. **B** Knee in 90 degrees of flexion so that pins may enter anatomical site in the femur. **C** Incision over lateral side of the femur to the periosteum prior to pulling sutures through.

3/32 in. Steinmann pins, are drilled either percutaneously through the anterior medial aspect of the tibia for the tibial reattachment, or through the anterior medial aspect of the joint line underneath the meniscus into the notch for the femoral reattachment (Figure 11–7, A). The knee must be flexed 90 degrees so that the suture passers will enter the anatomical insertion on the posterior medial aspect of the lateral femoral condyle (Figure 11–7, B). When proper position has been obtained, a skin incision is made over the pins on the posterior lateral side of the femur and dissected to the periosteum (Figure 11–7, C).

The suture from the inferior lateral portal is pulled into the knee joint and passed through the lateral pin while the medial suture is placed in the medial pin (Figure 11–8, A). Then both pins are removed from the joint. Prior to tying the suture over the periosteum of the anterior medial tibia or of the lateral femur, the torn cruciate ends are tucked into the avulsed bed (Figure 11–8, B and C).

Postoperatively the patient is placed in a hinged brace that is set initially at 60 degrees flexion. Over a 6-week period this flexion is progressively advanced, 10 degrees every 2 weeks. While the patient is wearing the brace, straight-leg raising and quadriceps exercising are encouraged from day 1. With the brace off, range-of-motion exercise is started, and once 30 to 110 degrees flexion has been obtained, isotonic exercises of the hamstrings with light weights are begun and progressed as tolerated. The hamstrings are emphasized because they do not produce stress on the repaired anterior cruciate ligament. Also, they play an important role in centering the tibia beneath the femoral condyle. Quadriceps isotonic exer-

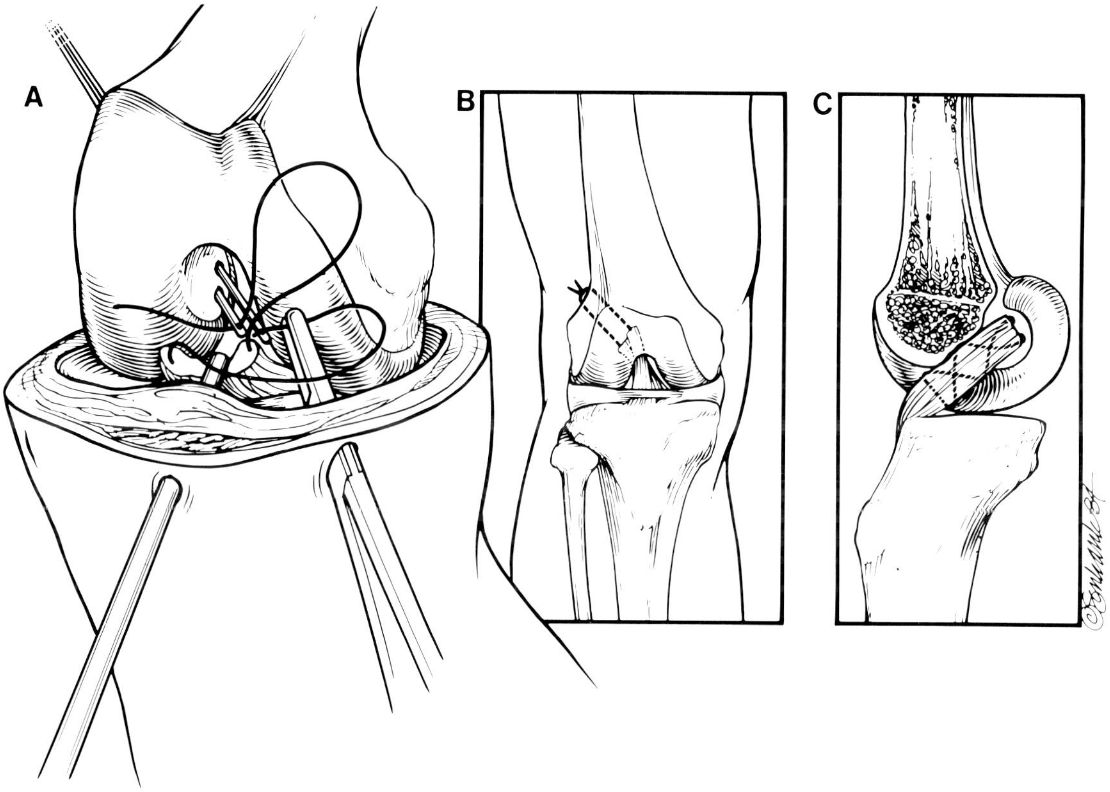


**Figure 11–8** **A** Sutures pulled into the joint and placed through the two pins. **B** and **C** Drawing showing anterior cruciate replaced into anatomical position and tied over periosteum.

cises are also begun with very light weights (3–5 pounds) in a short flexion arc not to extend beyond 30 degrees for the first 6 weeks out of the brace. This prevents anterior draw force on the tibia (22), thus protecting the unorganized collagen of the repaired anterior cruciate ligament. The two other exercises stressed in the rehabilitation program are bicycling and swimming. The bicycle should have the seat set to attain 30 degrees of knee flexion at the low point of the stroke. This provides anterior cruciate ligament protection and patellar motion, which nourishes the articular cartilage and prevents its deterioration. Swimming allows an antigravity environment for active range-of-motion and muscle exercises in a fluid medium resistive to all the lower extremity musculature.

Once the patient lacks only 10 degrees of extension, partial weight bearing is begun. The patient is maintained on a 9-month course of rehabilitation, and when the girth of thigh and calf muscles is equal to that of the opposite side, the patient may resume sporting activity, protected by a derotational brace. These knees are not tested with any type of Cybex machine during the first 9 months because maximum contraction of the quadriceps to obtain extension creates a nonphysiological stress upon the anterior cruciate ligament.

## Follow-up Study

Of the 19 patients reported here, only 1 was lost to follow up. All of the remaining 18 have resumed their daily activity without limitation. Of the eight who injured their knees participating in a sporting event, all have returned to their previous sport, with three playing football without the derotational brace that was advised. Only two have some intermittent pain with heavy work and one has occasional effusion.

Evaluating themselves, 94% felt that their knees were normal, even the patient with intermittent effusion. The remaining 6% felt they had improved with the surgery. Objectively, range-of-motion measurements showed 88% had full extension and only two patients who were 3 to 4 months postoperative lacked the last few degrees. All the patients that were over 1 year postoperative regained quadriceps and hamstring size as compared to the opposite leg. On clinical testing 83% showed improved Lachman and anterior drawer test results and 89% showed improvement in the pivot shift test (Table 11–4). These tests showed no deterioration in knee stability over the 5-year study.

The knee laxity tester developed by Cannon was used postoperatively to test the stability obtained with our repairs in 16 patients. Measuring the amount of anterior displacement from a pull of 20 pounds and from a pull of 40 pounds (Figures 11–9, 11–10) and also the amount of total sagittal displacement (Figure 11–11) showed an increased displacement over the normal opposite knee of only 1.5, 1.5, and 0.25 mm, respectively. When compared to Cannon's measurements in his patients (W. D. Cannon, personal communication) with unrepaired torn cruciate ligament (7.1, 8.6, and 7.6 mm, respectively), it became evident that arthroscopic repair of the torn anterior cruciate ligament resulted in significant improvement toward normal function. A rather impressive fact surfaced when measured displacement was plotted against length of time postoperatively. Studying Figure 11–12, we see no indication that with passage of time the stability of the repaired knee had deteriorated. Further evaluation both pre- and postoperatively using this tester is under investigation to correlate the results of the 40-pound pull with the findings on arthroscopic examination.

**Table 11–4** The Clinical Testing Before and After Surgery Shows 83% Improvement in Lachman, Anterior Draw, and 89% in Pivot Shift

| | MANUAL STABILITY TESTING | | | | | |
|---|---|---|---|---|---|---|
| PATIENTS | Lachman | | Pivot | | Anterior Draw | |
| INITIALS | Preop | Postop | Preop | Postop | Preop | Postop |
| LA | 2+ | NEG | 1+ | NEG | 1+ | NEG |
| BB | 1+ | NEG | 1+ | NEG | 1+ | NEG |
| MB | 2+ | NEG | 2+ | NEG | 2+ | NEG |
| CB | 3+ | LOST | 3+ | LOST | 3+ | LOST |
| MB | 1+ | 1+ | 1+ | 1+ | 1+ | 1+ |
| DB | 1+ | NEG | 1+ | NEG | 1+ | NEG |
| TB | 2+ | NEG | 2+ | NEG | 2+ | NEG |
| JC | 1+ | NEG | 1+ | NEG | 1+ | NEG |
| PH | 1+ | NEG | 1+ | NEG | 1+ | 1+ |
| RJ | 2+ | NEG | 2+ | NEG | 2+ | 1+ |
| DJ | 3+ | 2+ | 3+ | 2+ | 2+ | 1+ |
| DK | 1+ | NEG | 1+ | NEG | NEG | NEG |
| DM | 2+ | 1+ | 2+ | 1+ | 1+ | NEG |
| JR | 3+ | NEG | 3+ | NEG | 2+ | NEG |
| LR | 2+ | NEG | 2+ | NEG | 1+ | NEG |
| DR | 1+ | NEG | 1+ | NEG | 1+ | NEG |
| TW | 1+ | 1+ | 1+ | 1+ | 1+ | NEG |
| BZ | 2+ | 1+ | 2+ | 1+ | 1+ | 1+ |
| | 83% | | 89% | | 83% | |

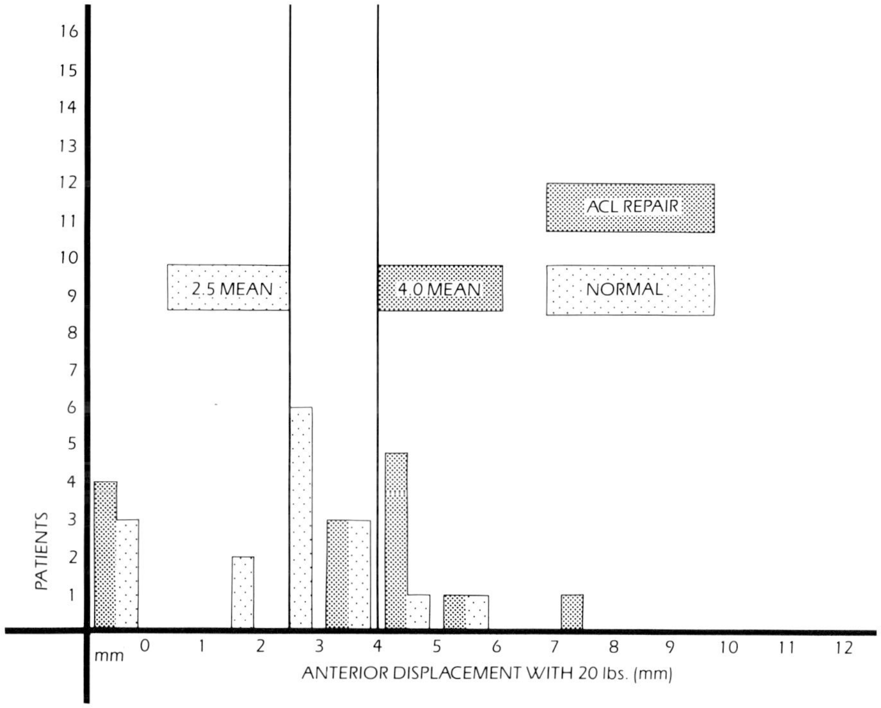


**Figure 11–9** The pre-anesthetic examination reveals that adduction and abduction tests were negative, but only able to perform one pivot shift. The Lachman test performed 12 times, with the anterior draw test performed in only four cases.

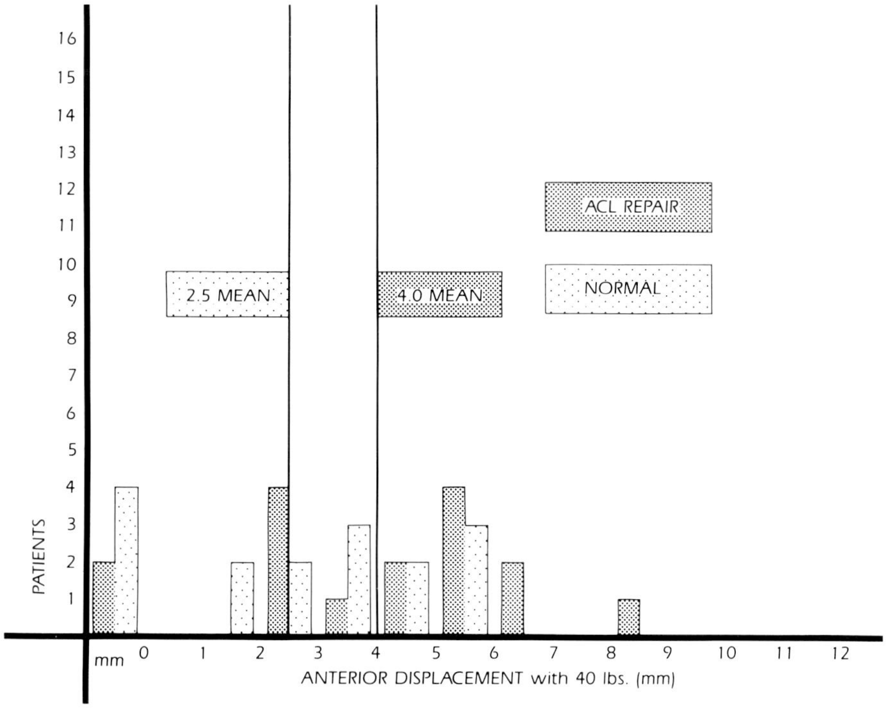


**Figure 11–10** Multiple symptomatic complaints in percentages for the acutely torn anterior cruciate.

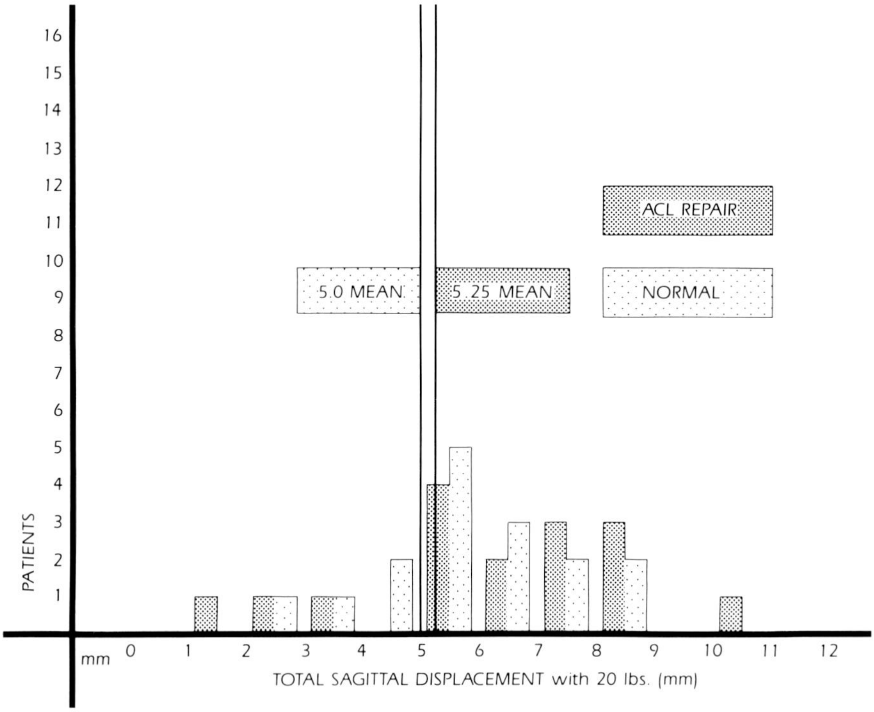


**Figure 11–11** Under general anesthesia the pivot shift and Lachman test was positive 100%, with the anterior draw positive 79%.

# Discussion

In the acutely injured knee with swelling and severe pain, when the physical examination produced little evidence of lateral instability but gave positive Lachman and pivot shift test results under general anesthesia, we concluded that an isolated tear of the anterior cruciate existed. Diagnostic arthroscopy is indicated depending on the age, occupation, activity level, and severity of dysfunction and instability. Although the early pioneers such as Watanabe et al. (24), Jackson and Abe (11), and Casscells (3) wrote that arthroscopy in the face of acute hemarthrosis was contraindicated, O'Connor (20) in 1974 solved the problem by irrigation with a Toomey syringe and using a 15-gauge needle to remove the clots. Over the past 10 years, technical advances in instrumentation and biomechanical skills have resulted in use of the arthroscope and a large-bore cannula to allow irrigation with copious amounts of saline. It now requires only a few minutes to evacuate the bloody effusion that is nearly always pathognomonic of ligamentous tears.

After resection of the voluminous synovium hypertrophied from the trauma, all compartments are easily visualized through the arthroscope, even the posterior recesses of the medial and lateral compartments that cannot be seen even in the open knee. This obviates the use of an arthrotomy incision to confirm the clinical impression and to determine the type of repair. Although many knees are treated conservatively, it has been noted that untreated tears, especially when associated with injured secondary restraints, lead to torn menisci and even articular cartilage damage due to the abnormal knee motion. The decision to operate in the high-risk group is very critical. It has been demonstrated that associated pathology such as chondral, osteal, and especially meniscal lesions can be accurately diagnosed and treated competently by arthroscopic techniques, thus decreasing the number of

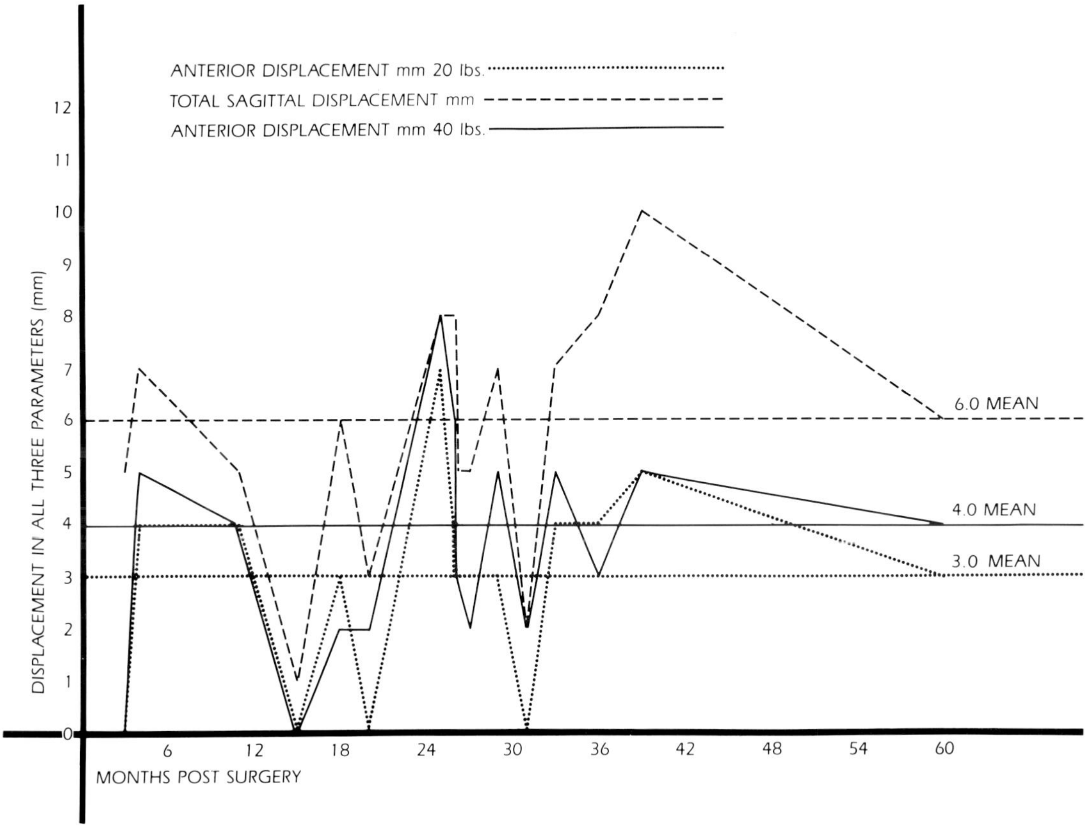


**Figure 11–12** The clinical testing before and after surgery shows 83% improvement in Lachman, anterior draw and 89% in pivot shift.

undetectable lesions. We believe that management of all torn menisci through the arthroscope is preferred, allowing removal of only the torn part and preventing the total meniscectomy necessitated by open arthrotomy.

In this series, tears of the anterior cruciate from the tibial and femoral insertions have been repaired successfully through the arthroscope. All patients resumed their preoperative activity and even competitive sports, with only two having minimal pain and effusion. Avoiding the long incision of the arthrotomy will result in less morbidity and a more rapid return to normal activities. Prolonged rehabilitation due to cutting the infrapatellar nerve, damaging the prepatellar bursa, and severing the muscles around the knee is avoided by the arthroscopic technique. No capsular incision is made, so that the patellar tracking is not altered and thus recovery time is short. The patient can be operated upon as outpatient or with a short hospital stay, thus decreasing considerably the cost to the patient.

Treatment of midsubstance tears is still controversial since the use of various graft materials under arthroscopic placement is being extensively investigated. A technique for arthroscopic repairs using multiple sutures with the appropriate drill guide and cannula system is on the horizon, awaiting development of better instrumentation. With these, sutures can be placed through the cruciate and retrieved on the tibial and femoral attachments rather than passing through the suture passer, which is technically difficult and time consuming. An internal stint of organic and nonorganic material may be used to augment the stability. If stability cannot be obtained due to extensive injury of secondary restraints, an extra-articular procedure can be used in conjunction. Morbidity from arthroscopic surgery alone or associated with extra-articular surgery is far less than that from open articular surgery. These techniques will be reported in the near future.

The immobilization and intense rehabilitation program after surgery is a very vital part of the management. Peripheral meniscoligamentous separation and some partial tears in the anterior cruciate ligament in the older nonathlete with a sedentary occupation and no desire to do any extracurricular activity or sports probably need immobilization and rehabilitation alone, proving the old adage that with immobilization and stabilization, it will heal.

The postoperative status of 18 patients was tested by various methods using manual techniques and the knee laxity tester. The results for knees with repaired anterior cruciate ligaments compared to normal knees were surprisingly good and correlated well with the patients' activity levels and self-assessments. This improvement was consistent and persisted throughout the observed period of 5 years, no deterioration being noted with the passage of time.

We propose to investigate further the use of mechanical testing devices to standardize measurement of the end results of our various methods of reconstruction. With a universally accepted method of evaluation and comparison, we can then attune our thinking and manual proficiency for the better treatment of the enigma, the acute ruptured anterior cruciate ligament.

## Summary

Treatment of acute tears of the anterior cruciate ligament has rapidly expanded in the past twenty years, but still the final answer has not been found. A method for arthroscopic repair of the torn cruciate has been presented here. Avulsion tears can be managed with this technique very effectively, but midsubstance tears still need vigorous investigation and development of new instrumentation and material for stints. The advantage for the arthroscopic approach over the open arthrotomy incision has been discussed, as well as the value of the arthroscope in the diagnosis and management of the torn meniscal lesion often associated with cruciate tears. The importance of a good rehabilitation program has been stressed, with emphasis on selected exercises from day 1 of repair. The results of the knee laxity tester have been reported with the proposal to search for a universally accepted method that will objectively measure the final results of various methods of repair for the torn anterior cruciate ligament.

### *References*

1. Andrews JR, Sanders R. A "mini-reconstruction" technique in treating anterolateral rotary instability (ALRI). Clin Orthop 172:93, 1983
2. Arnoczky SP. Anatomy of the anterior cruciate ligament. Clin Orthop 172:19, 1983
3. Casscells SW. Arthroscopy of the knee joint. A review of 150 cases. J Bone Joint Surg [Am] 53:207–298, 1971
4. DeHaven KE. Diagnosis of acute knee injuries with hemarthrosis. Am J Sports Med 8:9–14, 1980
5. DeHaven KE. Arthroscopy in the diagnosis and management of the anterior cruciate deficient knee. Clin Orthop 172:52,1983
6. Ellison AE. Distal iliotibial band transfer for anterolateral rotary instability of the knee. J Bone Joint Surg [Am] 61:330, 1979
7. Feagin JA, Curl WW. Isolated tears of anterior cruciate ligament: 5 year follow-up study. Am J Sports Med 4:95, 1976
8. Girgis FG, Marshall JC, Monejem ARS. The cruciate ligament of the knee joint: Anatomical, functional and experimental analysis. Clin Orthop 106:216, 1975
9. Groves, EW. The cruciate ligaments of the knee joint. Their function, rupture and operative treatment of the same. Br J Surg 7:505, 1920

10. Horns, JW. Simple contrast arthrography in abnormalities of the articular cartilage. Radiology 105:537, 1972
11. Jackson RW, Abe I. The role of arthroscopy in management of disorders of the knee: An analysis of 200 consecutive examinations. J Bone Joint Surg [Br] 54:310–322, 1972
12. Kennedy JC, Weinberg HW, Wilson AS. The anatomy and function of the anterior cruciate ligament as determined by clinical and morphological studies. J Bone Joint Surg [Am] 56:223, 1974
13. Liljedahl SO, Lindmall W, Wetterfors J. Early diagnosis and treatment of acute rupture of the anterior cruciate ligament. A clinical and arthrographic study of 48 cases. J Bone Joint Surg [Am] 47:1503, 1965
14. Liljedahl SO, Lindmall W, Wetterfors J. Roentgen diagnosis of the rupture of the anterior cruciate ligament. Acta Radiol 4:225, 1966
15. MacIntosh DL. The anterior cruciate ligament: "Over the top" repair. J Bone Joint Surg [Br] 56:591, 1974
16. Marshall JL, Arnoczky SP, Rubin RM, Wickiewicz TL. Microvasculature of the cruciate ligaments. Phys Sports Med, 7:87, 1979
17. Marshall, JL, Warren RF, Wickiewicz TC. Primary surgical treatment of anterior cruciate ligament lesions. Am J Sports Med 10:103, 1982
18. Mott WH. Semitendinosus anatomic reconstruction for cruciate ligament insufficiency. Clin Orthop 172:90, 1983
19. O'Connor RL. Arthroscopy in the diagnosis and treatment of the acute ligament injuries of the knee. J Bone Joint Surg [Am] 56:333, 1974
20. Parlov H. The radiographic diagnosis of the anterior cruciate ligament deficient knee. Clin Orthop 172:57, 1983
21. Paulos LE, Butler DL, Noyes FR, Grood ES. Intra-articular cruciate reconstruction. II: Replacement with vascularized patellar tendon. Clin Orthop 172:78, 1983
22. Paulos L, Noyes FR, Grood E, Butler DL. Knee rehabilitation after anterior cruciate ligament reconstruction and repair. Am J Sports Med 9:140, 1981
23. Warren RF. Primary repair of the anterior cruciate ligament. Clin Orthop 172:65, 1983
24. Watanabe M, Takeda S, Ikeuchi H. Atlas of Arthroscopy, 2nd ed. Isabu Shoin, Tokyo, 1969

# The Role of Exogenous Materials in Arthroscopic Management of Cruciate-Deficient Knees

# 12

Terry L. Whipple

In the past decade there has been intense interest in the diagnosis and treatment of injuries to the anterior cruciate ligament. Numerous tests have been described to improve on the traditional anterior drawer and Slocum tests by isolating more specifically the anterior cruciate ligament and demonstrating the clinical and functional instability that results from injury to this structure. The Lachman test, pivot shift, reverse pivot shift, jerk, and flexion-rotation-drawer tests each have respective merit, but none is necessarily pathognomonic of cruciate deficiency and immune from the false negative results because of the variety of associated injuries that may occur to other stabilizing structures about the knee. Similarly, numerous surgical procedures have been devised for correction of anterior and rotatory instabilities that may result from cruciate injury, but none is singularly and universally effective in every case, and none has consistently passed the tests of time and durability. Proponents and critics of the intra-articular and extra-articular repairs, reconstruction, and substitutions continue to wrestle with the relative advantages and disadvantages of each procedure, while still others design a variety of braces that incompletely protect the surgical patients postoperatively and treat those who decline or whose physicians denounce surgical treatment. The implication of this consternation is that the ideal, definitive treatment for cruciate-deficient knees has not yet been precisely identified and that additional research—both basic and clinical—is required. Not even the natural history of cruciate-deficient knees has been precisely described as the injury only recently has been well appreciated, although it surely has occurred with similar frequency for years. Despite the spectrum of functional instability, insecurity, or pain attributed to anterior cruciate injuries, a very small percentage of patients requiring total knee arthroplasty are found to be without this ligament.

Arthroscopic examination of acutely injured knees has focused attention sharply on all grades of injury to the anterior cruciate ligament from minor sprains to complete rupture. The incidence of associated meniscus injuries has established the anterior cruciate as an important protector of the menisci. With earlier diagnosis and a keener appreciation of the significance of cruciate injuries, it is proper that the quest continues for appropriate and timely surgical, as well as nonsurgical, treatment.

## Intra-articular Versus Extra-articular Reconstruction

Surgical treatment of cruciate-deficient knees can be divided generally into two categories:

1. extra-articular harnessing of the clinical instability
2. intra-articular repair or simulation of the ligament per se.

The first category is typified by the MacIntosh, the Ellison, and the Losee procedures, which reroute strips of iliotibial band about the lateral collateral ligament in various ways to tether the anterolateral corner of the tibia to the posterolateral region of the femur. These procedures are designed to arrest anterolateral rotatory instability by preventing shift of the iliotibial band anterior to the axis of knee flexion from 0 degrees to 30 degrees. These procedures have been generally effective in eliminating the pivot shift if not the functional symptoms of giving way and insecurity in knee extension, although it is generally agreed that they do not eliminate the positive anterior drawer sign. With time these repairs have stretched out, with worsening of the Lachman test. The arguable merit of attempting to obtain a dynamic restraint by basing the tether proximally on the tensor fascia lata muscle (Ellison) has not proved practical for many surgeons.

Transfer of the biceps anteriorly to Gerdy's tubercle and simple anterior transfer of the insertion of the iliotibial band (Johnson procedure) are other examples of attempts to apply extra-articular dynamic restraint to functional instability. More recently, Andrews (2) has devised a lateral extra-articular procedure that plicates the iliotibial band from Gerdy's tubercle and imbricates it to the lateral femoral epicondyle, using a Bunnel-type suture. The inherent weakness in all of these procedures is attributed to the inadequate strength of the transferred tissue, which is directly related to its cross-sectional area. The author has attempted to address this issue by splitting and braiding a similar width of iliotibial band together with an inelastic Dacron tape (41). The braid shortened the overall length of transferred tissue and at the same time increased the effective cross-sectional area per unit length.

Marshall et al. (23) reported successful repairs of midsubstance ruptures of the anterior cruciate ligament using multiple nonabsorbable sutures, but their results have not been reproducible. It is likely that their results were based on the combined strength of multiple sutures rather than actual healing of the ligament stumps. Hey-Grooves and Jones (15) devised ligament or tendon transfers through drill holes in the lateral femoral condyle to reconstruct the anterior cruciate ligament. MacIntosh improved on this technique anatomically by routing a portion of the quadriceps and patellar tendons over the top of the posterolateral femoral condyle. More recently, however, Clancy (11), Paulos (32) and their co-workers have repopularized the bone tunnel technique, emphasizing the importance of precise anatomical placement of the tunnel entrance at the anatomical origin of the anterior cruciate, high in the posterolateral wall of the intercondylar notch. They, too, utilized portions of the quadriceps and patellar ligament to reconstitute an anterior cruciate ligament, with Paulos (32) attempting to preserve the vascular supply to the graft to maintain viability of the tissue. Nicholas and Insall (28) transferred the iliotibial band through the joint, with a bone block for improved fixation.

These intra-articular reconstructions of the anterior cruciate consistently eliminate or substantially reduce scores on the pivot shift test for anterolateral rotatory instability. They have an advantage over the extra-articular procedures in that they also will reduce or eliminate scores on the anterior drawer and Lachman tests for instability in most cases by more closely simulating the structure and function of a normal cruciate ligament. They have a disadvantage as well: as intra-articular transfers, the grafts are subjected to a "hostile environment" of cathepsin, collagenase, and other proteolytic enzymes in the synovial fluid. The durability of extra-articular tissues in an intra-articular environment is questionable and unproven since these procedures enjoy only a few years follow-up at most.

Restoration of normal knee function and performance requires not only reliable stability, but also the absence of surface wear on articular cartilage (30). There is little subjective functional difference in the success of intra-articular reconstructive procedures compared with extra-articular stabilizing procedures. Both are initially successful and effective in eliminating anterolateral rotatory instability during normal daily activities, and in many instances during stressful working or athletic conditions. As the intra-articular procedures are more effective in reducing the anterior drawer and Lachman test results clinically, they would seem preferable, if only to reduce the amount of abnormal shear forces imposed on the articular cartilage. This is a critical factor in attempting to restore normalcy to an injured knee.

The anterior cruciate does not function in isolation, but in concert with other capsular structures in governing motion. The ligament complexes, menisci, and bone contours together provide primary and secondary restraints against abnormal motion. Effective reconstructions in the cruciate-deficient knee, therefore, should take into consideration the ligament's secondary function as a restraint against varus and valgus forces, hyperflexion and hyperextension, and traction, as well as its primary restraint against anterior and anterolateral instability. In this regard, the intra-articular reconstruction would appear again to have an advantage over the extra-articular procedures by more closely approximating normal anatomical form.

Although clincal testing in no way reproduces the functional forces to which the knee is subjected during normal and stressful use, ideal clinical testing does evaluate the knee in a passive state. Powerful muscle groups including the quadriceps, hamstrings, gastrocnemius, tensor fascia lata, and even the relatively small popliteus muscles are eliminated in clinical testing for instability, whereas they are extremely influential during functional situations. Functional or subjective results of surgical reconstructions in the cruciate-deficient knee, therefore, attest to the adequacy of these muscle groups as well as the surgically created restraints to abnormal motion (29, 31). Clinical testing for instability using mechanical devices as the best approximation of functional stress objectively favors intra-articular reconstruction over extra-articular transfers at 36 months after surgery (20). However, in the lives of young adult athletes who most commonly sustain injuries to the anterior cruciate ligament, 36 months is a relatively short-term evaluation of these procedures.

## Criteria for Reconstruction Materials

Noyes et al. (29) have indicated that strength and stiffness are the most important biomechanical features in the selection of a material to recreate cruciate ligament function. Strength refers to the ability to withstand tensile forces to the point of plastic deformation and ultimate failure. Stiffness connotes resistance to bending. Finite element analysis of bending a cylindrical structure, however, amounts to compressing one side of the cylinder and tensile loading of the opposite side. Therefore, the properities of strength and stiffness are related.

Noyes and co-workers (29) have demonstrated the relative strengths of commonly transferred biological tissues about the knee for anterior cruciate reconstruction (Table 12–1). These values are calculated from freshly harvested healthy cadaveric specimens. Similar testing of these structures months or years after intra-articular human implantation has not been done and is in fact implausible. Nevertheless, given the hostile enzyme environment of normal synovial fluid and the fact that transferred tissues—vascularized or not—undergo initial necrosis before revascularization, recollagenization, and remodeling, it is the ultimate strength of the transferred tissue long after recovery from the surgical procedure that would determine its suitability for cruciate reconstruction.

From the data available, based on tensile strength in the fresh state, the bone-tendon-bone composite of patella-infrapatellar tendon-tibia would appear to be the preferred choice of tissues for transfer. This tissue has proven suitable in clinical trials for intra-articular reconstruction of the anterior cruciate by Noyes et al. (29), Clancy et al. (11), and others with follow-up to approximately 6 years. (W. G. Clancy, 1984, personal communication). However, the measured width of the tissue tested to obtain these results, as indicated in Table 12–1, was 14–15 mm, which seems a substantial portion of infrapatellar ligament to sacrifice. In fact, Noyes (29) cautions that transfer of a major portion of the infrapatellar tendon may "compromise the delicate action of the quadriceps mechanism."

Many other factors besides strength and stiffness are important in the selection of appropriate tissue or material for the reconstruction of an anterior cruciate ligament. Durability has already been noted as a major concern. The hostile environment of synovial fluid may be the most critical factor in the demise of extra-articular tissues transferred into the joint. The possibility that a normal cruicate ligament, primarily composed of type I collagen, may harbor some unknown means of resistance to proteolytic enzymes not found in similar type I collagen of extra-articular structures has not been explored. On the other hand, because of devascularization the transferred type I collagen necroses after transfer and is replaced, at least temporarily during the remodeling process by type III collagen, which may be inherently less resistant to enzymatic degradation. Whatever the mechanism of enzymatic breakdown and whatever the factors that affect resistance, the substituted

**Table 12–1** Intra-articular Cruciate Reconstruction

| Tissue | Maximum load, (%) |
|---|---|
| Anterior cruciate ligament, young adult (1730 N ±269) | 100 |
| Bone/Patella tendon/Bone | |
| Central 14 mm | 175 |
| Medial 15 mm | 163 |
| Semitendinosus | 75 |
| Gracilis | 49 |
| Lata, 16 mm | 36 |
| Lata, 45 mm | 102 |
| Quadriceps-patella retinaculum-patella tendon | |
| Medial third of each structure | 21 |
| Central third of each structure | 15 |

Adapted from Noyes et al. (29).

tissue or material should offer the greatest possible tolerance to synovial fluid. Meyers (26) has demonstrated by arthroscopic examination consistent deterioration of transferred autogenous fascia lata one year after cruciate reconstruction.

The selected tissue for reconstruction must also offer durable mechanical stability. Stabilization procedures subject the transferred tissue to traction, bending, and twisting forces that may exceed the tolerance of its normal biological limits. Most procedures for stabilization of the cruciate-deficient knee require fixation of the transferred tissue to bone at one point at least, and this has proved to be a more critical consideration than was initially appreciated, especially for the intra-articular reconstruction techniques. Many of the acute failures of intra-articular cruciate reconstructions have occurred because of erosion of the grafts at the bone-graft interface, whether biological or nonbiological materials are employed for the reconstruction. This has been a particular problem with bone tunnels through the femoral condyle, where the graft material bends into a different axis, as opposed to the more gradual direction change in the "over the top" techniques of femoral fixation. Measures have been taken to minimize graft erosion at the bone-graft interface by altering the direction of bone tunnels and chamfering the edges. But the problem of erosion remains. The materials selected for reconstruction ideally should be resistant to abrasion which cannot be eliminated by surgical technique.

Finally, the issue of remodeling is a critical consideration in the selection of material for cruciate reconstruction. All free grafts, and long grafts remaining biologically attached at one end, undergo avascular necrosis after transfer. Revascularization of the tissue is a slow and tenuous process and may be difficult to achieve, at best. Vascular ingrowth from endosteal circulation, synovial proliferation, and fat pad circulation may each contribute variably to the graft, but complete revascularization requires months in human and primate studies, regardless of the material employed.

Vascularization does not imply strength or durability, however. The graft must be remodeled to an appropriate form and orientation of collagen bundles to tolerate the forces required of a cruciate ligament. This process also requires several months. Thus biological materials used for cruciate reconstruction will not withstand normal functional forces for many months after surgery, during which time the knee requires unusual protection, not only in consideration of the instability, but of the fragile remodeling of the graft as well.

Graft materials that depend on revascularization and remodeling should accommodate these biological processes by provoking minimal inflammatory responses, providing adequate interstitial space for host tissue ingrowth, and possessing adequate initial and lasting tensile strength to protect the joint and new tissue during remodeling stages.

## Surgical Considerations

It is difficult to improve on normal anatomy. Procedures that recreate or approximate normal form are likely to result in more normal function. This speaks in favor of intra-articular reconstruction of the cruciate-deficient knee but also emphasizes the importance of precise anatomical placement of the graft when an intra-articular procedure is used. Clancy and colleagues (11) have made a great contribution in emphasizing this point. Nonanatomical graft placement will either limit or inadequately control the knee's range of motion by altering the normal anatomical centers of rotation and end points of constraint. Inaccurate placement may also result in undue terminal stress on a graft and so limit its durability. Anatomical placement of the graft origin and insertion, furthermore, is less likely to result in impingement on the graft in the intercondylar notch during terminal extension.

For a relatively common disorder, a surgical procedure that is successful only at the hands of a select few surgeons is of limited value. The ideal procedure should give predictable and successful results when performed by most adequately trained surgeons. The best reconstruction procedure for cruciate-deficient knees, therefore, should be technically straightforward and relatively simple to perform. This will allow its broadest application for greatest patient relief.

In addition, a straightforward procedure will be less prone to complication and technical error. Minimizing the risk and sacrifice for the patient makes a procedure more commendable and increases the benefit-to-cost ratio. Complex dissection, prolonged operative time, inordinate pain, and prolonged hospitalization are obviously undesirable if equally good and long-lasting results can be obtained with a more simple procedure.

Cosmetic considerations should also be taken into account. An increasing number of women and girls are participating in competitive athletics, including jumping and pivoting sports such as basketball, softball, and field hockey. Consequently, there is greater incidence of injuries to the anterior cruciate ligament occurring in females. However many athletes, male and female, are body conscious and deserve consideration of the appearance of a surgical scar in an area as visible as the knee, especially if an equally good procedure can be offered without extensive surgical exposure.

With regard to the graft material used for cruciate reconstruction or joint stabilization, immediate secure fixation to bone is extremely desirable. Prolonged immobilization required for biological fixation or bony ingrowth into the graft material is detrimental to articular cartilage and other periarticular soft tissues. Capsular fibrosis, intra-articular adhesions, and chondromalacia all result from immobilization and are to the patient's disadvantage. In addition, muscle atrophy and bone demineralization, even reflex sympathetic dystrophy, commonly result from postoperative casting for sustained periods and require weeks of concentrated, often expensive efforts to reverse. Immediate secure fixation that will endure should allow early mobilization of the joint within a nonstressful range to avoid these undesirable side effects.

All of these considerations should influence the design and selection of a surgical procedure for stabilization or reconstruction of a cruciate-deficient knee to minimize complications and maximize stable function.

## Exogenous Graft Materials

Several of the aforementioned considerations of graft material and surgical technique for reconstruction of cruciate-deficient knees have aroused interest in the use of exogenous materials. In an unstable knee an intact and well-conditioned quadriceps extensor mechanism provides important additional stability to the joint during functional activities, especially in knee flexion. As the infrapatellar ligament appears to be the strongest autogenous tissue available for transfer, there is concern for the extensor mechanism if a substantial portion is harvested from an injured knee to reconstruct the anterior cruciate ligament. In addition to weakness of the tendon, donation of the medial third or more of the infrapatellar ligament effectively lateralizes the insertion of the extensor mechanism, thereby increasing the Q-angle, possibly disrupting patellofemoral dynamics and placing a greater anterior force on the lateral side of the tibia during quadriceps contraction.

The second strongest autogenous tissue is the iliotibial band, an important lateral stabilizer of the knee. More than 4 cm width of this structure are required for an adequate cruciate graft. Transferring that much of the iliotibial band would effectively eliminate closure of the defect at the donor site, with loss of its important stabilizing function laterally.

Since autogenous tissue inevitably undergoes necrosis, even when transferred as vascularized grafts, similar tissues harvested from young cadaver donors should be neither weaker nor more subject to avascular or enzymatic degradation. Ligaments, tendons, and bones are relatively hypocellular tissues composed mainly of collagen and so provoke very little antigenic reaction. Freeze-drying techniques used by tissue banks can make such tissues available in sufficient quantity and size, packaged as sterile implants according to desired specification.

The greatest advantage of this concept, of course, is that no intact tissue from an already compromised knee need be sacrificed to reconstruct the cruciate ligament. In addition, surgical exposure can be reduced considerably, along with its associated morbidity and pain, when graft material does not need to be obtained from the patient. This also reduces operating time, which helps to decrease risk of complication.

Yet allografts are no more resistant to enzymatic degradation than autogenous tissues and are subject to the same long-term remodeling processes described above. For these reasons interest in the use of synthetic materials as grafts or graft supplements has developed. Many synthetic materials are biocompatible, sterile, strong, durable, and can be readily available. They may possess more desirable biomechanical properties than the best biological tissues. They can also be manufactured to resist enzymatic or chemical breakdown. As such, they further fulfill many of the desired characteristics for a cruciate ligament graft, although they introduce unique problems and considerations as well.

## Synthetics

Synthetic materials employed to this date for anterior cruciate ligament reconstruction can be grouped into three general categories. Temporary and permanent scaffolds, the first two categories, are materials that provide temporary strength and stability while allowing—or perhaps inducing—host tissue ingrowth for ultimate ligament reconstruction. Prosthetic materials make up the third category. These grafts literally supplant the anterior cruciate ligament, and while host tissue may or may not invade the prosthetic structure, restraint against instability depends solely on the implant in late as well as early stages following reconstruction. These materials must be extraordinarily durable, literally capable of lasting a lifetime without fatigue, creep, or degradation through cyclic loading.

The scaffolding materials need not be as durable since the ultimate intent is to provide stability with biological tissue that remodels to provide strength and response to stress, much as the strength provided by a bone fixation plate is assumed by the regrowth and remodeling of osseous tissue. The implant may remain permanently, in which case its strength ideally should be subnormal to allow stress to be applied to the host tissue for remodeling purposes. Or the implant may be temporary, removed surgically when the biological tissue is sufficiently mature, or degrading spontaneously in situ, gradually transferring tensile stresses to the host tissue.

Finally, composites of synthetics or of synthetics and biological tissue may be used to modulate the biomechanical properties of any simple material to greatest advantage.

### Group I: Temporary Scaffolds

***Carbon Fiber*** Carbon fiber has been implanted for cruciate-deficient knees more than any other synthetic material. It was developed originally by D. H. R. Jenkins, Ch.M., of Great Britain (17) as a ribbon consisting of approximately 80,000 filaments of elemental carbon. Carbon is a primary element in biological tissues and is well tolerated by the host when implanted. It appears that fibroblastic response is stimulated or at least enhanced by carbon filaments implanted in extra-articular tissues, with fibroblasts proliferating rapidly to invade the implant and deposit new collagen along the carbon fibers.

The impressive tensile strength of carbon filaments suits it well for tensile loads required of the anterior cruciate ligament, but the material is extremely brittle and fragments easily (3–8). The filaments are ultimately separated by host tissue ingrowth, then become broken and ineffective. Theoretically, the invading tissue aligned along the filaments of carbon assumes the load-bearing role.

Carbon particles released may migrate to regional lymph nodes, as demonstrated in sheep studies (17). Although this is of great concern, there has not been any evidence of ill effects from the presence of carbon particles in regional lymph nodes, and the particles have not been demonstrated at more remote sites in in vivo studies (36, 43).

The brittleness of bare carbon filaments makes surgical handling difficult because they break so easily when bent. Therefore, Jenkins et al. ( ) and Weiss et al. (6–8) have resorted to coating the carbon with a gelatinous material to improve the handling properties. Multiple animal studies and human implantation in extra-articular tissues have proved carbon filaments to be well tolerated and very effective in stimulating fibrogenesis and restoring stability to lax joints (3, 4, 6, 8, 10, 12, 13, 18, 19, 27, 36, 40, 43).

***Coated Carbon Fibers with Polylactic Acid*** Hexcel Medical (Livermore, California) has developed a device consisting of carbon filaments coated with a polylactic acid polymer to improve handling properties and reduce carbon particle migration following surgical implantation. Alexander, Weiss, and Parsons ( ) have collaborated in the development as well as laboratory and clinical testing of this device to augment biological tissue grafting for cruciate-deficient knees. [As of June, 1984, over 700 reconstructive procedures with the Hexcel product had been performed, including extra-articular and intra-articular implantations (16).]

This carbon-polymer composite consists of nearly 10,000 individual carbon filaments that are approximately 8 μm in diameter. The polylactic acid is nonreactive in the host and is broken down and absorbed through the carbohydrate metabolism cycle in a matter of days after implantation. The carbon filaments are then exposed for host tissue ingrowth. Tensile strength to failure of the implant measures approximately 400 N. [Normal anterior cruciate strength is approximately 1700 N (29).] Implant strength can be increased by using multiple grafts. The implant has been extremely effective in clinical trials, restoring stability to joints and stimulating abundant, appropriately oriented fibrogenesis. The carbon-polymer composite has been approved by the FDA for clinical investigation.

In limited clinical centers intra-articular reconstruction for the anterior cruciate using this device is performed by wrapping several of the ribbons with autogenous fascia lata, fixing it distally to the tibia through a drill hole and proximally to the femur routed over the top of the lateral femoral condyle. Fixation to bone is achieved with an expandable carbon rivet, which is not entirely adequate. There is concern over intra-articular release of carbon particles which may become imbeded in synovium or articular cartilage and cause an abrasive effect on articular surfaces. This concern has not been substantiated in clinical or laboratory trials, nor has it been disproved (17, 27, 43). Despite the polymer coating, the carbon fibers remain difficult to handle surgically, with a high incidence of breakage and fraying, and the current mechanism for fixation to bone remains tenuous.

### Group II: Permanent Scaffolds

***Dacron*** Dacron is a synthetic polymer with proven biocompatibility through extensive use as surgical suture and vascular graft implants. Stryker Corporation (Kalamazoo, Michigan) has developed a ligament graft consisting of four braided Dacron tapes surrounded by a woven Dacron velour sleeve intended to promote host tissue ingrowth (Figure 12–1). As an augmentation that will ultimately be thoroughly invaded by host tissue to share tensile load, the graft will sustain approximately twice the load with half the elongation of a normal anterior cruciate ligament (35). Although Dacron has excellent fatigue strength, it is subject to abrasion at the bone interface when implanted as an anterior cruciate ligament through bony tunnels. Rupture of the device in animal and human trials has usually occurred at the entrance into bone and is attributed to friction wear.

Histological studies at 6 weeks in dogs show excellent bone ingrowth into the implant for biological fixation. At 20 weeks there is extensive fibrous ingrowth observed in the intra-articular portion of the graft when implanted as an anterior cruciate ligament. As with carbon fiber, surrounding the Dacron graft with autogenous fascia lata may enhance fibrous and vascular ingrowth.

The Dacron graft is easier to handle surgically than the carbon fiber or coated fiber materials but is not biologically degradable. Therefore, it may shield the host tissue from complete remodeling as the graft continues to bear most of the tensile loads.

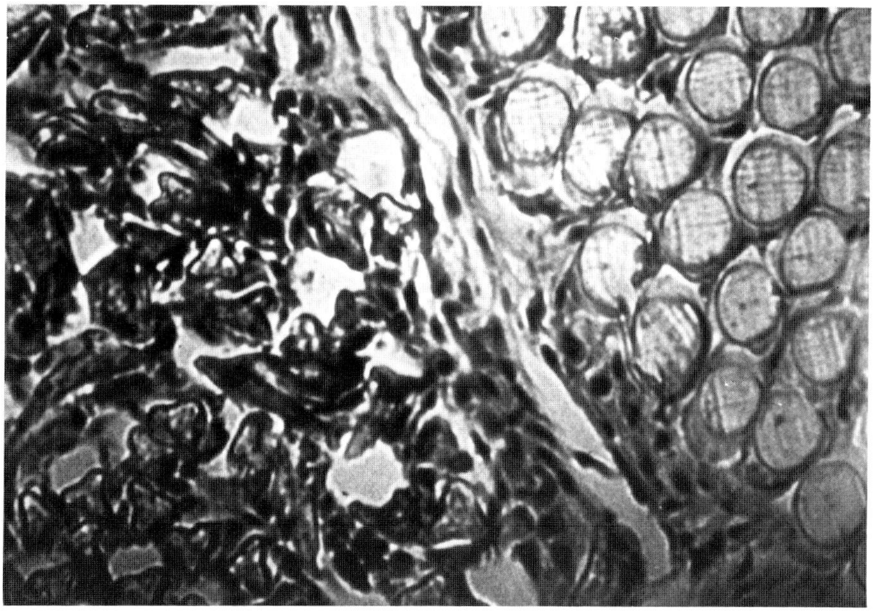

**Figure 12–1** Fibrous ingrowth into Dacron velour graft in dog model at 12 weeks.

***Dexon Dacron*** Dexon is the brand name of polyglycolic acid used for several years as delayed absorbable surgical suture and is well tolerated physiologically. This device consists of an inner Dacron core coated with polyglycolic acid. The rationale for the coating is not completely clear. In dog models in which the graft was implanted, the Dexon coating was predictably absorbed within 4 weeks, as is the case with Dexon suture (9). This exposes the central Dacron core, which is invaded by host tissue in like manner to that previously described. This device has not been extensively tested, and its relative merits must await further study.

***Dacron Velour-Fascia Lata Composite*** Woven Dacron velour readily accepts fibrous tissue invasion when implanted in humans as well as animal models. The loose weave design allows thorough interdigitation of capillary buds and collagen fibers in both intra-articular and extra-articular locations. This would seem to provide a rich vascular source for biological tissues implanted for cruciate ligament substitution.

Bassett has devised a two-stage procedure in which a Silastic rubber rod surrounded with a double-weave Dacron velour sleeve is implanted initially in the place of the anterior cruciate ligament (F. H. Bassett III, 1984, personal communication). After maturation of the vascularized fibrous connective tissue that invades the velour sleeve, the Silastic rod is removed and a fascia lata graft is pulled through the sleeve in the second stage of the procedure. Theoretically, the prepared vascular sleeve in close apposition to the graft will permit earlier and more thorough remodeling of the graft. The Dacron remains a permanent part of the ligament substitute but is not designed to take tensile loads. Thus ultimate stabilization depends on the remodeled biological tissue portion of the graft.

This technique has been employed in baboons with encouraging early results. Stress testing of harvested grafts after 1 year suggested that success would depend on the use of an ample width of fascia lata and demonstrated vascular invasion of the graft originating from the fibrous sleeve as well as endosteal vessels at each end. This procedure has not been employed in humans to date.

***Polypropylene Braid*** In connection with the 3M Company (St. Paul, Minnesota), Kennedy (33) developed a braided ribbon of polypropylene that has approximately the same strength as a normal human anterior cruciate ligament. The device measures 8 mm × 1.5 mm and is designed to be a ligament augmentation device (LAD) to supplement biological grafts for strength during the remodeling process. Extensive laboratory as well as clinical tests have proved the polypropylene material to be a well-tolerated implant that readily accepts host tissue ingrowth (33).

The surgical technique for this device varies from other permanent scaffolding material. It is implanted in the position of the anterior cruciate ligament along with a transfer of the middle third of the infrapatellar ligament and the quadriceps expansion over the patella, exiting the joint proximally over the top of the lateral femoral condyle, as described by MacIntosh. The polypropylene braid is only attached to bone distally. Theoretically this prevents stress shielding of the patellar tendon graft and allows the synthetic implant to seek its own effective length. This must assume that the flexible LAD will move passively in both directions to effectively shorten as well as lengthen. Prior to biological fixation of the composite, the maximum strength of the system is dependent on the patellar tendon and quadriceps expansion, which is incompletely protected by the unifixed LAD.

Kennedy performed this procedure in 144 patients (33). Preliminary results are pending publication but indicate more successful restoration of joint stability using the LAD than when the same procedure was performed on a parallel series of patients without the synthetic implants (J. H. Roth, 1984, personal communication).

### Group III: Ligament Prostheses

***Proplast*** In 1973 the FDA granted approval for implantation of the Proplast prosthetic anterior cruciate ligament, which is composed of several materials. The central core is an inelastic cord that is covered by strips of aluminum imbedded in a protein matrix skin. Each end is covered with carbon fiber to facilitate biological fixation, and the components are permanently bonded together by heat and pressure. The intra-articular portion is finally covered with Teflon to resist abrasive wear against bone edges in the intercondylar notch.

In clinical experience at multiple centers, this device has consistently failed. Although strong, it fatigues badly and eventually ruptures in its midportion. Most of these implants failed within 3 years of implantation. Its use is now essentially history.

***Gore-Tex*** This prosthesis is made of polytetrafluroethylene (PTFE) "expanded" into a structure of solid PTFE nodules interconnected by strong, highly oriented PTFE fibrils (W. L. Gore and Associates, Inc., Flagstaff, Arizona). The biocompatibility of PTFE has been established by the implantation of over a half million Gore-Tex vascular grafts (14). This polymer is inert and resistant to biochemical degradation. The fibrilar network provides ample porosity for host tissue ingrowth, although the graft is not intended to be dependent upon host tissue for any of its functional strength as a ligament replacement.

Gore-Tex has been extensively bench tested for biomechanical properties and proves to be adequately strong, resistant to creep, and resistant to fatigue failure under loaded cyclic bending situations. In sheep studies in which the material was implanted as an anterior cruciate ligament substitute, solid bony ingrowth with strong pull-out testing was demonstrated.

The prosthesis is designed with a loop at each end through which it is attached to cortical bone with self-tapping screws (Figure 12–2). The screw fixation is

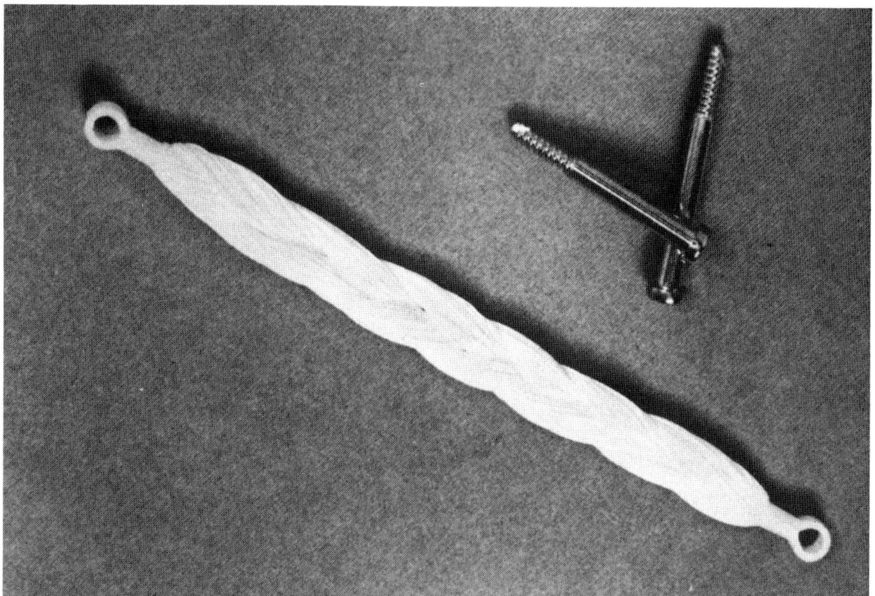

**Figure 12–2** Gore-Tex expanded PTFE prosthetic ligament with screws employed for ligament fixation.

intended to be temporary, however, as ultimate fixation is provided by host bone ingrowth. The graft interstices will accept fibrous tissue ingrowth along the intra-articular segment, although it is not anticipated this tissue will contribute appreciably to joint stabilization since the synthetic graft has an ultimate tensile strength of 5300 N, which far exceeds that of the normal anterior cruciate (14). Thus stress-induced realignment of fibrous tissue remodeling along the graft is unlikely.

Unfortunately, PTFE is not resistant to abrasion at the graft-bone interface. Fraying has been observed at this site in animal models. Clinical trials with Gore-Tex ligament grafts have been under way for over a year and short-term reports are expected soon.

***Xenografts*** The technology behind the Xenograft bioprosthesis (Xenotech Laboratories, Irvine, California) is the same as that which produced the porcine heart valve prosthesis. Thousands of such valves have been implanted successfully in humans without evidence of rejection or malfunction through millions of flexion cycles. The Xenograft is a bovine extensor tendon of nearly uniform dimensions, bifurcated at one end (Figure 12–3, A). It is a hypocellular structure of linearly oriented type I collagen fibers. The tendon is treated with glutaraldehyde under controlled conditions to cross-link lysine radicals on adjacent proteoglycan strands in the triple-helix collagen molecules with aldehyde bonds. These are strong chemical linkages that render the collagen bundles virtually immune to proteolytic enzymes. Such resistance makes this biological tissue a prosthetic implant that does not undergo remodeling after implantation (24, 25).

Tensile strength of the cruciate ligament replacement prosthesis exceeds 3000 N, two and one-half times that of normal young adult anterior cruciate ligaments. Created biologically to bear enormous tensile loads through flexion and extension, the stiffness and creep properties of this substance are excellent for cruciate replacement, but it does not resist abrasive forces against bony edges. That is a uniform disadvantage of all biological and synthetic materials for cruciate ligament reconstruction and is minimized but not eliminated by adequate surgical design.

The Xenograft has demonstrated host tissue ingrowth into its natural interstices in the dog model and has achieved strong biological fixation to bone if implanted in snug bone tunnels (Figure 12–3, B).

There have been approximately 200 cruciate ligament implants with the Xenograft performed in the United States and at least three times that number abroad (24). Teitge (37) has reported unacceptable clinical results due to synovitis and implant rupture in a 15-case series. Other reporters [Abbink and Kramer (1), Whipple (42), Springer, and Levitt (personal communication)] have had successful short-term experience with proper attention to surgical technique to avoid fraying and fragmentation of the implant at the entrance to bone tunnels. However wear particles from the graft may occur and evoke a proliferative synovial response. Clinical experience in excess of 3 years is not yet available.

## Arthroscopic Reconstruction

Recent advances in arthroscopic surgery have proved the value of this technique for successfully implanting anterior cruciate ligament grafts, either autogenous or exogenous (38, 42). The arthroscope affords excellent visibility of the entire intra-articular anatomy of an unstable joint for accurate diagnosis of injuries associated

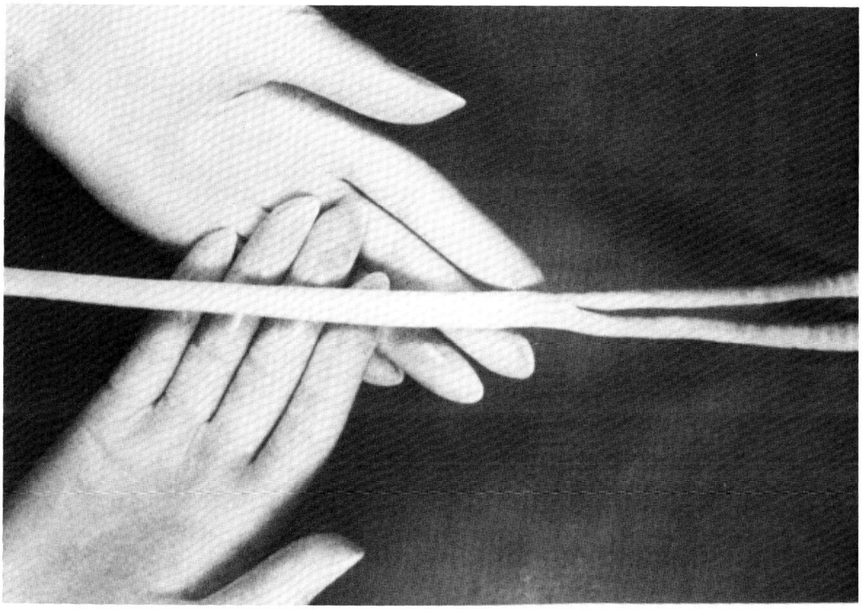

A

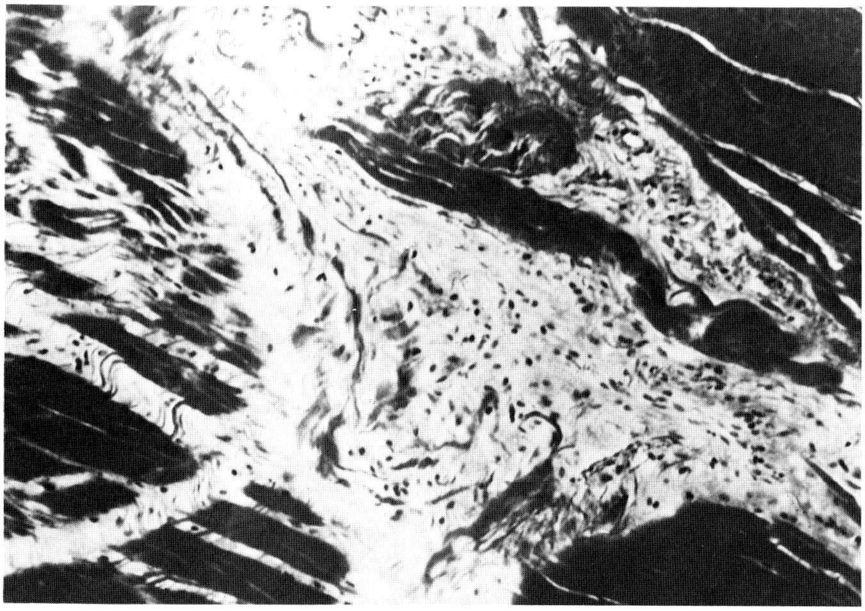

B

**Figure 12–3** **A** Xenograft bioprosthesis of gluteraldehyde-treated bovine tendon. **B** Bone ingrowth into prosthesis in dog model.

with rupture of the anterior cruciate ligament. The anatomical origin of the anterior cruciate can be precisely visualized arthroscopically, whereas it is extremely difficult to do so with an arthrotomy. Moreover, utilization of an appropriate ligament guide permits anatomical location of bone tunnels for intra-articular graft placement (Figure 12–4) and simplifies the procedure to allow reproducible results by any accomplished arthroscopist.

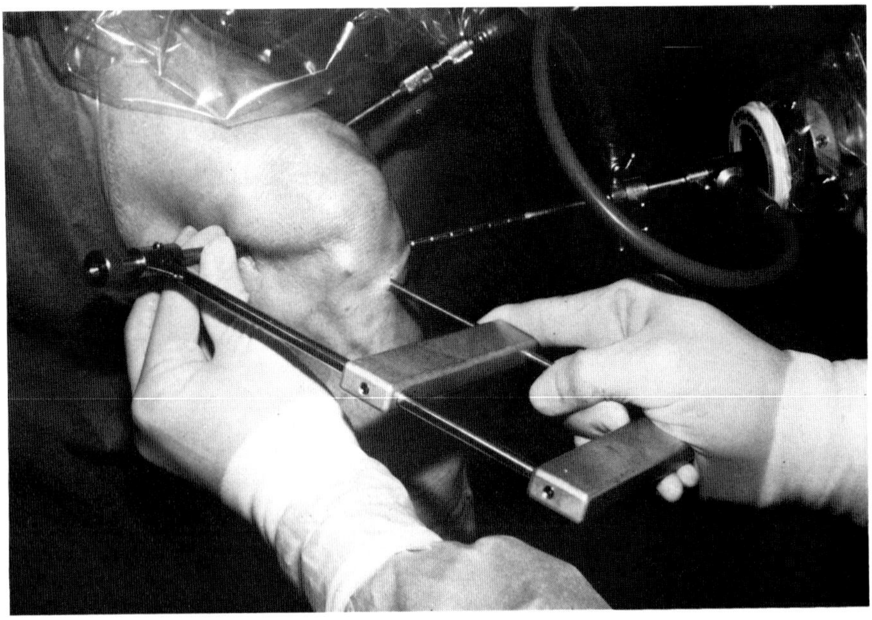

**Figure 12–4** Arthroscopic cruciate ligament guide used for precise placement of bone tunnels.

The technique consists of debriding the ruptured nonfunctional stumps of the anterior cruciate ligament but preserving any intact fibers that span the joint from normal cruciate origin to insertion. The appropriate centers of origin and insertion of the ligament are then located with the point of the ligament guide. Two Kirschner wires are drilled—one through the anteromedial metaphysis of the proximal tibia and another through the metaphyseal portion of the lateral femoral condyle, as near coaxially as possible—each entering the joint at the point of the ligament guide. The appropriate bone tunnels are created by reaming over each Kirschner wire through an incision about 20 mm in length. After chamfering of the edges of the bony tunnels on the intra-articular side, a graft can be pulled through the tunnels and across the joint. The instability is reduced with appropriate tension on the graft, and the graft is secured in place with staples or screws.

Any graft material may be implanted with such an arthroscopic technique, but the most obvious advantage of this procedure is the reduction in surgical morbidity by avoiding the arthrotomy in an already compromised joint. If exogenous materials providing durability and appropriate mechanical properties can be identified and produced, the need for surgical intervention to harvest autograft materials is also eliminated. Minimally invasive surgical techniques, therefore, represent a significant advance toward shorter periods of immobilization and earlier rehabilitation.

It is the potential to decrease the investment in time, dollars, pain, and side effects that accounts for the intense interest in the use of exogenous materials for cruciate ligament reconstruction. In consideration of the suboptimal results obtained with biological tissues for ligament reconstruction and the impressive results with synthetic materials for vascular reconstructive procedures and joint surface replacement, the interest in synthetic or semisynthetic grafting materials for ligament reconstruction has grown considerably.

The use of nonbiological or altered biological materials introduces a host of new problems and considerations, as noted. However, purely biological materials can pose limitations and problems of their own that to date remain unsolved. While still experimental, then, the implantation of nonbiological materials merits further investigation under the guidelines of safe and reasonable protocols. Strict monitoring of subject patients and unbiased reporting of results will in time prove the value of synthetic and semisynthetic materials. Meanwhile, refinement of the surgical technique for arthroscopic implantation of cruciate grafts, whether autogenous or exogenous, biological or not, will undoubtedly become a valuable adjunct in the surgical treatment of anterior cruciate-deficient knees.

## *References*

1. Abbink EP, Kramer FJK. Preliminary report on the use of xenografts in knee instability problems. In: Transactions of the 13th Annual Meeting of the Eastern Orthopaedic Association, 1982
2. Andrews JR, Sanders RA. A "mini-reconstruction" technique in treating anterolateral rotatory instability (ALRI). Clin Orthop 172:93–96, 1983
3. Alexander H, Parsons JR, Smith G, et al. Anterior cruciate ligament replacement with filamentous carbon. In: Transactions of the 28th Annual Meeting of the Orthopaedic Research Society, New Orleans, p 45, 1982
4. Alexander H, Strauchler I, Weiss AB, et al. Carbon-polymer composites for tendon and ligament replacement. In: Transactions of the Fourth Annual Meeting of the Society for Biomaterials, p 123, 1978
5. Alexander H, Weiss AB, Parsons JR, et al. Ligament and tendon replacement scaffolds. In: Transactions of the 11th International Biomaterial Symposium in Conjunction with the Fifth Annual Meeting of the Society for Biomaterials, 3:72, 1979
6. Alexander, H, Weiss AB, Parsons JR, et al. Ligament and tendon replacement with absorbable polymer-filamentous carbon tissue scaffold. In: Transactions of the 25th Annual Meeting of the Orthopaedic Research Society, p 27, 1979
7. Alexander H, Weiss AB, Parsons JR, et al. Canine patellar tendon replacement with a polylactic acid polymer-filamentous carbon degrading scaffold. Orthopaedic Review 1011:41–51, 1981
8. Aragona J, Parsons JR, Alexander H, Weiss AB. Soft tissue attachment of a filamentous carbon-absorbable polymer tendon and ligament replacement. Clin Orthop 160:268–278, 1981
9. Cabaud HE, Rodkey WG. Report to the American Academy of Orthopaedic Surgeons Knee Committee Seminar, 1983
10. Christel P, Buttazzoni B, Leray JL, Morin C. Tissue tolerance of carbon materials. In: Transactions of the First World Biomaterials Congress, p 474, 1980
11. Clancy WG Jr, Nelson DA, Reider B, Narenchania RG. Anterior cruciate ligament reconstruction using one-third of the patellar ligament augmented by extra-articular tendon transfers. J Bone Joint Surg [Am] 64:352–359, 1982
12. Forster IW, Ralis ZA, McKibbin B, Jenkins DHR. Biological reaction to carbon fiber implants. Clin Orthop 131:299–307, 1978
13. Goodship AE, Brown PN, Yeats JJ, et al. An assessment of filamentous carbon fiber for the treatment of tendon injury in the horse. Vet Rec March 8, 1980
14. WL Gore and Associates, Inc. Report, 1983
15. Hey Groves EW. Operation for the repair of the crucial ligaments. Lancet 2:674–675, 1917
16. Hexcel Medical. Memorandum, June, 1984
17. Jenkins DHR. The repair of cruciate ligaments with flexible carbon fiber. J Bone Joint Surg [Br] 60:520–522, 1978
18. Jenkins DHR, Forster IW, McKibbin B, Ralis ZA. Induction of tendon and ligament formation by carbon implants. J Bone Joint Surg [Br] 59:53–57, 1977
19. Jenkins DHR, McKibbin B. The role of flexible carbon fiber implants as tendon and ligament substitutes in clinical practice. J Bone Joint Surg [AM] 62:497–499, 1980
20. Kochan A, Markolf K, Amstutz H. Measurement of knee stiffness and laxity in patients with documented absence of the anterior cruciate ligament. J Bone Joint Surg 66A:242–253, 1984

21. Levitt J. Personal communication, July 1984
22. MacIntosh D. Personal communication, visiting professor lectureship, Duke University, Durham, North Carolina, 1977
23. Marshall JL, Rubin RM, Wang JB, et al. The anterior cruciate ligament. The diagnosis and treatment of its injuries and their serious prognostic implications. Orthopaedic Review 7:35–46, 1978
24. McMasters WC. Preliminary report, publication accepted by Clin Orthop, Summer, 1985
25. McMasters WC, Kougelas J, Liddle S, et al. Tendon grafting with glutaraldehyde fixed material. J Biomed Mater Res 10:259–271, 1976
26. Meyers JF. Arthroscopic examination following anterior cruciate reconstruction. Lecture presented at the Southern Orthopaedic Association Annual Meeting, St. Thomas, V.I., April, 1985
27. Minns RJ, Flynn M. Intra-articular implant of filamentous carbon fiber in the experimental animal. J Bioeng 2:279–286, 1978
28. Nicholas JA, Minkoff J. Iliotibial band transfer through the intercondylar notch for combined anterior instability. Am J Sports Med 6:341, 1978
29. Noyes FR, Butler DL, Paulos LE, Grood ES. Intra-articular cruciate reconstruction. Clin Orthop 172:71–77, 1983
30. Noyes FR, Grood ES, Butler DL, Malek M. Clinical laxity tests and functional stability of the knee: Biomechanical concepts. Clin Orthop 146:84–89, 1980
31. Noyes FR, Grood ES, Butler DL, Raterman L. Knee ligament tests: What do they really mean? Phys Ther 60:1578–1581, 1980
32. Paulos LE, Butler DL, Noyes FR, Grood ES. Intra-articular cruciate reconstruction. Clin Orthop 172:78–84, 1983
33. Roth JH, Kennedy JC, McPherson GK, et al. Long-term evaluation of the "ligament augmentation device" in the reconstruction of the anterior cruciate ligament. Paper presented at the Annual Meeting of the Canadian Orthopaedic Research Society, 1984
34. Springer S. Personal communication, July 1984
35. Stryker Corporation. Report, January, 1983
36. Tayton K, Phillips G, Ralis Z. Long-term effects of carbon fiber on soft tissue. J Bone Joint Surg [Br] 64:112–114, 1982
37. Teitge R. Paper presented at the Annual Meeting of the American Academy of Orthopaedic Surgeons Sports Medicine Society, Atlanta, 1984
38. Toft J. Dacron graft replacement of ACL. Arthroscopy Video Journal May, 1984
39. Weiss AB, Alexander H, Blazina M, Parsons JR. Ligament replacement with absorbable polymer-carbon fiber scaffolds—Early clinical experience. In: Transactions of the 13th Annual Meeting of the Eastern Orthopaedic Association, 1982
40. Weiss AB, Alexander H, Blazina M, Parsons JR. Ligament and tendon replacement about the knee with absorbable polymer-carbon fiber scaffolds—Early clinical experience. In: Transactions of the Third Congress of the International Society of the Knee, 1983
41. Whipple TL. Braided facia lata/Dacron composite for extra-articular cruciate reconstruction. Paper presented at the Annual Meeting of the Virginia Orthopaedic Society, Williamsburg, Va, 1982
42. Whipple TL. Arthroscopic reconstruction of the anterior cruciate ligament with bovine xenografts. Paper presented at the Annual Meeting of the American Academy of Orthopaedic Surgeons Sports Medicine Society, Anaheim, CA, 1984
43. Zichner L, Pruessner P, Bruckmann H. Tissue reaction to subcutaneous and intra-articular implantation of carbon powders. In: Transactions of the First World Biomaterials Congress, p 4.3.7, 1980

# Instrumentation and Operating Room Organization for Arthroscopy of the Shoulder

# 13

Richard B. Caspari

Shoulder arthroscopy has become of increasing value to orthopaedic surgeons as the techniques for performing this procedure have been delineated (5; L. L. Johnson, personal communication). Diagnostically, the entirety of the glenohumeral joint can be evaluated, allowing for the appreciation of subtle lesions such as tearing of the labrum and mild instability of the shoulder (4). More obvious disorders of the shoulder, such as rotator cuff tears, synovitis, rupture of the biceps tendon, and degenerative arthritis are also easily evaluated (1, 2). In rather predictable fashion, techniques for surgical arthroscopy of the shoulder are being introduced as skills with diagnostic arthroscopy become perfected. Initially, excisional types of surgical procedures such as removal of a torn labrum and debridement of the articular surfaces and synovectomy were performed (2). At the present time techniques for debridement of small rotator cuff tears, repair of Bankart lesions, and reconstruction for shoulder instability are being introduced by the author and also by L. L. Johnson (personal communication).

As with any arthroscopic procedure, training of personnel and organization of the operating room must be accomplished prior to performing the procedure itself. Whereas much of the instrumentation utilized for shoulder arthroscopy is transferable from our previous experience in the knee, some special instrumentation is also necessary.

## Operating Room Organization

Preoperative preparation on the part of all personnel is essential. For the orthopaedic surgeon, basic introduction to the techniques of shoulder arthroscopy is now routinely being covered in most arthroscopy courses. Shoulder models are available with replaceable intra-articular lesions of various types, allowing for training at a leisurely pace. A thorough review of the anatomy of the shoulder is also essential, and a dissection in the laboratory of one or more shoulders is most helpful. Several arthroscopists are now routinely performing procedures in the shoulder, and a visit to one of these centers is another means of obtaining information necessary to get started.

A program for training of ancillary personnel should be established. It is essential that the scrub nurse and circulating nurse be familiar with the various techniques and their roles at any time during the procedure.

Anesthesia personnel must also be introduced to the procedure as the patient will require intubation allowing for positioning on the patient's side. The anesthesiologist and his equipment will be positioned toward the foot of the table but in front of the patient. In this regard, it is easier following intubation to rotate the operating table rather than move the anesthesiologist and all of his equipment. Once the table is positioned and locked in place, the patient can be rotated onto his side with the operative shoulder uppermost and the body stabilized with a beanbag device or sandbags and kidney rests. Care should be taken to protect the patient's head and neck with an appropriate head rest. An axillary pad or roll will protect the opposite shoulder without compromising pulmonary function and allowing for aeration of the opposite lung. Bony prominences about the hips and knees should be padded.

Positioning of personnel and equipment about the operating table is arranged to allow for free access to the patient's shoulder by the surgeon without being compromised by the various lines and cables entering the operative field (Figure 13–1). Clear visualization of the television monitor is necessary for all personnel without turning or placing the neck or body in a contorted position. We have found that grouping the television monitor, light source, and power packs on a single table placed at the patient's head and angled at approximately 45 degrees to the patient's face fulfills the above criteria. A small Mayo stand is placed just above the patient's head and in front of the ancillary equipment table. This Mayo stand is included within the sterile draping and provides a convenient area to place tools that are in use during the procedure.

The patient's shoulder and arm are then sterilely prepared and draped to allow the arm to be moved freely about the operative field. If sophisticated shoulder arthroscopy is to be accomplished, a shoulder traction device will be necessary (Figure 13–2). Whereas manual traction can be applied by an assistant, this traction is inconsistent, and invariably the assistant will be in the way of the operative procedure. A traction device should allow for a sterile connection to the patient's arm and can be removed and reassembled during the operative procedure at the surgeon's discretion without compromising the sterile field. Traction should be limited to 15–20 pounds so as to avoid neuropraxia. In some procedures, it will be necessary to change the position of the shoulder while maintaining traction, and this mechanism should be a feature of the device.

Once the patient is prepped and draped and the shoulder is placed in traction, the surgeon assumes a position so that he has free access from the head of the operating table around to the posterior aspect of the shoulder. This will allow him to manipulate the instruments anteriorly and posteriorly simultaneously. The scrub nurse and Mayo stand are placed posterior to the patient at the level of the patient's waist.

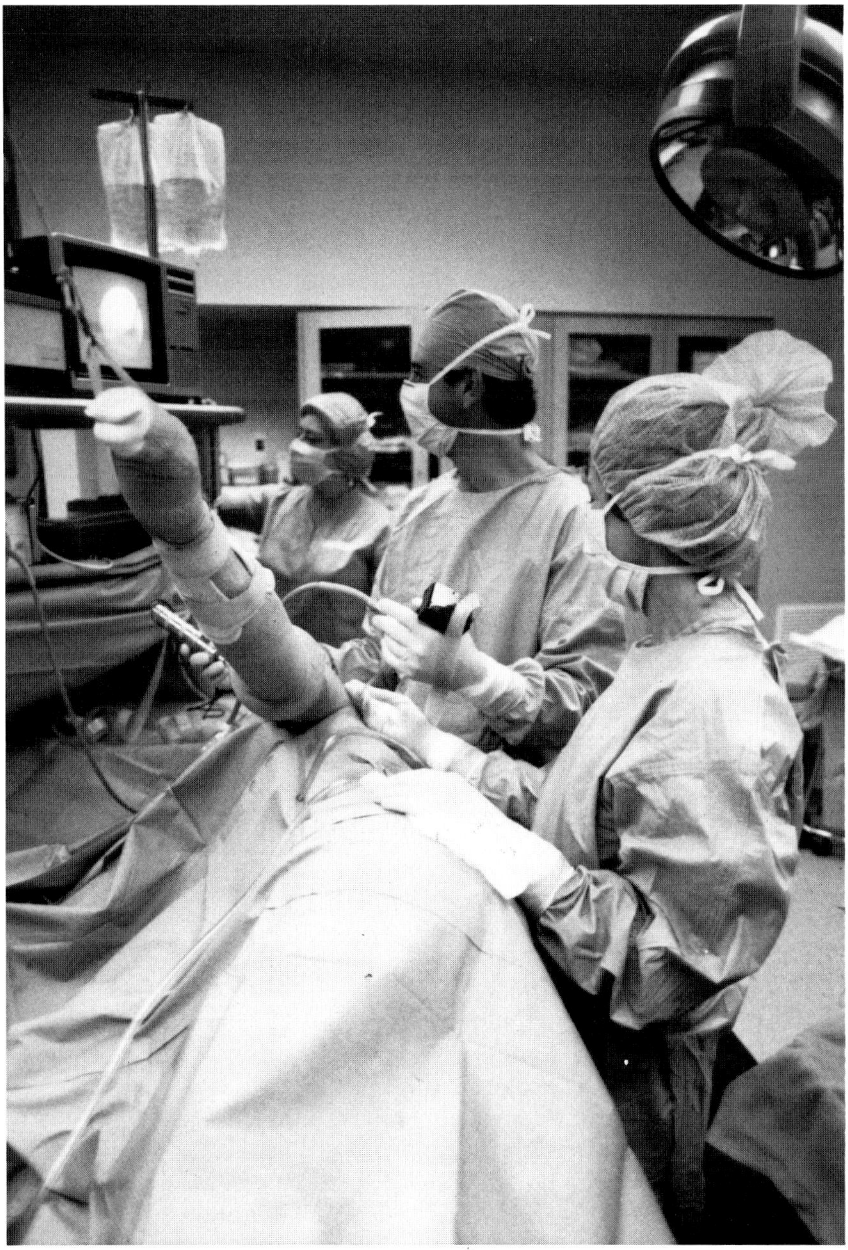

**Figure 13–1** Personnel and patient positioning for arthroscopic surgery of the shoulder.

## Techniques

The various portals to the shoulder have been well described and delineated anatomically (3). The posterior portal is the most common one used for visualization of the shoulder and is located 2 cm or one thumb's breadth below the posterior point of the acromion. The shoulder may be preinsufflated with saline by utilizing a spinal needle prior to actually inserting an arthroscopic trocar. A puncture wound is then made with a no. 11 blade and the arthroscopic trocar and cannula are directed toward the coracoid process anteriorly and into the glenohumeral joint. The backflow of saline confirms entry into the joint. The shoulder is then insufflated with

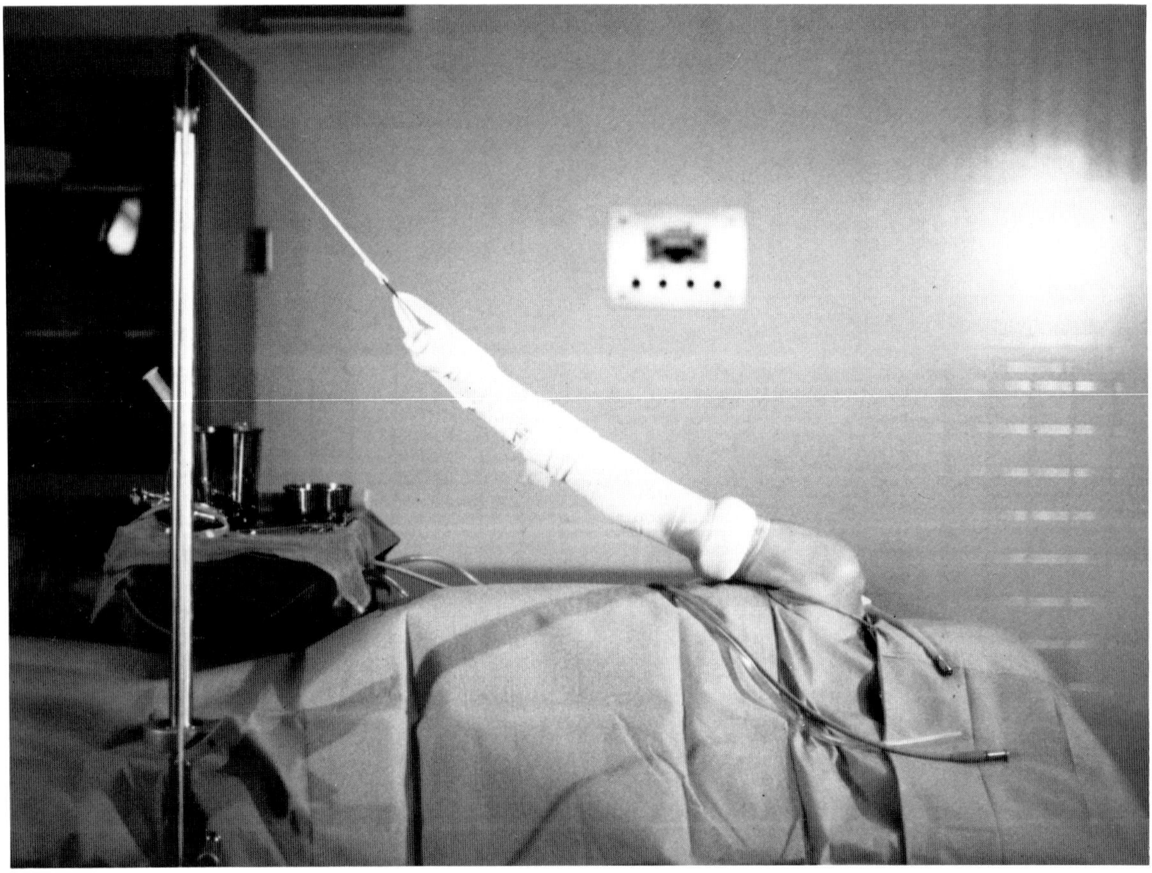

**Figure 13–2** Patient is placed in a traction device that allows for motion of the shoulder in all planes and for removal of the arm from traction while maintaining the sterile field.

saline via the side arm of the arthroscopic cannula, utilizing a syringe. Visualization of all of the intra-articular structures of the shoulder can be accomplished via this portal except for the very anterior face of the humerus and the infraspinatus and teres minor portion of the rotator cuff.

The superior or supraspinatus fossa portal is usually utilized as an inflow portal. The portal may be used, however, for visualization of the posterior compartment of the shoulder and allows for excellent examination of the posterior humeral head, the posterior glenoid recess, and the teres minor and infraspinatus portions of the rotator cuff. The portal is located at the lateral end of the supraspinatus fossa and is bounded anteriorly by the posterior margin of the clavicle, laterally by the medial border of the acromion, and posteriorly by the scapular spine. The cannula is introduced at this location at approximately a 30-degree angle from the horizontal plane and traverses the muscle bellies of the trapezius and supraspinatus muscles. The cannula enters the shoulder joint just suiperior and posterior to the glenoid neck. From this position it can be conveniently tucked into the posterior recess, well out of the way of the arthroscope and operative instruments.

The anterior portal is used primarily for operative instruments and is located just lateral to the coracoid process. Any entry medial to the coracoid places the musculocutaneous nerve in jeopardy and therefore should be avoided. The anterior portal may be obtained directly by placing a spinal needle through the anterior aspect of the shoulder, observing its entry into the joint. The course of the needle can then be reproduced with a cannula. Entry into the joint should be observed arthroscopically and be in a triangle bounded by the biceps tendon, the margin of the humeral head, and the anterior margin of the glenoid. The portal may also be obtained indirectly by advancing the arthroscope to the point on the anterior capsule where entry is desired. The arthroscope is removed from its cannula, and a Steinmann pin is passed through the arthroscopic sheath, puncturing the anterior structures of the shoulder. The arthroscopic sheath and Steinmann pin are then separated and the arthroscope is replaced in its cannula. The blunt end of the Steinmann pin is then visible in the shoulder. A cannula is then worked over the Steinmann pin until it enters the joint, and then the pin is removed.

The soft tissue structures that encompass the shoulder are quite thick, and therefore, once a portal is satisfactorily obtained, it should never be lost. The cannula should always remain in position, or if it is to be removed, a Wissinger rod (L. L. Johnson, personal communication) or a Steinmann pin should be substituted for the cannula prior to its removal so that the portal is not lost (Figure 13–3).

## Instrumentation

As with most arthroscopic procedures, shoulder arthroscopy has evolved from a diagnostic modality to a surgical modality with increasingly sophisticated techniques. A standard 30-degree fore-oblique arthroscope in the 4.5- to 5-mm range is utilized. The shoulder is a fairly large joint and allows easy access with an arthroscope of this size. Instrumentation for diagnostic arthroscopy is not different from that in the knee and primarily utilizes the hook probe, which must be long enough to access the joint through a cannula. Most diagnoses can be made, however, by direct visualization alone. If diagnostic arthroscopy is to be followed by

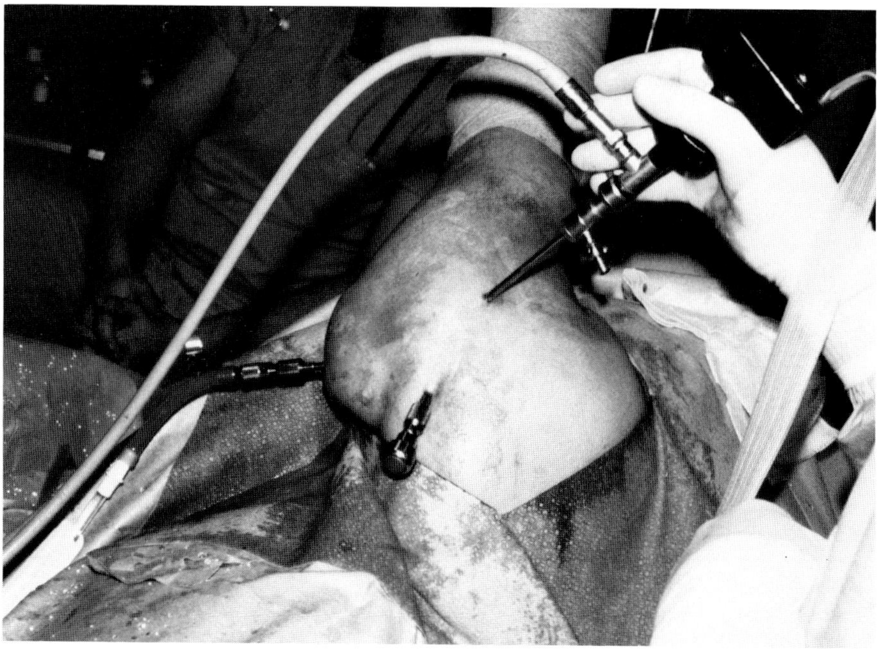

**Figure 13–3** Anterior, posterior, and superior portals are necessary for arthroscopic surgery of the shoulder.

an arthrotomy, it is sometimes helpful to avoid establishing an anterior portal and avoid the leakage of saline into the soft tissues anteriorly, which makes dissection quite difficult (N. Small, personal communication).

Surgical arthroscopy of the shoulder has primarily been excisional in nature. To this end the most useful surgical tools have been the grasping forceps for removal of loose bodies and a power shaving system for the debridement of a torn labrum or small rotator cuff tear and for synovectomy of the shoulder.

Some specialized instrumentation has been developed in response to specific needs for arthroscopic surgery of the shoulder. The Wissinger rod system mentioned previously allows for interchangeability of cannulas without losing the arthroscopic portal. A system of cannulated trocars with cannulas has also been developed for the same purpose. A universal cannula system has also been introduced that can be used interchangeably for arthroscopic power instrumentation and inflow. Beath pins or K-wires with eyes at either end have been utilized to suture a detached labrum back to the glenoid neck. An intra-articular stapling device has also been developed for this same purpose. The stapling device is also used to fix the anterior capsule to the glenoid neck for repair of an unstable shoulder.

Instrumentation and techniques continue to be developed to accomplish other procedures as well. The operative technique and instrumentation for repair of a dislocating shoulder with an extra-articular ligamentous graft is presently being clinically tested. Finally, bursoscopy is being explored and decompression of the coracoacromial arch has been accomplished by sectioning the coracoacromial ligament with an electrocautery device, with acromioplasty being performed with an abrader to remove bone.

## Summary

To become skilled arthroscopists of the shoulder, we must in many ways become beginners again. Most of the principles, however, that we learned in the knee are transferable to the shoulder, making this task much easier. A thorough understanding of the anatomy of the shoulder is mandatory. Operating room organization and training of paramedical personnel is essential. Most of the instrumentation and operative techniques utilized in shoulder arthroscopy are the same as in the knee. Some new and specialized techniques and instrumentation are being introduced for the shoulder to solve problems specific to this joint. The orthopaedist and his team must first learn the basic skills for arthroscopy of the shoulder and then in the laboratory work out the nuances of these new techniques prior to offering them to patients. When approached in this organized manner, shoulder arthroscopy can be accomplished successfully.

### *References*

1. Andrews JR, Carson WG. The arthroscopic treatment of glenoid labrum tears in the throwing athlete. Orthop Trans 8:44, 1984
2. Caspari RB. Shoulder arthroscopy: A review of the present state of the art. Contemp Orthop 4:523–530, 1982
3. Caspari RB, Whipple TL, Meyers JF. The Neviaser portal for shoulder arthroscopy. Paper presented at Annual Meeting of the Arthroscopy Association of North America, New Orleans, 1984
4. McGlynn FJ, Caspari RB. Arthroscopic findings in the subluxating shoulder. Clin Orthop 183:173–178, 1984
5. Wiley AM, Older MWJ. Shoulder arthroscopy: Investigations with a fiber optic instrument. Am J Sports Med 8:31–33, 1980

# Arthroscopy of the Ankle

# 14

Douglas L. Gollehon
David Drez, Jr.

As surgeons become more familiar with the technique of ankle arthroscopy, its use for diagnostic and surgical purposes will become much more widespread than has been true in the recent past. When arthroscopic examinations of cadaveric ankles were first begun in Japan (2, 3) and here in the United States (1) the investigators found it extremely difficult to maneuver the scope and obtain adequate visualization. These first authors wrote that ankle arthroscopy was so difficult as to not be practical for routine use. Unfortunately, the ankle has not changed; arthroscopic visualization remains difficult to achieve. To minimize difficulties encountered when we first begin arthroscopic procedures for ankle problems, we should become familiar with arthroscopic approaches, techniques to aid in visualization, and pitfalls we may encounter.

## History and Physical Examination

### History

Patients presenting with ankle problems should have a careful history taken, followed by a thorough physical examination. Questions during the first visit center around mechanism of initial injury, treatment, and chronologic sequence of problems since the major injury. Establishing the mechanism of injury helps focus attention on painful structures most likely to have sustained primary damage, thus allowing us to differentiate these from secondary problems which have developed over time. Since postinjury treatment and rehabilitation have tremendous influence on the final outcome of ankle injuries, the exact regimen undergone needs to be carefully elicited. This treatment may have significantly altered the location of major pain points, further confusing the presenting problem. As the chronologic order of injuries, treatment, and therapy is discussed, character and location of the pain can be clarified and exacerbating activities identified.

### Physical Examination

The physical examination is divided into functional and static portions, the functional part starting while the patient is standing. Gait pattern during normal walking and slow jogging is observed, with any malalignment or abnormalities being noted for further examination. Next the patient is asked to do a full squat and then jump, first on the unaffected and then the affected side. This provides a great deal of information on range of motion and functional use of the ankle.

The second part of the examination is carried out with the patient seated. Initial observation for swelling and deformity is followed by gentle palpation of suspected areas of pathology. The patient actively moves the ankle through a full range of motion while palpation for crepitation or abnormal joint motion is carried out. Subsequently, the ankle, hindfoot, and midfoot joints are placed through passive ranges of motion while palpation for crepitation is continued. At this point testing for ankle stability using anterior drawer and varus stress tests is performed.

After the history and physical examination, radiographs to demonstrate the involved areas should be taken and evaluated for arthritic changes, bony injuries, ligamentous calcification, avulsions, loose bodies, and degeneration consistent with ankle instability. In the case of acute injuries, careful evaluation of the talar dome is necessary to exclude osteochondral fractures. After completion of this thorough evaluation, a diagnosis can usually be established for the majority of ankle problems, and treatment with a combination of immobilization, mobilization, and rehabilitation can be started. There will always be a small percentage of patients whose ankle problems cannot be diagnosed, even with this complete evaluation. These patients who need further evaluation and those needing surgical intervention for ankle problems can benefit from arthroscopic evaluation or surgery.

## Indications

Intra-articular ankle problems needing further diagnostic evaluation or surgical intervention have in the past presented difficult treatment problems since arthrotomy was the only direct method of satisfying these needs. Fortunately, arthroscopy can now be used instead of arthrotomy for both diagnosis and surgery in the ankle, avoiding the morbidity associated with an open procedure. Common indications for ankle arthroscopy are listed in Table 14–1.

**Table 14–1** Indications for Arthroscopic Examination and Surgery of the Ankle

| |
|---|
| 1. Posttraumatic hemarthrosis |
| 2. Osteochondral fractures or loose bodies |
| 3. Persistant posttraumatic symptoms |
| 4. Posttraumatic or inflammatory arthritis |
| 5. Osteochondritis dissecans |
| 6. Undiagnosed synovitis |
| 7. Articular surface evaluation prior to reconstructive procedures |

Patients with posttraumatic hemarthrosis of the ankle most frequently have chondral or osteochondral fractures; however, when significant injury to the joint capsule and surrounding ligaments has also occurred, extravasation of blood into the soft tissues will prevent a tense hemarthrosis. Acute osteochondral fractures or more chronic injuries producing loose body formation usually result from fracture of the talar dome. As the patient sustains pronation or supination ankle forces, the lateral or medial talar dome will impinge against the tibia and fracturing will occur if the ligaments do not first rupture. This mechanism is much the same as seen with tibial plateau fractures. These fracture fragments often rotate or displace from their beds and demand surgical intervention, which can be carried out nicely by arthroscopic means.

We frequently have patients with a history of previous ankle injuries who continue to have pain or symptoms of popping and instability, and in whom we are unable to demonstrate any abnormalities on radiographs. Rehabilitation of these patients will be aided by arthroscopic evaluation to establish a precise diagnosis. When patients with the above symptoms are examined we often find changes of early articular surface degeneration consistent with posttraumatic arthritis. These ankles as well as those with inflammatory arthritis may be helped temporarily by a thorough lavage and debridement of osteophytes and inflammed synovial tissue.

When osteochondritis dissecans of the talar dome is diagnosed, evaluation of the articular surface and, if indicated, debridement, drilling, and loose body removal can be accomplished arthroscopically. Occasionally, arthroscopy of the ankle will be used to obtain biopsy material and make a diagnosis when an undiagnosed and persistent synovitis is present.

We may also want to use arthroscopic evaluation to provide more information on the condition of the articular surfaces in those patients with chronic instability who are considering a reconstructive procedure. This will allow us to advise the patient more intelligently and also will help the patient to make a more educated decision regarding surgery, rehabilitation, and future activities.

# Procedures

## Portals

Multiple arthroscopic portals, three anteriorly and two posteriorly, can be used for ankle arthroscopy (Table 14–2). However, during any single operative procedure, one or two portals should be adequate to visualize the entire joint, with further portals needed only for triangulation of surgical instruments. Either the anterolateral, anterocentral, or anteromedial portal (Figure 14–1) will provide excellent visualization of the anterior compartment of the ankle joint, but the concave talar dome does not allow passage of the arthroscope into the posterior compartment from the anterolateral or anteromedial portals as frequently as from the anterocentral approach (Figure 14–2). When visualization of only the articular surfaces is needed,

**Table 14–2** Arthroscopic Portals Used for Ankle Arthroscopy

| ANTERIOR PORTALS | POSTERIOR PORTALS |
|---|---|
| Anterolateral | Posterolateral |
| Anterocentral | Posteromedial |
| Anteromedial | |

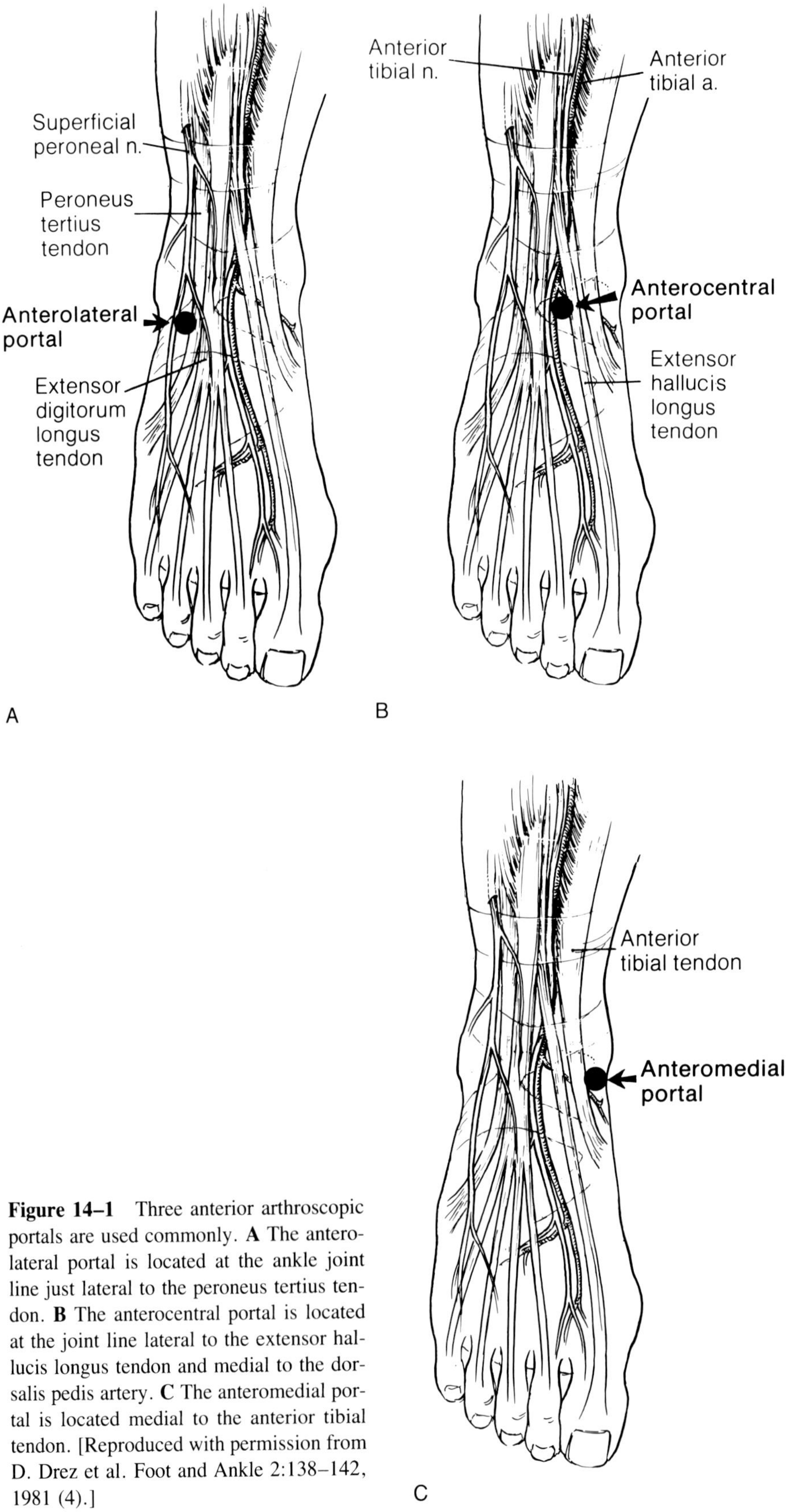


**Figure 14–1** Three anterior arthroscopic portals are used commonly. **A** The anterolateral portal is located at the ankle joint line just lateral to the peroneus tertius tendon. **B** The anterocentral portal is located at the joint line lateral to the extensor hallucis longus tendon and medial to the dorsalis pedis artery. **C** The anteromedial portal is located medial to the anterior tibial tendon. [Reproduced with permission from D. Drez et al. Foot and Ankle 2:138–142, 1981 (4).]

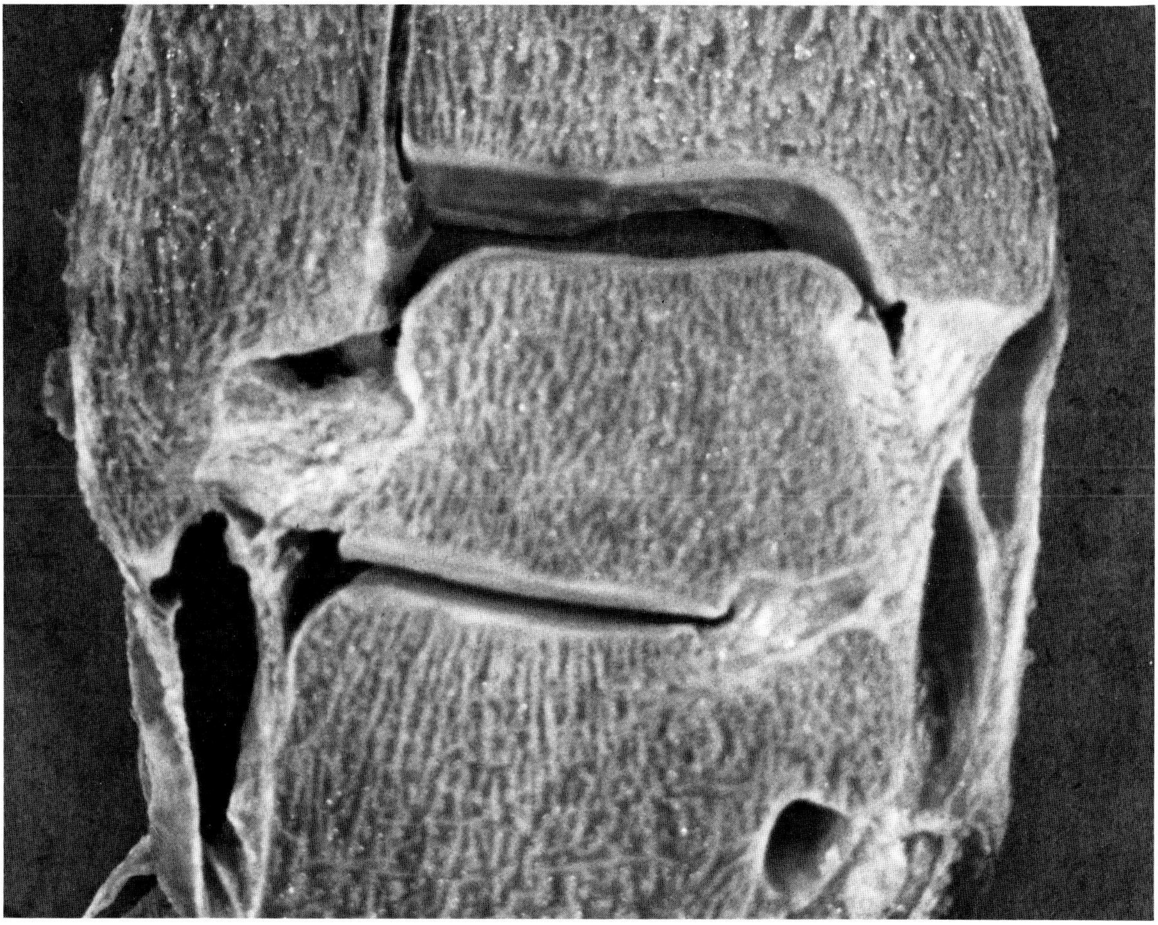

**Figure 14–2** The normal talar dome is concave in shape, making advancement of the arthroscope from the anterior to posterior compartment difficult when the anterolateral or anteromedial portals are used.

the anteromedial or anterolateral portals will provide the most complete views of the medial or lateral articular surfaces, respectively; however, when the entire joint needs to be evaluated for diagnostic purposes, the anterocentral portal is best since it gives good visualization of the anteromedial and anterolateral aspects of the joint, as well as generally allowing advancement of the sleeve and trochar over the talus for visualization of the posterior compartment. Use of the posterolateral and posteromedial portals (Figure 14–3) may be necessary when pathology is localized to the posterior compartment of the joint or when it is impossible to advance the arthroscope over the dome of the talus. These posterior approaches must be done with the patient in the prone position, so the surgeon should be prepared to turn the patient if visualization of the posterior compartment from the anterior portals is impossible.

## Technique

Ankle arthroscopy is carried out in the operating room under general anesthesia to ensure optimal operating conditions, including full muscle relaxation. Before the procedure begins, careful planning for the arthroscopic approach should

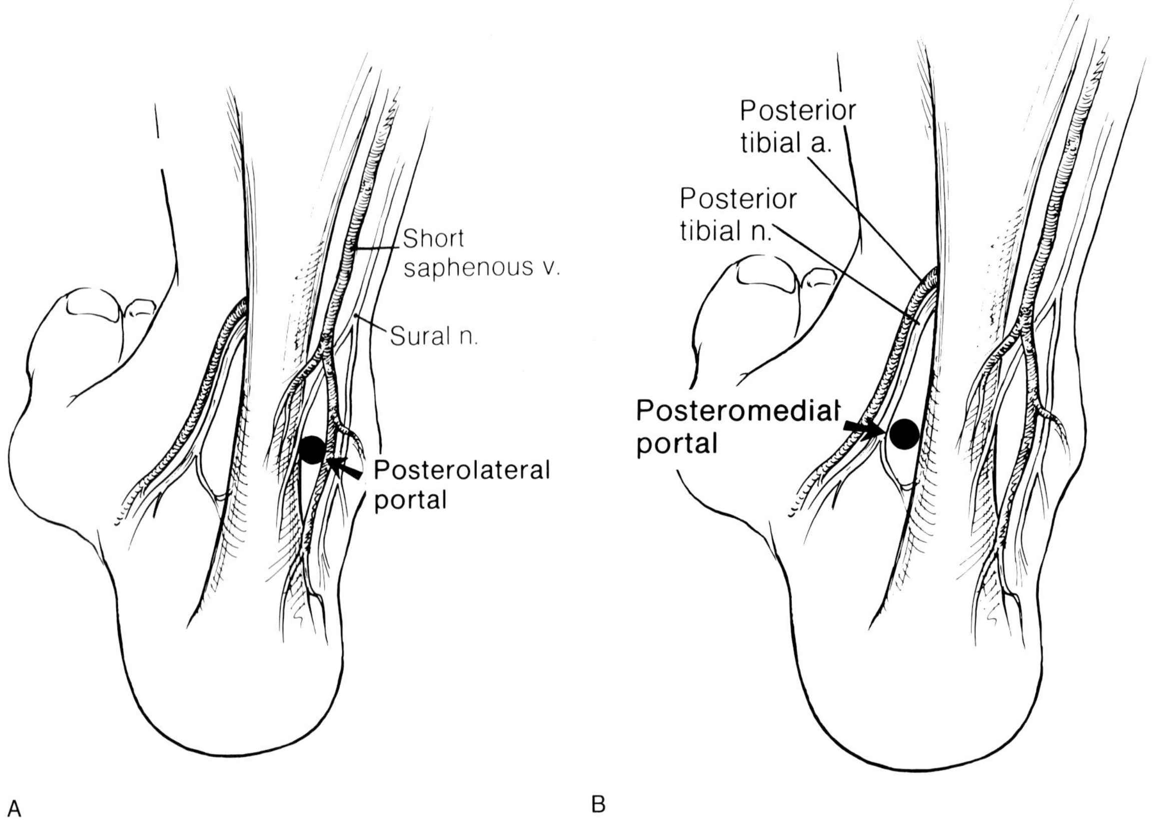


**Figure 14–3** Two arthroscopic portals are commonly used posteriorly. **A** The posterolateral portal is located at the joint line lateral to the Achilles' tendon and medial to the peroneal tendons. **B** The posteromedial portal is located at the joint line medial to the Achilles' tendon and lateral to the neurovascular bundle. [Reproduced with permission from D. Drez et al. Foot and Ankle 2:138–142, 1981 (4).]

be done. Extra-articular anatomy, either anterior or posterior (Figure 14–4) is outlined so portal placement will carry the least risk of injury to surrounding structures and provide optimal visualization of the pathology. This is much more crucial in the ankle than the knee since the important anatomical structures are so compactly arranged about the ankle.

By plantar and dorsiflexion of the foot, the anterior joint line is located, a needle is placed into the joint, and saline is instilled to provide distension. At the site of the proposed arthroscopic portal, a small skin incision is made, and a hemostat is used to separate subcutaneous tissue from the skin to the joint capsule, moving the important surrounding structures away from the portal itself. While a saline-filled syringe is used with the previously placed needle to maintain firm joint distension, the sleeve and sharp trochar are passed to the joint capsule, angled toward the midline, and with a firm twisting motion, are felt to pop into the joint. The sharp trochar is then exchanged for the blunt one, and with the ankle held in plantar flexion and using firm pressure, the sleeve and trochar are passed over the central portion of the talar dome into the posterior compartment. Saline inflow is switched from the needle to the sleeve, the arthroscope is placed, and examination of the ankle joint is begun.

As the arthroscope is moved across the back of the joint from lateral to medial, the lightly colored synovial folds and fat pad of the posterior compartment should be examined and probed (Figure 14–5). Angulation of the field of view

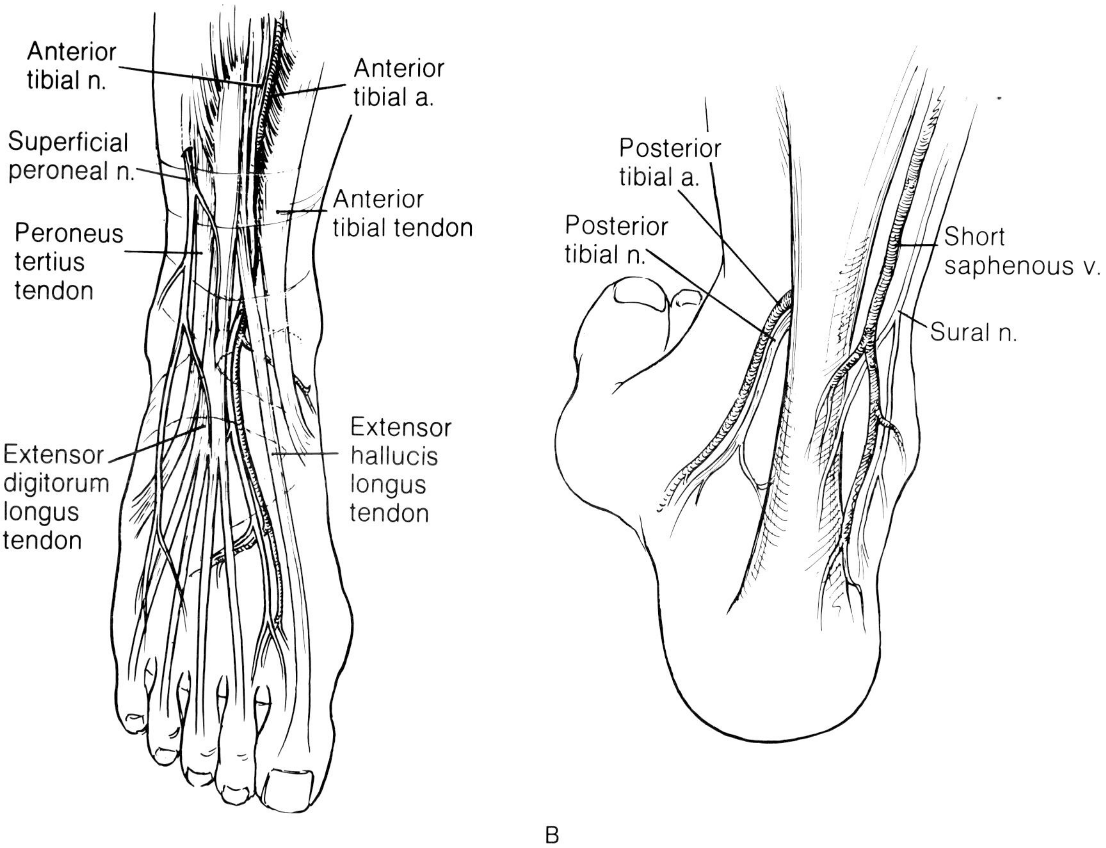


**Figure 14–4** The extra-articular anatomy, both anterior and posterior, should be reviewed during preoperative planning. **A** The anterior extra-articular structures outlined prior to placing arthroscopic portals include the anterior tibial and extensor hallucis longus tendons, the dorsalis pedis artery, and the extensor digitorum communis and peroneus tertius tendons. **B** The posterior extra-articular structures outlined include the borders of the Achilles' tendon medially and laterally, the posterior tibial artery, and the peroneal tendons. [Reproduced with permission from D. Drez et al. Foot and Ankle 2:138–142, 1981 (4).]

brings the medial talomalleolar space and articular surfaces into view (Figure 14–6). Advancing the arthroscope further anteriorly will cause the scope to "jump" into the anterior compartment, so a sweep from the posteromedial side of the joint to the posterolateral side should be done to continue the examination of the posterior compartment. With the arthroscope positioned in the posterolateral corner of the joint, rotation of the scope brings the tibiofibular articulation into the visual field (Figure 14–7). This joint should be examined visually while either a probe is used or manual stress is applied in an attempt to demonstrate any abnormal widening of the ankle mortise (Figure 14–8). By maneuvering the arthroscope anteriorly and changing the field of view, the lateral talomalleolar space and articular surfaces come into view and should be examined from the edge of the talar dome (Figure 14–9) down to the anterior talofibular ligament (Figure 14–10). After the ligament has been probed, visualization of the anterior synovial wall and neck of the talus can be accomplished by maneuvering the arthroscope across the front of the joint

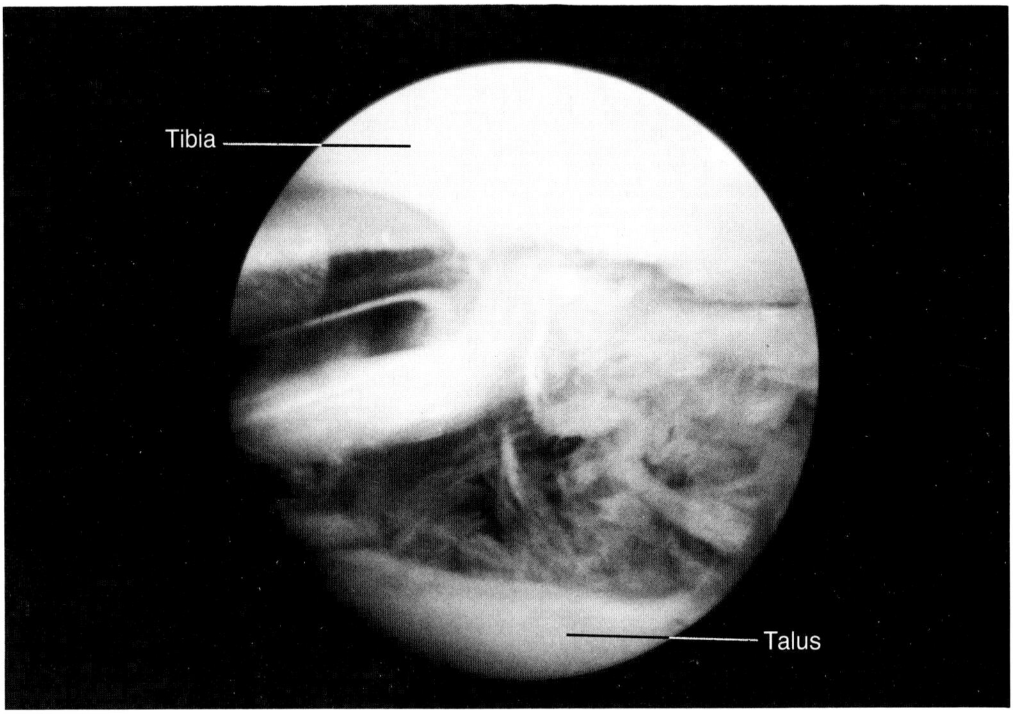


**Figure 14–5** The posterior synovial wall of the ankle is lightly colored with multiple folds and capsular bands.

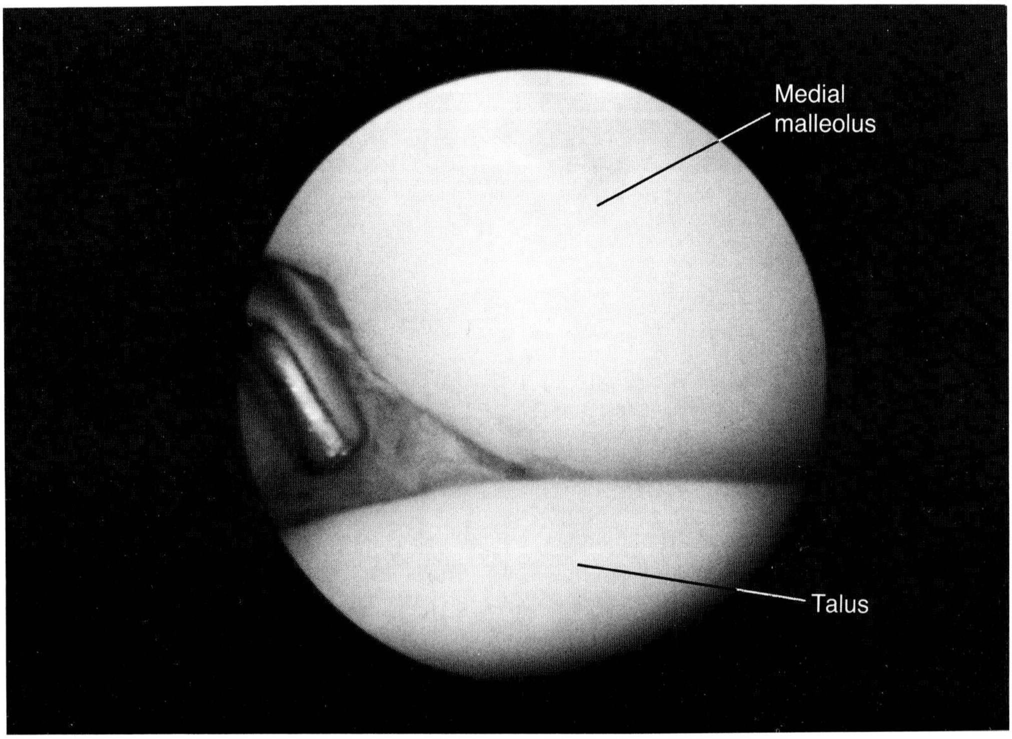


**Figure 14–6** The medial talomalleolar articular surface can be evaluated visually and probed to determine cartilage integrity.

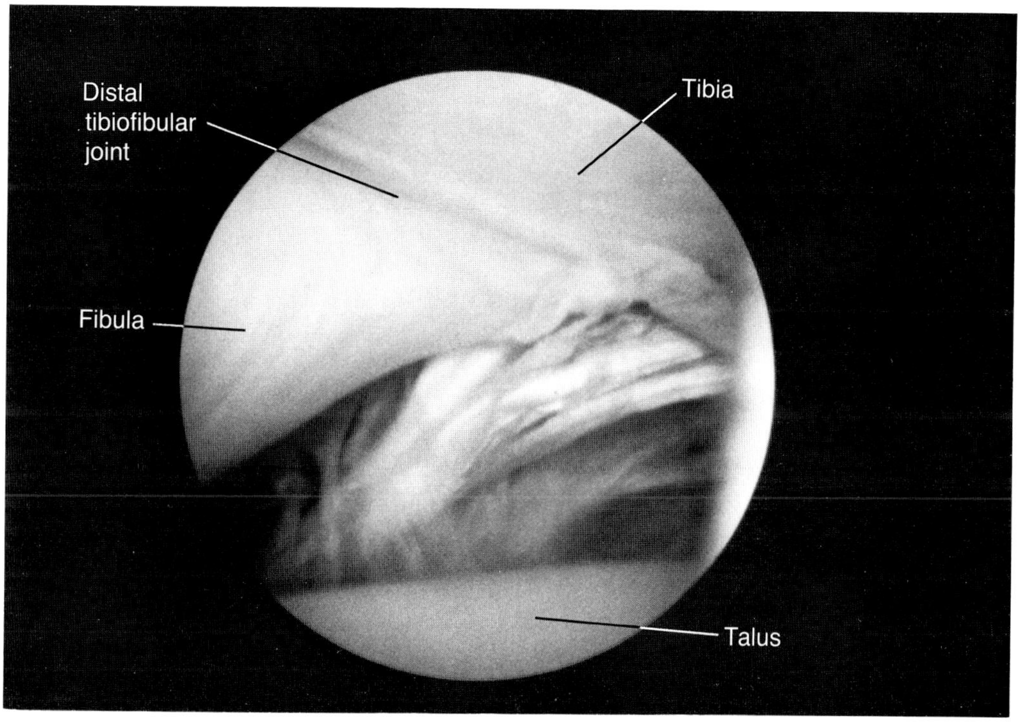


**Figure 14–7** The distal tibiofibular joint frequently has capsular and synovial folds about it that should not be mistaken for abnormal tissue.

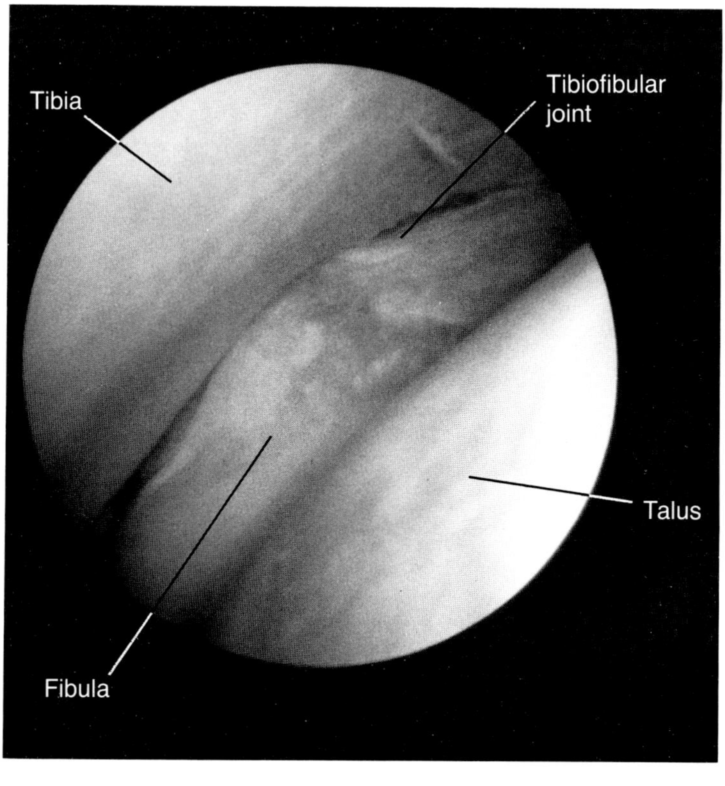


**Figure 14–8** The entire distal tibiofibular joint can be visualized while probing is done or manual stress is applied to evaluate the competance of the tibiofibular ligaments.

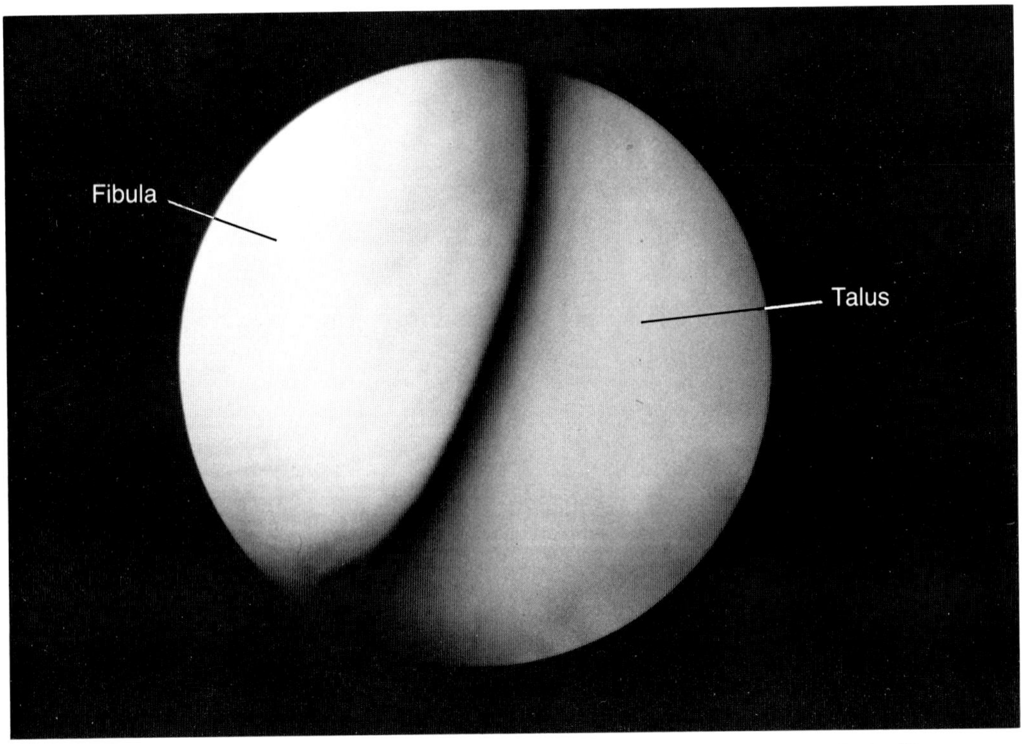


**Figure 14–9** The lateral talomalleolar articulation should be symmetrical with no more than 2–3 mm of space between the articular surfaces.

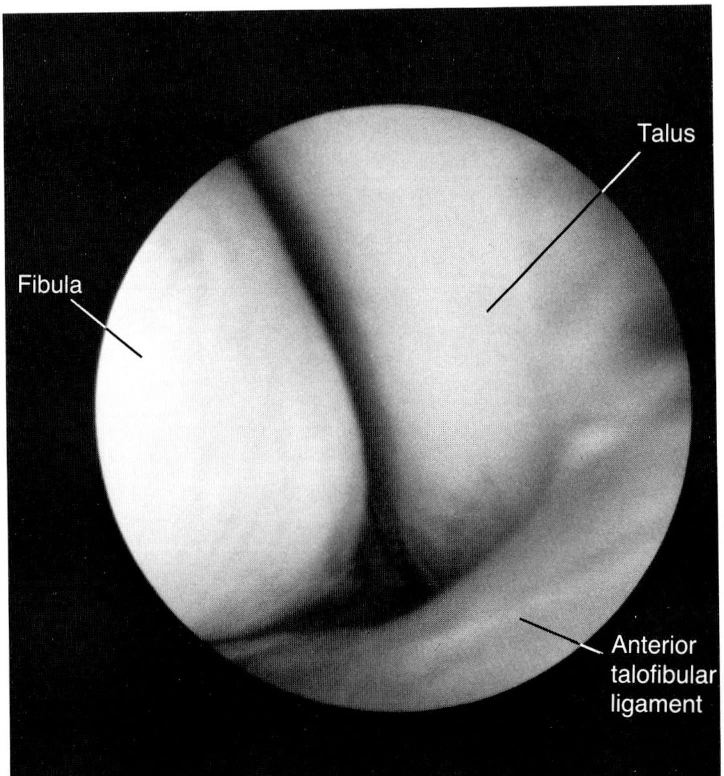


**Figure 14–10** The anterior talofibular ligament can be easily seen while a probe is used to test its attachment and competance.

toward the medial side (Figure 14–11). The articular surface of the anterior aspect of the medial malleolus will come into view and can be examined and probed (Figure 14–12).

During the procedure continuous saline inflow under pressure is used, with care taken to use as few arthroscopic portals as possible since visualization will be lost if adequate fluid pressure in the ankle cannot be maintained.

## Postoperative Care

At the completion of the procedure, the joint is drained of saline and a pressure dressing is applied from the toes to knee. During the first 24 hours after surgery, the patient is encouraged to elevate the leg but also is allowed to ambulate with the use of crutches, taking partial weight on the involved side unless articular surface damage has been diagnosed at surgery. The pressure dressing is removed 48 hours after surgery, band-aids are applied to the arthroscopic portals, and weight bearing to tolerance is begun if no contraindications are present. Rehabilitation is started with active and active-assisted range of motion of the ankle. Once the preoperative range of motion has been regained and no joint swelling remains, strengthening is started and rehabilitation progresses to endurance and activity phases as the patient improves. If articular surface damage was found at surgery, the patient should progress through a normal rehabilitative program, but no weight bearing is allowed on the involved side for 6 weeks from the date of surgery.

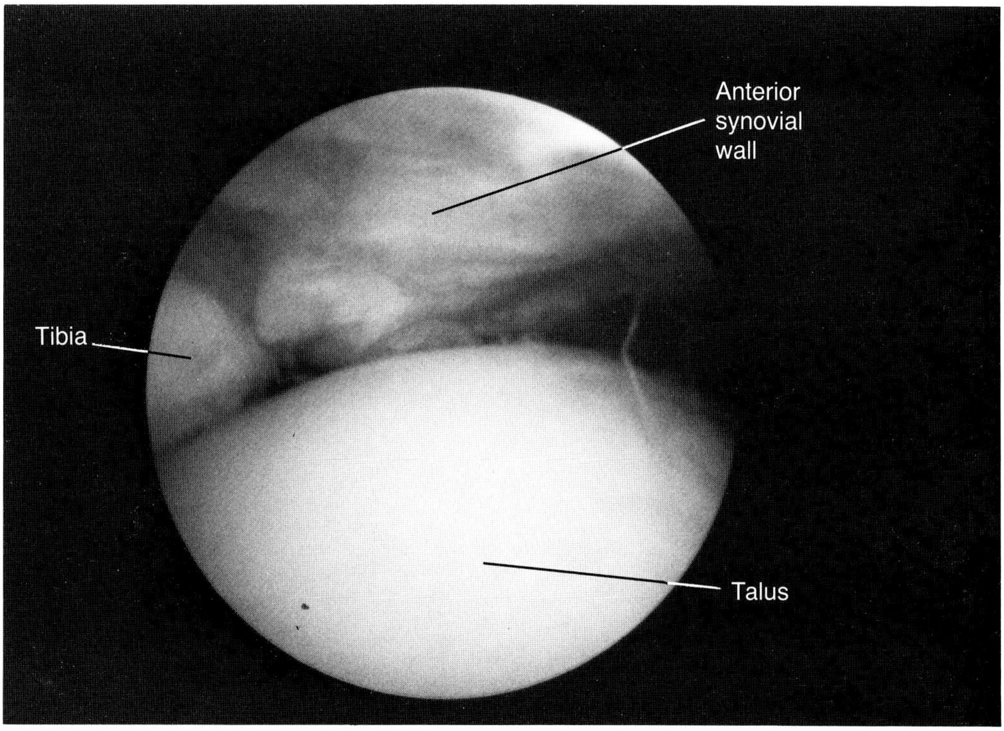


**Figure 14–11** The anterior compartment synovial wall can be evaluated for synovial changes, and a search for loose bodies or osteophytes along the neck of the talus should be done.

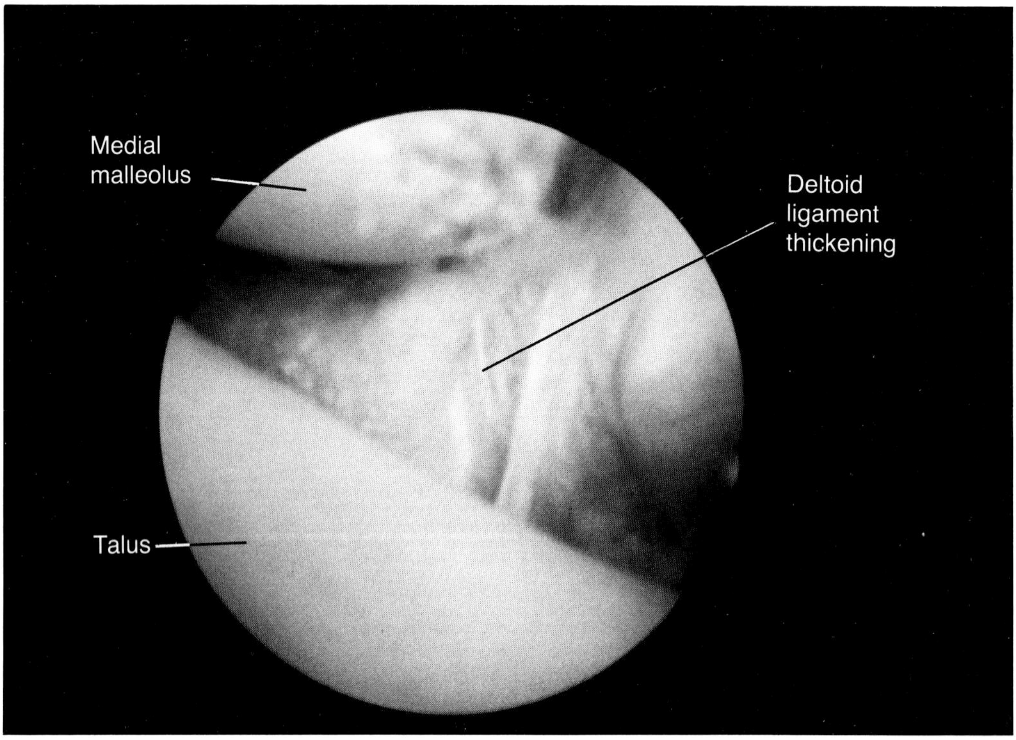


**Figure 14–12** The capsular thickening of the deltoid ligament and the medial malleolar articular surface can be evaluated for damage and probed.

## Complications

Due to the small size and tightness of the ankle joint, instrument breakage is the most frequently encountered problem during surgery. This problem is minimized by keeping the joint firmly distended and taking great care during instrument manipulation. Other potential problems, such as damage to surrounding vital structures and infection, are encountered no more frequently than with arthroscopic knee or shoulder surgery, as long as appropriate care is taken during the procedure. During extended procedures a considerable amount of saline extravasation into surrounding tissues occurs. Although concern for possible development of a compartment syndrome in the leg is appropriate, this has not been observed since the fluid generally rapidly reabsorbs with use of the pressure dressing.

## Summary

Ankle arthroscopy is extremely useful to aid in the diagnosis of certain complex ankle problems and provides a means of surgical treatment for other lesions. When care is taken with preoperative planning and during surgery, a large number of common ankle problems can be safely assessed and treated arthroscopically. Acute problems such as hemarthrosis and osteochondral fractures can be evaluated and treated in this manner. When chronic problems such as osteochondritis dissecans, arthritic conditions, old articular fractures, or vague and persistent posttraumatic symptoms are encountered, the articular surfaces may be precisely evaluated arthroscopically and appropriate treatment can be carried out. Arthroscopy of the ankle may also be used to evaluate the articular surface prior to reconstructive procedures and to assess and biopsy synovial tissue when chronic undiagnosed synovitis is present.

Ankle arthroscopy affords a tremendous decrease in morbidity when compared with arthrotomy and in addition does not limit our ability to perform appropriate surgical procedures for many ankle problems.

## *References*

1. Burman MS. Arthroscopy or the direct visualization of joints. J Bone Joint Surg 18:669–695, 1931
2. Chen YC. Clinical and cadaver studies on the ankle joint arthroscopy. J Jpn Orthop Assoc 50:631–651, 1961
3. Chen YC. Arthroscopy of the ankle joint. Arthroscopy 1:16, 1976
4. Drez D, Ghul J Jr, Gollehon DL. Ankle arthroscopy: Technique and indications. Foot and Ankle 2:138–142, 1981

# Arthroscopic Reconstruction for Chronic Lateral Instability of the Ankle

# 15

Richard B. Hawkins

One of the exciting aspects of arthroscopic surgery is its application to everyday problems facing the orthopaedist. For example, early in the development of arthroscopy, it became possible to extract a loose body from the knee without resorting to the traditional arthrotomy incision with its attendant morbidity, scarring, and hospital stay, not to mention discomfort to the patient. More recently, reconstruction of the anterior shoulder ligaments for chronic dislocation has been performed on an outpatient basis, using three small portal wounds and thereby avoiding a somewhat formidable surgical approach to the shoulder joint.

The purpose of this chapter is to report on recent developments in arthroscopic technique as applied to a common everyday orthopaedic complaint—that of chronic lateral instability of the ankle. Orthopaedists for decades have been improving upon ways of stabilizing weak lateral ankle structures, usually by tendon transfers using part or all of the peroneus brevis to provide a combined dynamic and static reinforcement of the lateral ankle. With the advent of ever-smaller arthroscopic surgical tools, it is now possible to treat ankle instability by a combined capsulorrhaphy-tenodesis procedure, by stapling the anterior talofibular ligament and lateral capsule into the vertical surface of the talus just anterior to the fibula.

## Biomechanics

The ankle, because of its geometry and ligamentous support, is a supple and strong joint for locomotion. Nevertheless, it is prone to injury from a variety of mechanisms, most commonly from an excessive plantar flexion and inversion stress. In this position, the anterior talofibular ligament is aligned nearly parallel to the long axis of the tibia (7, 12). In plantar flexion and inversion, the anterior talofibular ligament is loaded by inversion and internal rotary movements (3, 5). A number of biomechanical studies of the ankle have measured increased ankle motion after sectioning of the various ligaments (1, 2, 8, 9, 11). The results showed that injury to the anterior talofibular ligament allows anterior and medial displacement of the talus. Inversion of the talus was also observed with the foot in excessive plantar flexion. Other studies using radiographic techniques have shown that the anterior talofibular ligament does not contribute very much to the varus tilt of the talus (4, 12), unless injury has also occurred to the calcaneofibular ligament (6, 13). Still another experimental study of the ankle under loaded conditions showed significant increases in rotation without simultaneous increase in varus angulation after dividing the anterior talofibular ligament (10). A recent biomechanical study (8) found the anterior talofibular ligament to be a primary stabilizer of the ankle, indicating that it provides significant resistance to varus tilt of the talus in all positions of flexion. The authors noted that because the increased motions of the talus are relatively small after sectioning of the anterior talofibular ligament, many ankles that are chronically symptomatic following ankle injury may have increased talar instability secondary to insufficiency of the anterior talofibular ligament, which is undetectable by clinical or radiographic evaluation.

## Patient Selection

As in all orthopaedic procedures, careful patient selection and preoperative assessment is of paramount importance. The lateral ankle sprain is among the most common of all athletic injuries, and most heal uneventfully with traditional conservative approaches to treatment. And yet there are some patients who develop chronic instability problems, usually after several severe lateral ankle sprains.

As always, the history is most important. The patient with clinically significant lateral ankle instability will describe a progression of events over months or even years, indicating ever-increasing laxity of the ankle. Minor provocations such as stepping off a curb or stepping on a small stone lead to a significant varus injury to the ankle.

In the office or clinic, it is frequently possible to detect a positive "anterior drawer test." The examiner's hand, grasping the heel, can slide the entire foot forward at the tibial talar joint, using the opposite hand to anchor the lower leg. Many of these patients will have an increased "talar tilt" test radiographically. When inversion stress is applied, the talus appears to tilt out from underneath the lateral aspect of the tibia and even sublux medially. Usually this test is quite subtle unless the calcaneofibular ligament is torn in addition to the anterior talofibular ligament.

## Arthroscopic Technique

The general technique for ankle arthroscopy will be presented in Chapter 16. We prefer to perform outpatient surgery under general anesthesia, using a thigh tourniquet, as in all extremity surgery, and a leg-holding device applied to the midcalf. It is important to avoid undue pressure over the proximal calf near the fibular neck, which could lead to peroneal palsy. For ankle ligament reconstruction we have found portal placement to be exceedingly important. An 18-gauge needle is used to establish an anteromedial portal just anterior to the saphenous vein and medial to the anterior tibial tendon. As saline is instilled through a 30-cc syringe, the ankle dorsiflexes. Another 18-gauge needle localizes an anterolateral portal through which the Dyonics 2.2-mm needlescope is introduced. Although a larger 4.0-mm arthroscope can be used to visualize the ankle joint, we have found it technically difficult to gain exposure in the lateral gutter near the tip of the fibula unless the smaller 2.2-mm arthroscope is used. A 3.0-mm water inflow cannula is then inserted in the anteromedial portal already established by the first 18-gauge needle. The saline bag is suspended at least 1 meter above the ankle, providing sufficient head of pressure for distension of the joint for the surgical procedure.

The diagnostic part of the procedure commences. Patients with chronic lateral instability of the ankle will often show a relative laxity or "ballooning" of the entire lateral capsule and anterior talofibular ligament when viewed from an anterolateral portal. Cadaver dissection is an important prerequisite to performing this procedure and will reveal that the lateral capsule and anterior talofibular ligament are contiguous structures that are in reality quite thin in comparison to the thick deltoid ligament medially. An increased synovitis is often present in patients with chronic lateral instability. Frequently, articular cartilage defects are seen at the medial corner of the joint where the corner of the talus has struck the tibia at the medial aspect of the plafond during a subluxation or inversion stress. Articular cartilage loose bodies may be aspirated through the arthroscope in these cases.

Arthroscopic stapling repair for chronic lateral instability is simply a shortening or tightening of the lateral capsule and anterior talofibular ligament (Figure 15–1). A 6- or 8-mm diameter area on the vertical surface of the talus is abraded

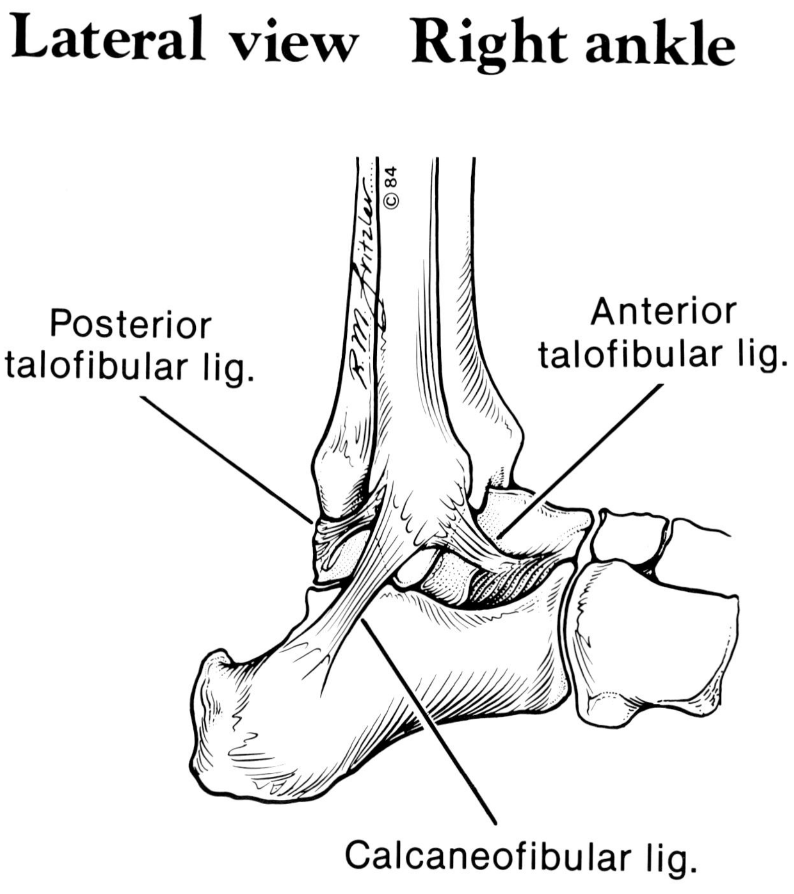


**Figure 15–1** Lateral view of right ankle demonstrating ligamentous structures.

about 1 cm anterior to the tip of the lateral malleolus. An accessory portal is established with an 18-gauge needle about 1 cm distal to the anterolateral portal used for the arthroscope. The abrasion is done with the Dyonics Small Joint System. A 2.8-mm abrader tip is used to denude articular cartilage down to bleeding bone. The 2.8-mm synovial resector is then used to remove soft tissue and debris so that a smoothly tapered surface is created about the same size as the staple. Finally a small-sized arthroscopic staple, from the Instrumentmakar Ligament and Capsular Repair System, is inserted from an accessory portal chosen so that the staple will enter the talus at a right angle. The two tines of the staple surround and gather capsule and ligament tissue and are lined up with the prepared bed on the talus, bringing the foot to neutral position to allow sufficient tightening of the lateral structures. After insertion of the staple with a mallet, the impactor-extractor device is unscrewed (Figure 15–2).

No sutures are used. All portals are left to close secondarily for minimal scarring, after infiltrating them with 0.25% bupivacaine and epinephrine solution to minimize postoperative bleeding and discomfort. Postoperative radiographs are shown on Figure 15–3. A bulky dressing is applied, followed by a posterior plaster splint and an elastic bandage. Five days later the initial dressings are removed in

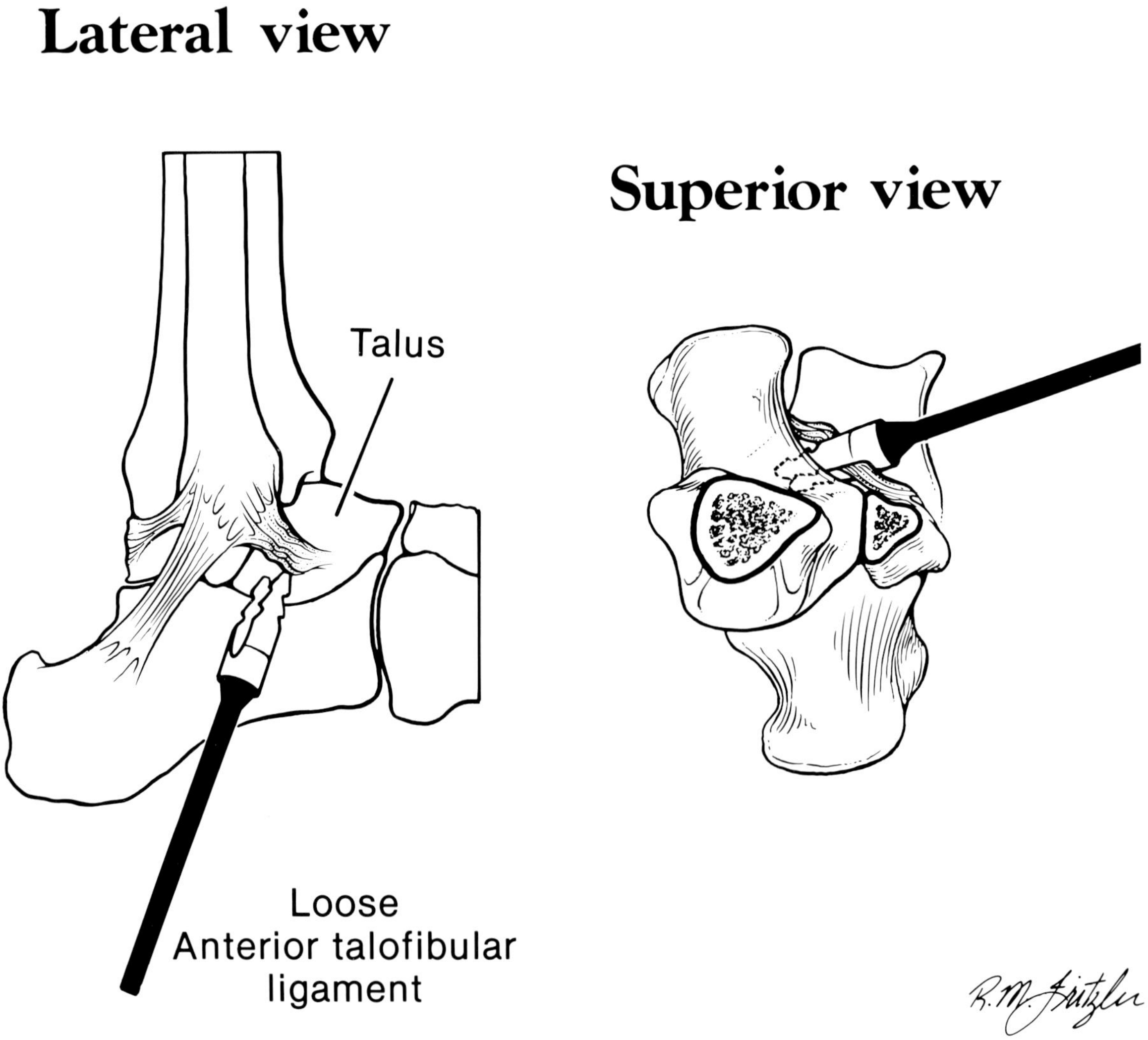


**Figure 15–2** Lateral view (left) and superior view (right) of staple insertion.

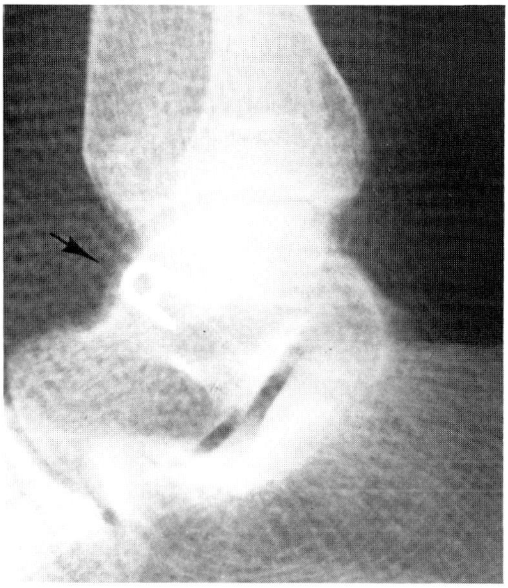

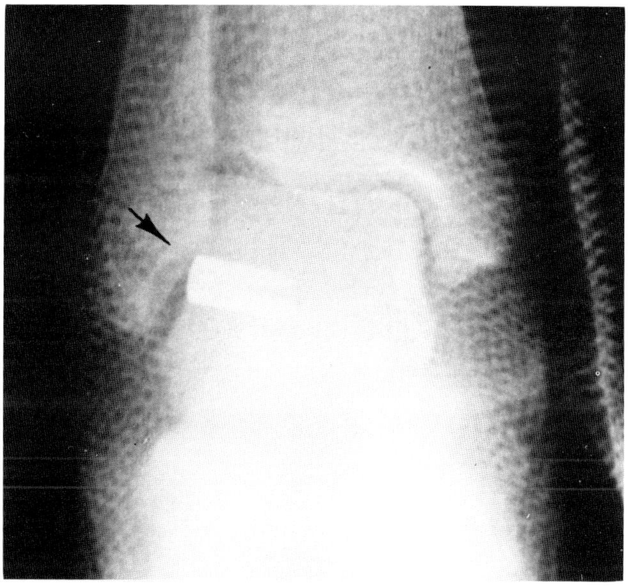

A B

**Figure 15–3** Postoperative radiographs show position of staple.

the outpatient department and a fiberglass walking cast is applied. The patient is encouraged to discard crutches when comfortable, usually at about 10 days. After 6 weeks the cast is removed and range-of-motion and strengthening exercises are begun. An elastic pull-on support or aircast is recommended for sports for the first few months.

Initially, we carried out second-look arthroscopies at 3 months and removed the staple. We found that an intense fibrous tissue reaction had occurred, correcting the lateral ankle instability quite adequately. In fact, viewing down into the lateral gutter was difficult. Extraction of the staple required a cutdown incision over the staple head. The staple was generally so imbedded in bone, ligament, and scar that it was difficult to find and remove. In the most recent series of cases over the past 18 months, the staples have been left in place, to be removed only if they should cause future symptoms.

Early results have been quite promising, with greatly improved stability that allowed patients to return to normal activities and functional levels, including sports. No patient has yet wished to have additional open surgery for lateral reconstruction.

## Case Report

D.A., a 28-year-old self-employed building contractor, presented with a complaint of chronic "giving out" of the left ankle. The first injury had occurred during high school with an inversion stress during running. Marked swelling of the lateral ankle had lasted nearly a week. Over 10 years he had had innumerable episodes of ankle sprain, associated with transient disability. His work as a contractor involved walking on uneven terrain, and his major complaint was a feeling of instability in the ankle. He had learned to avoid perching on roofs for fear his ankle would give out.

Clinical evaluation confirmed a 3-plus positive anterior draw test and varus instability. Stress radiographs showed talar tilt of 16 degrees compared to 4 degrees in his normal ankle (Figure 15–4).

At the time of outpatient arthroscopy of the ankle, loose cartilage debris was aspirated from the joint and a surface defect was seen at the medial plafond on the tibial surface. A stapling reconstruction was carried out.

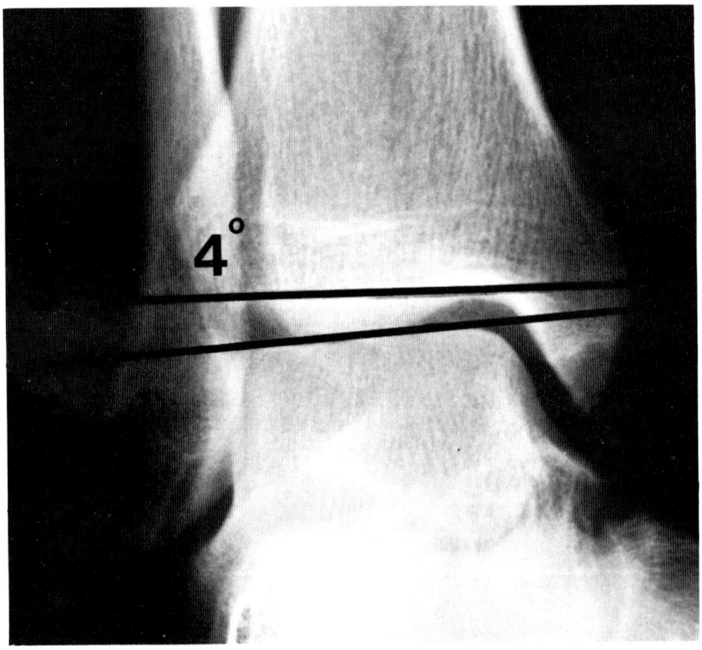


A

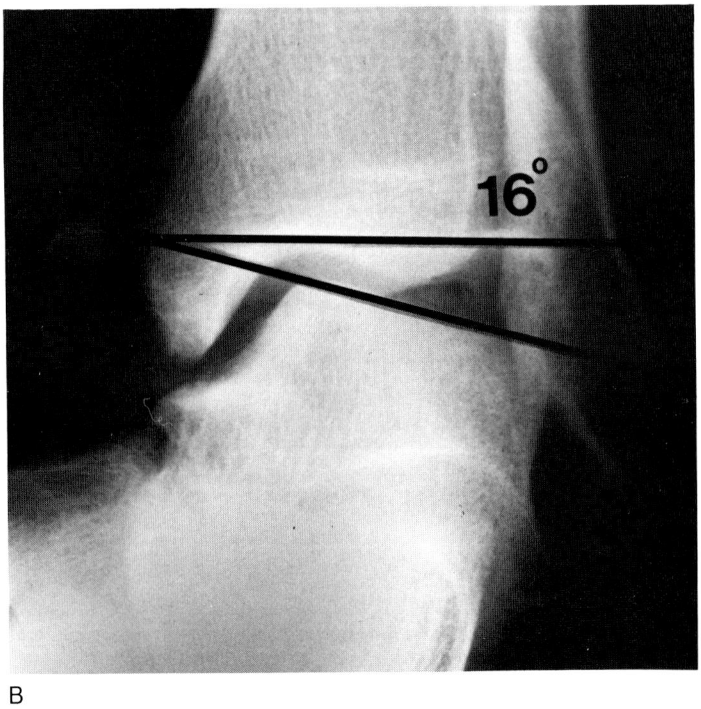


B

**Figure 15–4** Stress radiographs comparing 4-degree talar tilt of normal right ankle (**A**) to 16-degree tilt of unstable left ankle (**B**).

Eighteen months later he was clinically asymptomatic. In fact, he had resumed climbing on roofs and playing softball, using a soft elastic brace for protective support. His follow-up stress x-ray showed improvement, despite persistence of varus instability of 11 degrees, indicating probable damage to the calcaneofibular ligament.

## Summary

We have presented a preliminary report on a limited number of patients with chronic lateral instability of the ankle treated with arthroscopic stapling reconstruction. Longest follow-ups are 3 years, so the results over the long term are not yet known. Early results have been quite encouraging, however, with improved functional stability of the ankle.

The principle of secure fixation of ligaments to exposed bone surfaces with staples is a well-accepted and effective technique familiar to orthopaedists for many years. What is changing is that microsurgical techniques can be adapted to common orthopaedic problems. As in most outpatient arthroscopic procedures, there is a high degree of patient acceptance of the procedure. Discomfort is minimal and some patients have not even filled out their prescription for analgesic medication. The period of disability is relatively short and rehabilitation rapid. As in most arthroscopic surgical procedures, the key to success is careful forethought, planning, and teamwork. Instruments of the correct size are most important, as is precise surgical technique.

## *References*

1. Anderson KJ, LeCocq JD. Operative treatment of injury to the fibular collateral ligament of the ankle. J Bone Joint Surg [Am] 36:825–832, 1954
2. Anderson KJ, LeCocq JD, LeCocq EA. Recurrent anterior subluxation of the ankle joint. J Bone Joint Surg [Am] 34:853–860, 1952
3. Brostrom L. Sprained ankles. I. Anatomic lesions in recent sprains. Acta Chir Scand 128:483–495, 1964
4. Chrisman OD, Snook GA. Reconstruction of lateral ligament tears of the ankle. An experimental study and clinical evaluation of seven patients treated by a new modification of the Elmslie procedure. J Bone Joint Surg [Am] 51:904–912, 1969
5. Freeman MAR. Instability of the foot after injuries to the lateral ligament of the ankle. J Bone Joint Surg [Br] 47:669–677, 1965
6. Glasgow M, Jackson A, Jamieson AM. Instability of the ankle after injury to the lateral ligament. J Bone Joint Surg [Br] 62:196–200, 1980
7. Inman VT. The Joints of the Ankle, pp 3–10. Williams & Wilkins, Baltimore, 1976
8. Johnson EE, Markolf KL. The contribution of the anterior talofibular ligament to ankle laxity. J Bone Joint Surg [Am] 65:81–88, 1983
9. Leonard MH. Injuries of the lateral ligament of the ankle. A clinical and experimental study. J Bone Joint Surg [Am] 31:373–377, 1949
10. McCullough CJ, Burge PD. Rotary stability of the load-bearing ankle. An experimental study. J Bone Joint Surg [Am] 62:460–464, 1980
11. Pennal GF. Subluxation of the ankle. Can Med Assoc J 49:92–95, 1943
12. Rubin G, Witten M. The talar-tilt angle and the fibular collateral ligaments. A method for the determination of talar tilt. J Bone Joint Surg [Am] 42:311–326, 1960
13. Ruth CJ. The surgical treatment of the fibular collateral ligaments of the ankle. J Bone Joint Surg [Am] 43:229–239, 1961

# Arthroscopy of the Elbow

# 16

James R. Andrews
William G. Carson, Jr.

Arthroscopy, while most commonly used to diagnose and treat various disorders of the knee, is now being applied to smaller joints including the elbow (1–4). However, great attention to detail is required in performing this arthroscopic examination, particularly when entering the elbow joint. Introduction of arthroscopic instruments into the knee requires passage only through a thin retinacular area and allows generous distances from neurovascular structures. The elbow, however, requires arthroscopic instruments to be placed through deeper muscle layers and in proximity to important neurovascular structures. The need for attention to detail is crucial. In this chapter we present our technique of arthroscopy of the elbow, both diagnostic and surgical, and review the arthroscopic anatomy of the elbow.

## Indications

Because arthroscopy of the elbow is a relatively new advancement, the indications for its use are still being developed. At this time we feel elbow arthroscopy is indicated in the following situations:

1. Extraction of loose bodies
2. Evaluation and debridement of osteochondral lesions of the capitellum and radial head
3. Debridement and lysis of adhesions in posttraumatic or degenerative processes about the elbow

4. Partial synovectomy in rheumatoid disease
5. To establish a diagnosis in the chronically painful elbow when other etiological processes have been ruled out.

The above indications most readily apply to chronic processes about the elbow. Arthroscopy of the elbow in the acute setting is less clearly indicated. However, arthroscopy in the acute setting might be used to evaluate fractures of the capitellum, the radial head, or olecranon.

## Technique

Although the use of local anesthesia has been described for arthroscopy of the elbow (4), the authors prefer general anesthesia to afford complete muscle relaxation and comfort of the patient. The patient is placed supine on a routine operating table, and the forearm is placed in a prefabricated wrist gauntlet that is connected to an overhead pulley and suspended with a rope that is tied off at the end of the operating table. The entire arm is allowed to hang freely over the side of the table with the elbow flexed approximately 90 degrees (Figure 16–1). This positioning

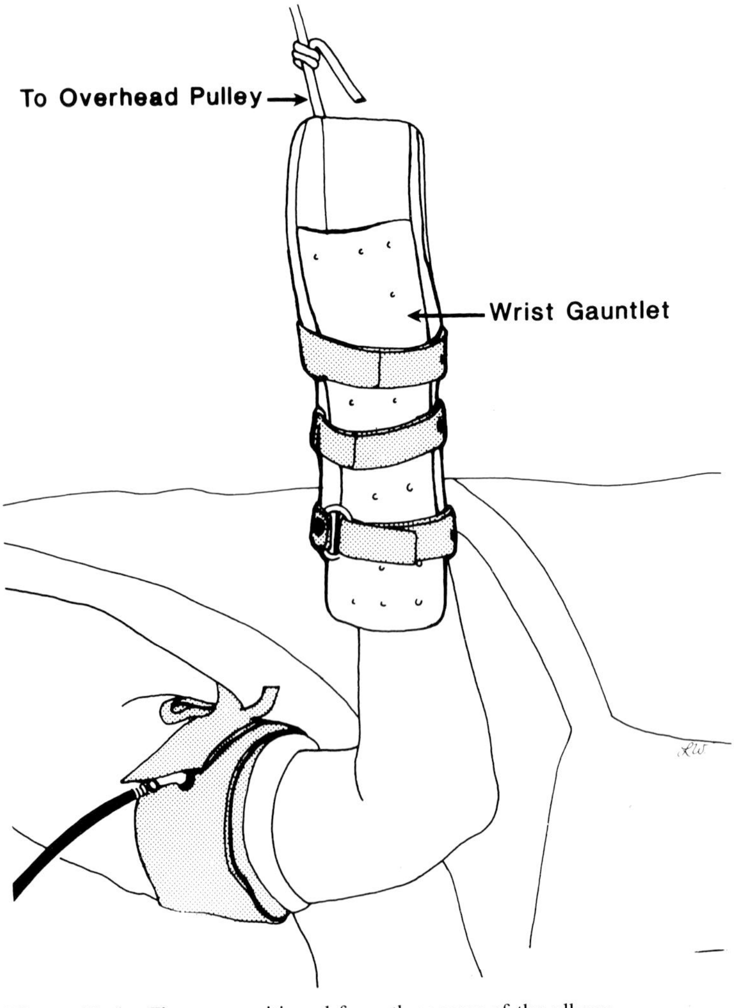


**Figure 16–1** The arm positioned for arthroscopy of the elbow.

provides excellent access to both the medial and lateral aspects of the elbow, and the forearm may be freely pronated and supinated. In addition, with the elbow flexed 90 degrees, the important neurovascular structures located in the antecubital fossa are placed in maximum relaxation. A tourniquet is routinely used for control of hemostasis, and the entire arm, including the hand, is draped in a sterile fashion after routine sterile preparation has been performed.

The bony landmarks of the elbow are outlined on the skin with a pen prior to the initiation of the procedure. Extravasation of fluid during the arthroscopic procedure prevents marking these structures during the procedure. The lateral structures to be identified are the radial head and the lateral epicondyle, and the medial structure to be identified and marked is the medial epicondyle. The three most commonly utilized arthroscopic portals for the elbow are the anterolateral, the anteromedial, and the posterolateral portals.

## Anterolateral Portal

The anterolateral portal is used as the initial entrance into the elbow joint. The general principle of inserting arthroscopic instruments into the smaller joints, such as the elbow or ankle, is to achieve maximum capsular distension at the time the instruments pass into the joint. This distension is provided by injecting saline through an 18-gauge needle at the initiation of the procedure. After the initial arthroscopic portal is established and the arthroscope is in place, fluid injection directly through the arthroscopic cannula will provide continued distension.

To inject saline into the elbow, the easiest location to insert a needle in a reproducible fashion is the lateral aspect directly between the lateral epicondyle, the olecranon tip, and the radial head. This location is the one most often used for aspiration of the elbow. The instruments will traverse only skin, a thin subcutaneous layer, the anconeus muscle, and the capsule. Once the joint is maximally distended through this approach, the actual anterolateral arthroscopic portal is established. With the elbow flexed 90 degrees, locate this portal approximately 2 cm distal and 1 cm anterior to the lateral epicondyle, just anterior to the radial head (Figure 16–2). Establish the portal by inserting an 18-gauge needle prior to placing the larger arthroscopic instruments. Palpation of the radial head is facilitated by pronating and supinating the forearm. This arthroscopic portal is somewhat more distal and anterior than the usual approach used for aspiration of the elbow, as just described. Aim the 18-gauge needle directly toward the center of the joint with the elbow flexed 90 degrees. This is done with the elbow joint maximally distended. Additional saline is injected through the needle into the elbow joint with the use of intravenous connecting tubing and a 50-cc syringe. Verification of entrance into the elbow joint is confirmed by observing for free back flow. Once this is confirmed, the elbow joint is further distended and the larger arthroscopic instruments and cannulas are now introduced. Maximum distension displaces the antecubital neurovascular structures anteriorly and gives one more space above the bony epicondyles to place appropriate instruments. Insert the larger instruments, closely observing the angle of the needle, and make a small skin incision for insertion of the arthroscopic cannula and sharp trocar into the elbow joint. Aim directly for the center of the joint and stay close to the bony landmarks of the lateral epicondyle and the radial head. When the tip of the sharp trocar is at the level of the joint capsule, exchange a blunt trocar for the sharp trocar and enter the joint capsule. The arthroscope is then inserted. We have found it helpful to connect a hand-held camera to the arthroscope for ease of visualization and videotape documentation. Continuous irrigation and drainage tubes are then applied to the arthroscopic inflow and outflow connectors, and inflow is maintained by the use of overhead bags of

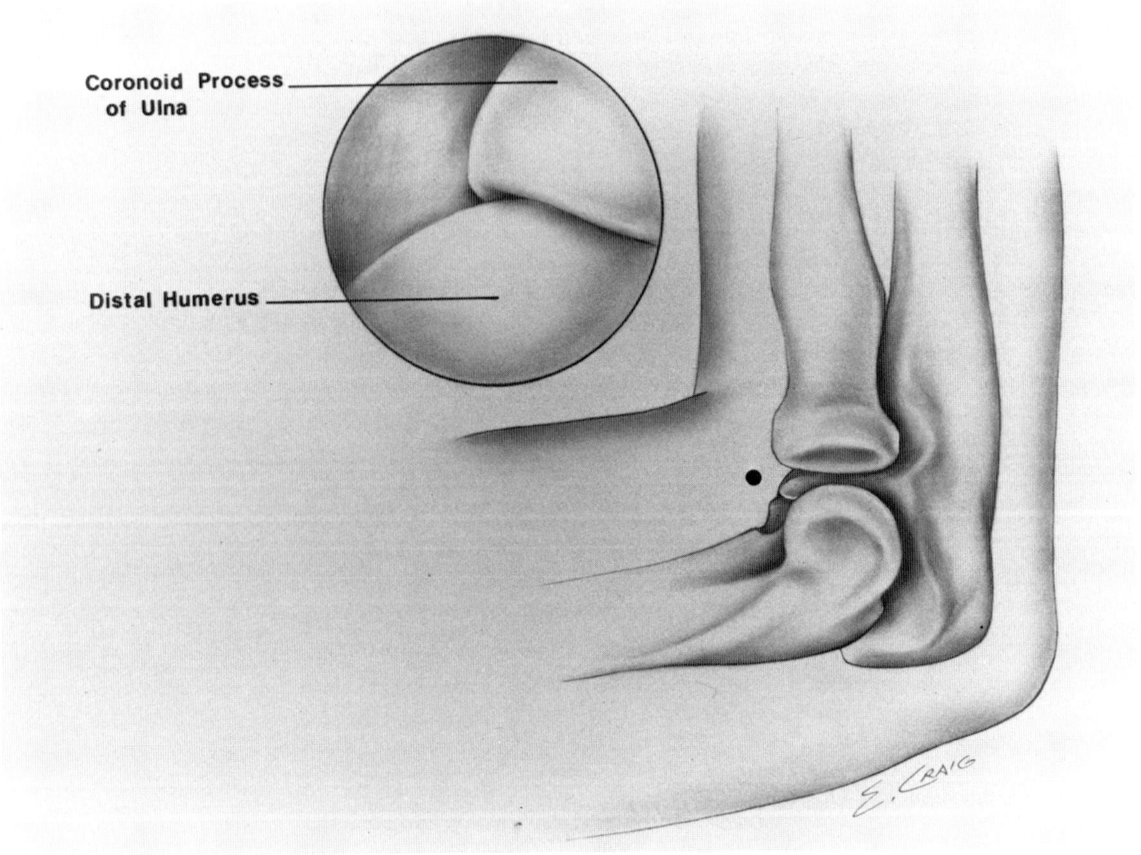


**Figure 16–2** The anterolateral portal is established approximately 2 cm distal and 1 cm anterior to the lateral epicondyle. Arthroscopic anatomy as seen through this portal includes the distal humerus and coronoid process of the ulna.

normal saline. Although smaller arthroscopes, such as the 2.7-mm needle arthroscope, have been used successfully for arthroscopy of the elbow (4), the authors have found that the larger 4-mm, 30-degree angled arthroscopes offer superior visualization and can be safely inserted through the anteromedial, anterolateral, and posterior portals by using the technique previously described (1–3).

Intra-articular structures of the elbow that may be visualized through the anterolateral portal are the distal humerus and trochlear ridges and the coronoid process of the ulna (Figure 16–2). Flexion and extension of the elbow will help to visualize the coronoid process of the ulna, and extension of the elbow will provide a better view of the medial and lateral trochlear ridges and the trochlear notch of the distal humerus. By slowly retracting the arthroscope and angling the 30-degree arthroscope toward the radial head, small portions of the radial head may be visualized from this anterolateral portal.

## Anteromedial Portal

After the arthroscope is in place through the anterolateral portal, additional instruments may now be placed in the anteromedial portal under direct visualization provided by the arthroscope already in place. The anteromedial portal is made by placing an 18-gauge needle approximately 1 cm anterior and 2 cm distal to the medial epicondyle, aiming directly toward the center of the joint with the elbow flexed 90 degrees (Figure 16–3). Confirmation of the needle's entrance into the elbow joint is provided by direct visualization by the arthroscope already in place. Carefully observe the needle passing just above the medial epicondyle and inferior to the antecubital structures that are displaced anteriorly, both by the position of the elbow in flexion and by the constant distension. Make a small skin incision and insert the arthroscopic cannula and sharp trocar. The sharp trocar is inserted to the level of the capsule and the blunt trocar is used to enter the elbow joint. With many of the newer arthroscopic systems, the inflow cannulas and arthroscopic cannulas are interchangeable, and thus, once the anteromedial and anterolateral portals are established, one may exchange instruments between these portals.

Most arthroscopic surgical procedures performed on the elbow are performed for pathological processes located over the lateral aspect of the elbow, such as loose bodies or osteochondritis dissecans of the capitellum. The anteromedial portal provides superior visualization of the lateral structures, and thus it is necessary to be familiar with the insertion of both anterolateral and anteromedial portals.

The structures that may be seen from the anteromedial portal are the capitellum and the radial head (Figure 16–3). Visualization of the radial head is facilitated by pronating and supinating the forearm. At times the annular ligament

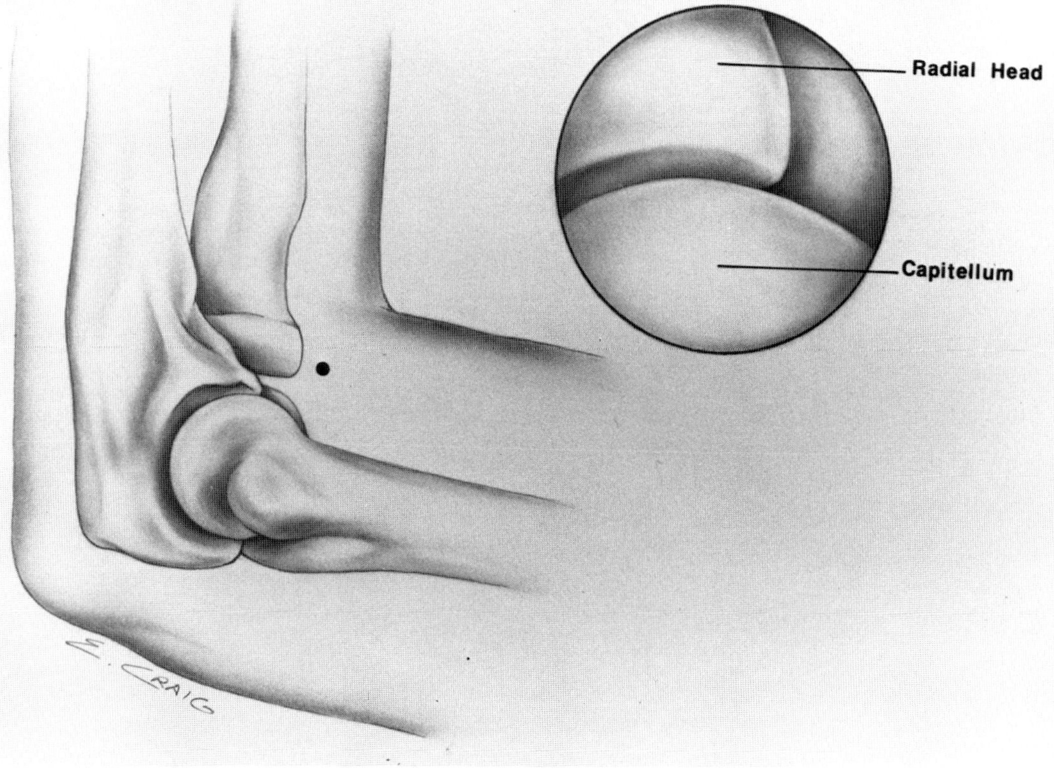


**Figure 16–3** The anteromedial portal. Instruments enter the skin approximately 2 cm distal and 1 cm anterior to the medial epicondyle. The arthroscopic view includes the capitellum and radial head.

coursing over the radial neck may be visualized. By slowly retracting the arthroscope and directing it toward the ulna, the coronoid process may be visualized through this anteromedial portal.

## Posterolateral Portal

The third arthroscopic portal that may occasionally be required in evaluation of the elbow joint is the posterolateral portal. The entrance point of this portal is approximately 2 cm proximal to the olecranon tip, just posterior and superior to the lateral epicondyle near the lateral margin of the triceps muscle (Figure 16–4). This portal is most readily established by extending the elbow to relax the triceps muscle and inserting an 18-gauge needle and aiming for the olecranon fossa. Inflow is injected, and once backflow is confirmed and entrance into the posterior aspect of the elbow is verified, a skin incision is made and the instruments are introduced. The two major areas to be visualized from the posterolateral portal are the olecranon fossa, located over the posterior aspect of the distal humerus, and the tip of the olecranon (Figure 16–4). Flexion and extension of the elbow will help to visualize the various portions of the distal humerus.

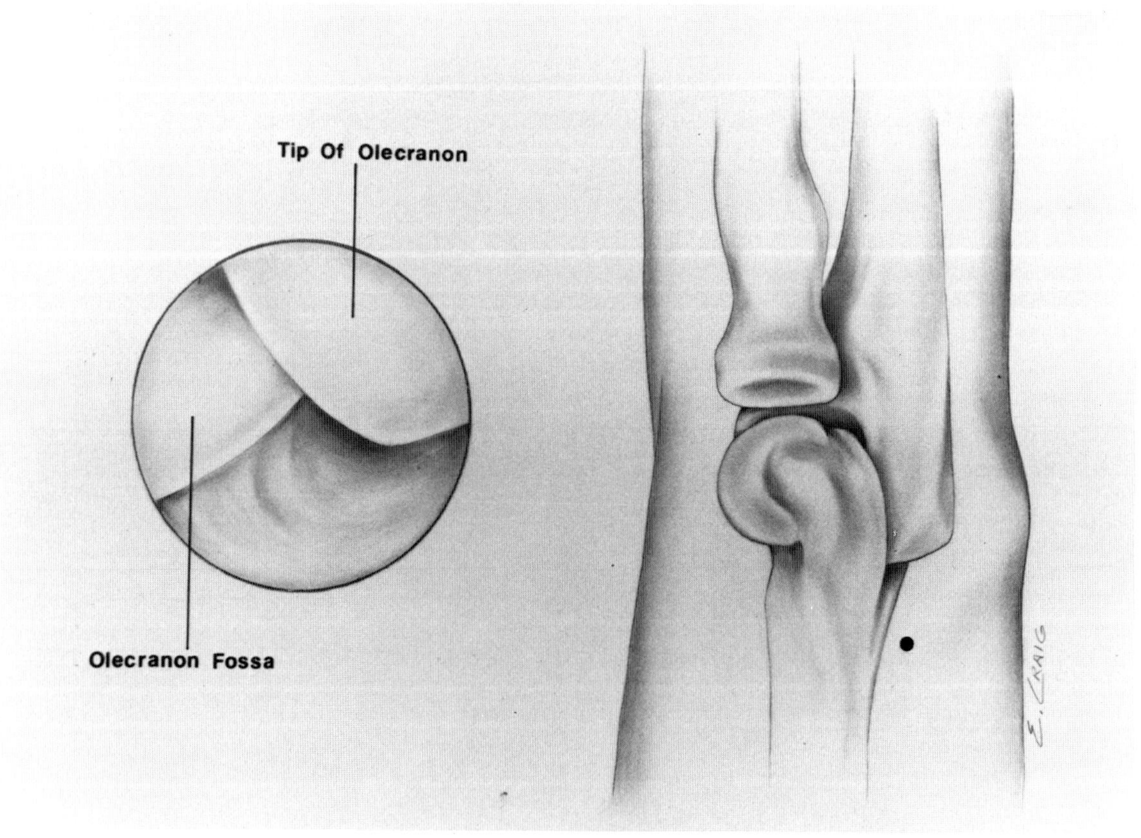


**Figure 16–4** The posterolateral portal is established with the arm extended to visualize the tip of the olecranon and the olecranon fossa. Instruments enter the skin through the posterolateral portal approximately 2 cm proximal to the olecranon tip just posterior and superior to the lateral epicondyle.

The operative arthroscopic instruments commonly used for the knee may also be used in the elbow and include such instruments as motorized suction instruments, knives, punches, and graspers. As previously stated, if surgery is to be performed on processes involving the lateral side of the elbow, the arthroscope is usually placed through the anteromedial portal and the instruments through the anterolateral portal. For pathology located on the medial side of the elbow, the arthroscope is placed anterolaterally and the instruments anteromedially. At the completion of the arthroscopic procedure, soft dressings are applied to the elbow and immobilization is usually not required. Early motion of the elbow joint is usually initiated as soon as pain permits.

## Pathology

Arthroscopy of the elbow has been performed on 24 patients at the Hughston Orthopaedic Clinic in Columbus, Georgia. The average age at the time of the arthroscopic examination was 27 years. Of this group of 21 males and 3 females, the most common pathological entities seen were loose bodies associated with osteochondritis dissecans of the capitellum (6 cases), isolated loose bodies (4 cases), and osteochondritis dissecans of the capitellum (3 cases). A preliminary study of 12 patients who underwent surgical arthroscopy of the elbow demonstrated that removal of loose bodies produced the best subjective and objective results (1). The only complication in this preliminary series was a transient median nerve palsy caused by the extracapsular extravasation of a local anesthetic.

## Discussion

For arthroscopy of the elbow to be a safe and effective procedure, a systematic and reproducible arthroscopic examination technique needs to be developed. The authors conclude that the technique and the identification of anatomical structures described earlier provides a safe and reliable means of performing an arthroscopic examination of the elbow. Attention to detail, especially when establishing the various portals, is essential to perform a safe arthroscopic examination and to avoid damage to nearby neurovascular structures. We have found that the 4-mm, 30-degree angled arthroscope provides an excellent visualization of the intra-articular structures of the elbow and can be used in a safe fashion. The use of the smaller 2.7-mm arthroscope has been described (4); however, the field of view is markedly reduced from that of the larger 4-mm arthroscopes. The diameter difference between the 4-mm arthroscope and the 2.7-mm arthroscope is only 1.3 mm. If the surgeon is concerned about injuring nearby neurovascular structures with only a 1.3-mm margin of error, then an instrument of any size, no matter how small, should probably not be placed in this area.

To verify that these larger instruments can be safely inserted into the elbow joint, the authors have performed cadaveric dissections over the various arthroscopic portals of the elbow (2). Steinman pins were placed through the three arthroscopic portals, and then, layer by layer, dissection was carried out and the underlying anatomy was examined. It was noted that in establishing the anterolateral portal, the arthroscope was seen to pass through the extensor carpi radialis brevis, and as the arthroscope entered the skin, it was approximately 12 mm from the radial nerve. As the arthroscope passed above the radial head and lateral epicondyle and entered the elbow joint, it came within 7 mm of the radial nerve. In establishing the anteromedial portal, the arthroscope pierced the tendinous portion of the pronator teres and entered through the radial aspect of the flexor digitorum superficialis. When the instruments coursed through these muscles, the median nerve was approximately 1 cm lateral to the arthroscope, with the brachial artery just lateral to the median nerve. As the instruments passed deeper and closer to the joint capsule of the elbow, the instruments passed within 6 mm of these same neurovascular structures.

Because of the proximity of these important structures, the surgeon must be attentive to technical detail when establishing the arthroscopic portals and inserting the various instruments. With the elbow flexed at 90 degrees and adequate distension maintained at the time of the insertion of the instruments, the neurovascular structures will be displaced anteriorly, and there will be adequate area above the medial and lateral humeral epicondyles in which to insert the various instruments.

The only complication in the author's preliminary series of elbow arthroscopies was a transient median nerve palsy caused by the extracapsular extravasation of local anesthetic placed into the elbow joint following the arthroscopic procedure. Because the instruments pass in such close proximity to neurovascular structures and an early postoperative neurovascular assessment is of obvious importance, we feel that the injection of a local anesthetic into a smaller joint such as the elbow is contraindicated.

In conclusion, the authors find that 1) attention to detail is essential to perform a safe and reproducible arthroscopic examination, especially when establishing the anteromedial and anterolateral portals; 2) arthroscopy of the elbow is an effective diagnostic procedure and visualization of intra-articular structures is accomplished quite readily; and 3) operative elbow arthroscopy appears to be effective in treating certain pathological processes about the elbow.

## *References*

1. Andrews JR, Carson WG. Arthroscopy of the elbow. Paper presented at the Annual Meeting of the Arthroscopy Association of North America, New Orleans, 1984
2. Andrews JR, Farrell J, Carson WG. Arthroscopy of the Elbow. Videotape no. VT-119. American Academy of Orthopaedic Surgeons, Chicago, 1983
3. Carson WG, Andrews JR. Arthroscopy of the elbow. In: Andrews JR, Carson WG, Zarins B (eds) Symposium on Throwing Injuries. WB Saunders, Philadelphia (to be published)
4. Johnson LL. Diagnostic and Surgical Arthroscopy, pp 390–399. CV Mosby, St. Louis, 1981

# The Necessity for Research in the Development of Arthroscopic Surgery

# 17

Terry L. Whipple

The first step to knowledge is to know that we are ignorant.

Cecil

## Definitions

Research is nothing more than observation: setting the stage for events and recording in detail what happens. Properly setting the stage, however, may be a particularly formidable task. The observer's primary interest may be in the spontaneous event, in which case the stage must be set with perfection to duplicate naturally occurring situations. On the other hand, he may be interested in the stage itself, the appropriate setting of which will result in a desired or anticipated event. Research, then, is the observation of cause and effect relationships, and whether the researcher is seeking the cause or the effect, it is his challenge to set the appropriate stage for events to occur.

Retrospective investigations also seek cause and effect relationships. These inquiries require stage setting, too: defining the players, the circumstances, the setting, and the timing so that some pattern of events becomes obvious. The quality of a research effort, whether retrospective or prospective, depends greatly on the creation of the stage on which events are to transpire, the tightness of the script to eliminate extraneous influence, and only then, the accuracy of the observations made.

Development is the creation of a means to accomplish certain events. If a cause and effect relationship is defined, and the cause is unavoidable or the effect is undesirable, one may be able to intervene in some way to influence the natural course of events. The means with which to accomplish this can be developed only after diligent study of the relationship between the cause and the effect.

Development then is based on research. With knowledge of naturally occurring cause and effect relationships, a new technology or a new technique may require unique instrumentation or environmental manipulation to achieve a desired conclusion from given circumstances; development of an appropriate means of intervention must occur.

## Perspective

In 1806, three years before his death, Philip Bozzini first developed a device for inspecting the internal anatomy of body cavities through a speculum. Reflecting the light of a candle with a mirror, Bozzini's "Lichtleiter" enabled him to examine the rectal and female urogenital tracts.

In 1853 A. J. Desormeaux developed a more sophisticated endoscope, the gasogene lamp, which reflected the light from burning turpentine and alcohol through a system of mirrors and lenses. Cystoscopy was born; Desormeaux had the credit. When Thomas Edison invented (developed) the incandescent lamp in 1880, Leopold von Dittel in Vienna incorporated that new technology into a cystoscope. Max Nitze and R. Kutner cleverly combined two technologies in 1890, using photographic equipment and a cystoscope with an incandescent lamp to photograph the inside of the urinary bladder. Physicians were now in a position, with new instrumentation, new technology, new techniques, and a background of careful observations, to intervene in the course of disease processes in the bladder and urethra. Research had lead to development, development had permitted additional research, and the latter research, in turn, permitted the development of a new science, new techniques to alter the natural course of urinary tract disease.

Thirty years later Professor M. Takagi in Tokyo developed an arthroscope. His interest was stimulated by the incidence of tuberculosis that commonly resulted in ankylosis of the knee. Observing that early diagnosis and treatment could often avert this complication, he sought a means to inspect the joint directly with minimal morbidity. Concurrently and independently, Bircher in New York observed that too often the clinical diagnostic accuracy in disorders of the knee was not confirmed at surgery and, like Takagi, sought a better mode of examination and diagnosis with acceptable risk and morbidity. He used a laparoscope instead of a cystoscope, and a gas medium instead of saline. By 1925 Kreuzer had developed an arthroscope that was similar to the new smaller version of Takagi's and was appealing for earlier diagnosis of lesions in the meniscus at a time when Smillie and Watson-Jones were reversing the trend of partial meniscectomy and recommending total meniscectomy for internal derangement of the knee.

Until around 1930, very little research had been done in the field of arthroscopy, but considerable development in technology had occurred. Heustinx challenged the procedure advocated by Bircher in an article written in March, 1937:

> How can anyone venture to introduce a luminous object into a knee joint in an effort to look between the articular surfaces, which cannot be separated. Even at arthrotomy it is impossible to see the posterior horn of the meniscus if the knee joint is not sufficiently open. How, then, could one expect to see it in a closed joint. This is quite impossible. Moreover, this procedure is more dangerous than an exploratory arthrotomy.

Was this true? Was this procedure developed by both Takagi and Bircher more dangerous than an arthrotomy? The research began as Sommer and Vaubel in Germany performed a series of arthroscopic examinations for tuberculosis and compared them with a series of cases examined for diagnosis by arthrotomy. They arrived at the following conclusions: arthroscopic examination and tissue biopsy proved accurate, more convenient, better tolerated, and more easily repeatable than did diagnostic exploratory arthrotomy. They had set the stage differently for the diagnosis of tuberculosis of the knee and recorded their results and consequences for comparison.

Vaubel went further. Recording every experience with the arthroscope, he found the procedure of value for five purposes:

1. The identification of pathological changes within the knee
2. The differential diagnosis between gonarthrosis of the knee and polyarticular arthritides
3. To monitor the progress of disease by repeated examinations
4. As an aid in intra-articular surgery in conjunction with arthrotomy
5. To study the biology of joints and enhance the understanding of their complex structure-function relationships.

This last application was a major thrust in the application of arthroscopy for research purposes. The biomechanics of the knee and its physiological responses to disease came under scrutiny through the arthroscope.

Takagi was recording his observations in applications other than knee disorders as well, using his arthroscope to examine the neural defects in patients with spina bifida and to detail and document the intraoral movements during speech training following cleft palate operations. Although used in only a few centers throughout the world, the arthroscope had become a jealously defended instrument for investigation as well as clinical application. Its advantage for documenting conditions and events with minimal invasion, risk, and morbidity was indisputable, but it represented a radical departure from traditional surgical means of exploration. The research for which it was used had to be convincing, tightly controlled, and defensible to challenge. The instrumentation had to be developed for greater reliability, optical perfection, and electrical isolation. It was in an atmosphere of criticism, if not contempt, that the few champions of the idea of minimally invasive diagnostic procedures for joint disorders continued their pursuits. Adequate technology in optics and illumination was a long time coming, and orthopaedic peers were skeptical of the idea that keyhole examinations had merit.

Research and development in any field is, by its very nature, a defensive business. It is always difficult to challenge traditional concepts and practices. New knowledge can be unsettling, and those who would propose new techniques in any field must prove themselves and the validity of their work. Every doctoral thesis must be "defended," every synthetic must be tested, every mathematical theory must be proved.

There is security in tradition, and thus there is an element of loneliness in the lives of pioneers who push back the frontiers of any discipline, science, or geographic boundary. Such men live and work with the burden of public scrutiny. This has been the case throughout history.

Christopher Columbus sailed west to test a theory, to prove an idea, to set a stage for events he believed would occur and to research the consequences. Lewis and Clark explored the great rivers of the Midwest, documenting the lands, the peoples, and the resources they encountered for the first time. These explorations were research exercises as much as any probe into the unknown and the unfamiliar, in a disciplined way for the sake of new knowledge and information. What fools were Galileo, Copernicus, Darwin, men with perseverance and conviction, who repeatedly set stages and recorded observations until the "discoveries" of some of the world's simple mysteries were reinforced with enough data to be convincing.

Through such painstaking advances do science and medicine grow; good but imperfect practices are set aside. The iron lung of the 1950s is a museum piece today, replaced by plastic positive-pressure ventilators. The crippling tragedies of polio are now essentially history thanks to the tireless laboratory efforts of Salk and Sabin. From the development of space-age materials, research animal laboratories, and the indefatigable energies of men like Sir John Charnley, there is finally incredible relief available to those who suffer the constant pain and premature debility of end-stage rheumatoid and degenerative arthritis. But consider the once radical idea of replacing biological tissues, which must provide mobility, stability, and durability, with metal, ceramic, or plastic.

Change does not come easily. But such are the contributions of men who had the courage to accept criticism and the stamina to walk always up hill, in pursuit of something better.

Probing this minimally invasive diagnostic concept for disorders of the knee, Masaki Watanabe published an atlas of arthroscopic observations in 1957 with artists' renderings of his observations, and in 1969 with photographs, again reporting that an adequate and useful examination could be achieved. The application of the arthroscope to rheumatology was reported by Robles Gil from Mexico in 1967 with his experiences in 60 cases. Arthroscopy provided the basis for prognosis and the evaluation of treatment regimens in rheumatoid patients. He studied the efficacy of chemical synovectomy and intra-articular steroid treatments by examining subjects arthroscopically before and after treatment. By serendipity, Gil observed that his patients all derived secondary benefit in pain relief and mobility attributable to the lavage of their joints during the course of arthroscopic examination; no small contribution.

In the United States Ward Casscells broke with tradition. In 1971 he reported his experience with 150 arthroscopic examinations of the knee, endorsing the procedure as a valuable diagnostic aid for lesions of the meniscus, articular cartilage, and synovium. The diagnostic accuracy would facilitate appropriate treatment planning.

In 1972 Robert W. Jackson in Toronto, Canada, reported the clinical value of 200 arthroscopic examinations of the knee. A meticulous surgeon and diligent observer, Jackson defined and justified the following indications for diagnostic arthroscopy:

1. Ill-defined pain as the sole symptom in adolescents in whom some local pathology can be present but is not otherwise readily apparent
2. Symptoms inconsistent with or contradictory to objective findings
3. Persistent symptoms after previous surgical treatment
4. Knee lesions in professional athletes, for whom an early diagnosis is of economic importance
5. Impediments to adequate evaluation by history, physical examination, radiographs, and arthrography
6. The need for direct tissue inspection for prognosis or treatment planning
7. Cost-effective confirmation or refutal of diagnoses in litigation or compensation cases.

Of tremendous additional importance was the demonstration by numerous authors of the value of confirming a diagnosis that might require surgical intervention prior to resorting to the expense and morbidity of arthrotomy.

John Joyce of Philadelphia undertook the organization of the International Arthroscopy Association, convinced that arthroscopic methods were of decided value to patients, but at the same time fully aware that appropriate applications and convincing demonstrations of the merit of the technique to the orthopaedic community would require educational coordination and an organized forum through which information could be shared and disseminated. This was the first attempt at providing peer-controlled quality assurance in the clinical application of these "new" arthroscopic techniques.

The development continued. As fiber optics technology permitted the design of improved instrumentation, Richard O'Connor developed an operative arthroscope through which he initiated the practice of removing portions of torn menisci under arthroscopic control. This was a logical evolutionary step. If visibility was so good, if diagnosis was so accurate, and if the morbidity of this minimally invasive technique was so reduced, why could not the surgeon manipulate pathological tissues within the joint by incision, excision, fragmentation, or cauterization if the appropriate instruments were available?

Surgeons could and they did. Through countless hours in the morgue and anatomy laboratory, combined approaches were developed for knee arthroscopy using ENT instruments to excise portions of the menisci. After the lead of O'Connor, pioneering surgeons like Johnson and Metcalf collected initial clinical series of arthroscopic meniscectomies, reporting their results at the International Arthroscopy Association Meeting in Denver in 1976. Patients undergoing partial meniscectomy were monitored closely and with anticipation. Although Robert Jones had advocated in 1909 that only the torn portion of the meniscus should be removed, this had not been the clinical practice for over 50 years because of the influence of Watson-Jones and Smillie for total meniscectomy. The emerging premature incidence of osteoarthritis following total meniscectomy gave credence to the concept of partial meniscectomy. The clinical investigators with arthroscopy then set the stage with partial meniscectomies and awaited the eventual satisfactory and encouraging results and decreased morbidity these patients enjoyed, although long-term results are not yet available.

## Projections

It is astonishing that as recently as a decade ago, only a handful of surgeons throughout the world were attempting surgical procedures under arthroscopic control. Arthroscopy's rapid proliferation, as well as its ascent into the forefront of orthopaedics today, is a testament to its effectiveness. Probably no other development in orthopaedic surgery, with the exception of joint replacement, has revolutionized treatment of joint disorders as much as arthroscopy. In addition to meniscectomy, fragmented articular cartilage and osteophytes are debrided from degenerative joints, abrasion has supplanted drilling of subchondral bone in repairing full thickness surface defects, and rheumatoid synovectomy and lateral retinacular release are commonplace. Arthroscopic techniques are used for the management of intra-articular fractures, and now, even for cruciate ligament reconstruction.

What lies ahead for arthroscopy is subject to imagination—imagination directed and nurtured by appropriate research and development. Areas such as understanding the mechanisms of healing in articular tissues, the physical and chemical basis of degenerative joint disease, the structural and functional relationships of intricate joint anatomy and how to preserve them, and the virtually untapped area of treatment of synovial diseases are all worthy of exploration. Research in these subjects is the obligation and the privilege of scientists and surgeons who pose questions for the sake of answers and seek answers for the sake of knowledge.

But quality research can be expensive. The time, energy, and resources invested in an investigation do not always yield the anticipated results. Yet it is important that even disappointing results be reported. Any legitimate observation from an appropriately designed experiment is of value. For if research is conducted not for the sake of profit or ambition, but for the sake of legitimate answers to legitimate questions, even the undesirable results represent progress.

We must be careful not to invest too much emotion in research endeavors lest emotion taint the results and sway the reporter's objectivity. Ulterior motives may disqualify an investigation because of a vested interest in the outcome. For this reason scientific inquiries should not be left exclusively to industry, which is always profit motivated. Rather it is our responsibility as trustees of the patient's interests to work within the scientific community to assure that medical research—even though sponsored or proposed by industry, as is often the case—remains pure and unbiased.

It is also important to progress that every worthwhile idea gain expression. An idea is worthless unless brought to fruition, and that is not always achieved by the originator of the idea. Unless ideas are shared through the scientific forum and publication, many stand a very good chance of dying on the vine. Thus research must not be sequestered or guarded under cloak for personal gain, but should be broadcast and discussed openly so that unfinished and immature ideas might be cultivated and nourished by communal wisdom and experience. Watanabe is probably the single greatest contributor to the development of arthroscopy and arthroscopic surgery as we know it today. No one has failed to benefit from giving him credit for his brilliance, ingenuity, and innovative developments. Recognition is due to any one who contributes to the advancement of medical science and should never be withheld. But neither should it be sought in its own right.

Participation in research can take several forms: the identification of problems, the engineering of an investigational protocol, critique of and consultation on the experimental design, or the actual conduct of an experiment and observation of results. One may contribute to the analysis of data, the organization and publication of results, the planning of the next level or tangent of inquiry, and for those who haven't the time or facilities for any of the above, financial participation is always available. Research and development in arthroscopic surgery, as much as any other field, are the governors of its progress. They are the calculated organization that seeks understanding, improvement, and perfection.

It has been my privilege during the last three years to coordinate the efforts of two research organizations: The Research Committee for the Arthroscopy Association of North America, and Orthopaedic Research of Virginia. Both of these organizations are stimulating and exciting. The Research Committee of the AANA has established as its charge and challenge the development of a means by which worthwhile ideas pertaining to arthroscopic surgery gain expression, encouragement, and the opportunity for development and enhancement. This has been a rewarding experience, with encouraging support from cooperative leaders, imaginative practitioners, and generous representatives from science and industry. Yet in a sense, this effort is nothing more than the fundamental care and feeding of the original ideas of Takagi, Burman, Watanabe, and the imaginative others who were brilliant in the initial stages of this emerging field.

Arthroscopic surgery, for all its painfully long embryonic development, has finally come to fruition with unquestionable success. The public demands it for comfort and convenience; the economy justifies it for earlier return to function, productivity, and overall cost effectiveness; and physicians endorse it as a more precise surgical modality with decreased risk and morbidity. Given the privilege of opportunity, physicians, academicians, and pure scientists, through participation in research and development on any of the aforementioned planes, can contribute to the improvement of patient care and the enhancement of understanding and treatment of common as well as rare orthopaedic disorders. Such a satisfying contribution of energy and resources will surely become a rewarding investment in arthroscopic surgery from our generation.

## Acknowledgments

I should like to acknowledge the works of Masaki Watanabe and H. R. Eikelaar, from which the historical review for this manuscript was taken.

# Index